Health Informatics

This series is directed to healthcare professionals leading the transformation of healthcare by using information and knowledge. For over 20 years, Health Informatics has offered a broad range of titles: some address specific professions such as nursing, medicine, and health administration; others cover special areas of practice such as trauma and radiology; still other books in the series focus on interdisciplinary issues, such as the computer based patient record, electronic health records, and networked healthcare systems. Editors and authors, eminent experts in their fields, offer their accounts of innovations in health informatics. Increasingly, these accounts go beyond hardware and software to address the role of information in influencing the transformation of healthcare delivery systems around the world. The series also increasingly focuses on the users of the information and systems: the organizational, behavioral, and societal changes that accompany the diffusion of information technology in health services environments.

Developments in healthcare delivery are constant; in recent years, bioinformatics has emerged as a new field in health informatics to support emerging and ongoing developments in molecular biology. At the same time, further evolution of the field of health informatics is reflected in the introduction of concepts at the macro or health systems delivery level with major national initiatives related to electronic health records (EHR), data standards, and public health informatics.

These changes will continue to shape health services in the twenty-first century. By making full and creative use of the technology to tame data and to transform information, Health Informatics will foster the development and use of new knowledge in healthcare.

More information about this series at http://www.springer.com/series/1114

Amit Acharya • Valerie Powell
Miguel H. Torres-Urquidy
Robert H. Posteraro
Thankam Paul Thyvalikakath
Editors

Integration of Medical and Dental Care and Patient Data

Second Edition

Springer

Editors
Amit Acharya
Marshfield Clinic Research Institute
Center for Oral and Systemic Health
Marshfield, WI
USA

Miguel H. Torres-Urquidy
Centers for Disease Control
and Prevention
Atlanta, GA
USA

Thankam Paul Thyvalikakath
Department of Restorative Dentistry
Indiana University School of Dentistry
Indianapolis, IN
USA

Valerie Powell
Robert Morris University
Moon Township, PA
USA

Robert H. Posteraro
Texas Tech University Health Sciences
Centre - School of Health Professions
Lubbock, TX
USA

ISSN 1431-1917 ISSN 2197-3741 (electronic)
Health Informatics
ISBN 978-3-319-98296-0 ISBN 978-3-319-98298-4 (eBook)
https://doi.org/10.1007/978-3-319-98298-4

Library of Congress Control Number: 2018961016

This Springer imprint is published by the registered company Springer Nature Switzerland AG
The registered company address is: Gewerbestrasse 11, 6330 Cham, Switzerland

Preface

Integration of Medical and Oral Healthcare: Eliminating the Medical Dental Divide

The first edition of this book was introduced by Dr. David Nash's preface entitled Dentistry is Medicine-Oral Medicine. He described the Gies Report of 1926 and its conclusions and recommendations based upon the times he described the 1994 World Health Organization report Oral Health in the Twenty-First Century. He described the Institute of Medicine's report Dental Education at the Crossroads of 1995 and organized dentistry's and dental education response to maintain the status quo. All of these writings suggested that the "status quo for the profession puts it on a path towards stagnation and decline." A recent editorial in the JADA in November 2017 suggested the need for dentistry to respond, faced with the changes already occurring in the twenty-first century and those on the way. The controversies and discussions over healthcare in general designed to improve access, decrease costs, and improve health will eventually impact oral health. Interprofessional education is now entering a phase of interprofessional practice. In 2011, I attended a meeting sponsored by ADEA on interprofessional education. Dr. Don Berwick, head of Institute for Health Improvement (IHI), spoke of meaningful use and triple aim, the subject of a chapter in this new edition. Other than the ADEA leadership and staff, I was the only dentist in attendance. Since then, the Commission on Change and Innovation (CCI) has published its findings, and now a second CCI is underway. The need for changes highlighted by Dr. Nash in his preface and his extraordinary paper entitled "The Band Played On" published in 1993 has only increased. Yet, if the Gies Report was to be released today, it would be as relevant as it was in 1926. In fact, my suggestion for a new Gies Report in 2006 has recently been conducted. Entitled the Gies Report for the Twenty-First Century, a series of papers have been published in the *Journal of Dental Education* in August and September 2017. While erudite, they are hardly provocative in directing dental education toward a more integrative role in healthcare. They point out that almost 70% of dental school curriculum is devoted to restorative dentistry. The potential changes on the way in oral health delivery of care based upon the economics and potential of dentists to widen their scope of practice and provide some primary care management of their patients' chronic diseases speak to the future possibilities. Dental education produces good clinicians who have a solid understanding of oral health but often a more limited perspective on overall health. Research efforts in most dental schools have decreased, and the practice and delivery of oral health to people is still hampered by lack of access, lack of insurance and integration with general healthcare.

Add to this the Cascada Declaration, calling for oral health to be a branch of medicine, the first ever Surgeon General's Report on Oral Health in 2001, the 2016 update by the surgeon general suggests that oral health integrates with primary care medicine and calls for greater integration of oral health and primary care medicine by physicians and dentists, and we have a moment for adaptive rather than technical change. Heifetz and Linsky point out in their book *Leadership on the Line* that adaptive leadership deals with problems that are not amenable to authoritative expertise or standard operating procedures. Adaptive challenges require experiments, new discoveries, and adjustments from numerous places in the organization, community, and yes, profession. Critically, adaptive change requires moving away from the status quo and loss for someone or some group. Consider the issues surrounding licensure by examination, that includes live patients in the US, experiments such as portfolio exams and OSCE exams exist, but the politics of the examination community is rocked by potential for huge loss in values, in culture, and maybe even in money. The tensions over dental therapists are rocking state legislatures. Ever since the first dental school was founded in the United States in 1840, dentistry and medicine have been taught as—and viewed as—two separate professions. This must change for true integration to occur. Kassebaum and Tedesco in a paper, "The 21st Century Dental Curriculum: A Framework for Understanding Current Models," have pointed out the challenges and opportunity for dental education to deal with changing scientific, social, and economic circumstances in order to move forward.

Advances in oral biology and craniofacial research are poised to produce new diagnostic and therapeutic options that will change the future character of dental and oral health practice. It is happening now. Medical treatments of surgical diseases exist today, and oral health is not immune, as silver diamine fluoride varnishes, and other advances begin to find a place in practice. What will be the tipping point? The establishment of the National Institute of Dental and Craniofacial Research as the third NIH institute was the result of the high percentage of WWII recruits who failed the requirement of seven upper and lower front teeth enabling the pulling of the pin from a hand grenade. Overall health and oral health remain separated by education, practice, and insurance coverage. Lack of integration is even evident in discussions of contemporary scientific advances. Any discussion of the human microbiome usually omits the major potential contribution of the oral microbiome. Gut microflora are highlighted in these discussions but rarely is the oral microbiome mentioned. Oral health is associated with procedures only, not science.

This second edition discusses some attempts to change course. The barriers between oral health and primary care are being chipped away with programs of integrated medical dental practice at regional healthcare systems like Kaiser Permanente Northwest and Marshfield Clinic Health System. The second editions present a case study on one such integrated care delivery model being focused on Marshfield Clinic Health System. Integrated oral and general health record computer systems are essential for these efforts. Integrated insurance coverage is another way to foster integration. Movement away from solo practice and the evidence that good oral health promotes good general health and reduces overall costs are other factors conducive to change. Our Harvard Initiative to Integrate Oral Health and Primary Care Medicine is based on the economic advantages. The Health Resources Service Administration (HRSA) has highlighted the importance of oral health in primary care by supporting grants to foster integration.

We need more than words now to accomplish integration. Pilots have existed for some time. I would suggest two that have had an impact. The first was the program at Yale Medical School in the 1930s. Dentists were admitted to the medical school to enhance their understanding of overall health and value of research. Although short-lived, due to WWII, this program produced some amazing people like Dr. Lester Burkett, the founder of oral medicine at the University of Pennsylvania, and Dr. Seymour Kreshover, who led the National Institute of Dental Research to prominence. Another such pilot is the oral and maxillofacial surgery-MD-general surgery program instituted at Harvard and the Massachusetts General Hospital in 1971 by Dr. Walter Guralnick. This acknowledged that rotations in medicine and surgery were not as good an education and training as completing the medical degree and doing general surgery at a more appropriate level of responsibility. This enabled expanded scope for many trainees that carried over into practice. What started as one program now is followed by almost 60. Moreover, the American College of Surgeons which originally considered only dual-degree individuals for membership now admits qualified single-degree oral and maxillofacial surgeons. So, the whole specialty has been elevated and acknowledged as well. This could happen to dentistry.

This volume speaks to the relationships between oral health and systemic health and vice versa and presents a handful of chapters that discuss such contact points from an informatics perspective. It is a call for the profession to consider altering its scope of practice, enlarging its interest in overall health, and moving away from procedures only to diagnosis and prevention. This goal is important to the health of the world's populations. This second edition of the book presents the case for integration well.

Walter Guralnick Distinguished Professor of Oral and Maxillofacial Surgery
Harvard School of Dental Medicine
Boston, MA, USA

Bruce Donoff

Integrating Medical and Dental Care: The Role of Informatics in Solving This Challenge

The intimate relationship between oral and systemic health makes the integration of medical and dental care essential. Epidemiological studies are continually advancing our understanding of this relationship, as evidenced by links between poor oral health and multiple systemic conditions, such as cardiovascular disease, respiratory diseases, and adverse birth outcomes. For instance, periodontal disease contributes to poor metabolic control in diabetics, placing these patients at risk of increased health complications. Diabetes, in turn, exacerbates periodontal infection and inflammation. This bidirectional nature is common to many oral-systemic disease relationships. Further, oral signs and symptoms can also indicate underlying systemic conditions and aid in their early detection. Viral diseases, such as HIV, herpes, and HPV, affect mucosal membranes, and corresponding lesions may first be seen in the mouth. Sjogren's syndrome can cause excessive dry mouth and enlarged parotid glands, signs that could help diagnose this autoimmune disorder. These examples demonstrate the value of integrating dental and medical care to manage oral and systemic health in a holistic manner. As many oral and systemic diseases, such as periodontal disease, cardiovascular disease, and diabetes, rise in prevalence and related healthcare costs increase, adopting an integrated approach becomes even more compelling.

As Dr. Bruce Donoff points out in his preface, many changes are needed to fully integrate dental and medical health systems effectively. Medicine and dentistry have evolved independently of each other, resulting in significant structural and operational differences among the professions. Integrating the two professions involves more than just colocating medical and dental providers. At its heart, integrating medicine and dentistry hinges on successfully merging information relevant to each of the two domains—the core focus of this book.

First, we must understand what information is important to medical and dental care providers, respectively. Such information needs to be structured, presented, and communicated in a way that provides meaning and value to clinicians. Lack of or difficulties in effective cross-communication can result in frustration, ambiguous shared health information, data collection redundancies and errors, and uncoordinated patient care. These communication issues can partially be addressed with a fully integrated and carefully designed electronic health record and communications approach.

How could real-time data access for a joint population of patients benefit both medical and dental providers? Consider, for example, a diabetic patient visiting a dental office for a regular checkup and prophylaxis. The dental hygienist, aware of the patient's health history, would like to know the patient's glycated hemoglobin level (HbA1c). High HbA1c levels signify uncontrolled diabetes and may require the hygienist to adapt the periodontal management and treatment plan. Typically patients have a hard time recalling test results from prior physician appointments. Wouldn't it be wonderful for the dental hygienist to effortlessly locate and review the patient's most updated medical health information and see the patient's most recent lab results? Consider, too, an obstetrician whose pregnant patient complains of bleeding and sore gums, but is afraid to see a dentist. The practitioner would like to contact a dentist to review and discuss this patient's case. A dental disease risk assessment tool for pregnant patients could be embedded into the electronic health record that would help the obstetrician understand the patient's oral health needs. And, wouldn't it be expedient for the obstetrician to contact a dental provider through the health system's electronic record? The two clinicians could team up to manage the patient's periodontal problems and her concerns with dental treatment during pregnancy. Supported by a seamless information and communication infrastructure, these healthcare providers can collaborate to ensure the mother is as healthy and disease-free as possible in time for the arrival of her newborn child.

With the shift from paper-based to electronic systems in healthcare, the integration of medical and dental data has already received increased awareness and support. Recently, the US Department of Defense (DoD) awarded a $4.3 billion contract to fund the Defense Healthcare Management System Modernization (DHMSM) program. Specifically, the funding supports the development of a new electronic health record (MHS GENESIS) that integrates medical and dental information into a single record. This streamlined electronic record system will give clinicians a complete picture of their patient's health through an interoperable, integrated medical and dental management system and promise to improve clinical decision-making and care outcomes for over nine million military personnel.

Other examples of operational systems that integrate medical and dental information can be found at the Veterans Administration, HealthPartners in Minnesota, and the Marshfield Clinic Health System, one of the largest private group medical practices in Wisconsin. At Marshfield, physicians and dentists can access and share patient medical and dental diagnoses, hospital data, radiographs, and prescription information. In addition, the Marshfield Clinic has implemented clinical decision support systems (CDSS) that use medical and dental data in the electronic health record to generate reminders and alerts. For example, the dental CDSS uses an algorithm that evaluates the patient's risk for diabetes or prediabetes based on selected medical data. If certain criteria are met, the dental CDSS generates an alert that notifies the dental provider to perform a blood glucose test at the dental appointment. This level of integration enables real-time decision support for diabetes management and disease prevention and illustrates the advances that medical and dental data integration can help foster. This book illustrate an integrated care delivery case study which provides a framework for action for others and how it can serve as important practical laboratory for what works and what does not.

Tremendous opportunities exist for the further integration of medical and dental data. However, realizing those opportunities requires that we overcome several challenges. For instance, we need to be able to connect a patient's health information across many clinical domains, care settings, and organizations. In the absence of patient-specific identifiers, this requires sophisticated patient-matching algorithms with high sensitivity and specificity. Second, we need to determine which information is relevant for which type of provider under which circumstances.

Modern digital infrastructures, such as health information exchanges, have been tremendously successful in aggregating patient information. However, for the clinician, accessing this information is akin to drinking from a firehose. The deluge of information needs to be distilled into manageable streams useful to clinicians. Third, standards for communicating information both within and across clinical disciplines need to evolve. While some well-developed and integrated standards exist, more work needs to be done in this area. (For instance, SNOMED now includes a subset of terms for dental diagnoses.) Fourth, new standards, such as Fast Healthcare Interoperability Resources (FHIR), need to be leveraged to effectively and efficiently aggregate patient information. Last, standards on privacy, security, and confidentiality that govern how patient information is shared and managed between the two professions require formulation and support.

If we surmount these challenges to integrating health information across medicine and dentistry, we can advance healthcare delivery significantly—for the betterment of the patient. Without data integration, successful interdisciplinary team approaches for optimal holistic care will continue to be difficult to implement. We owe it to our patients to provide them with high-quality, safe, efficient, and effective total body care. To do this, we must rethink how we care for our patients as a team of healthcare providers, not as individual practitioners. Can we achieve this vision? Read on! This book offers a thorough exploration of the integration of medical and dental data and provides examples and models as to why this work is essential for the future of healthcare.

Titus K. Schleyer
Clem McDonald Professor of Biomedical Informatics
Indiana University School of Medicine
Research Scientist, Regenstrief Institute, Inc.
Indianapolis, USA

Heather L. Taylor
PhD Student, School of Public Health, IUPUI
Indianapolis, USA

Editors' Preface

After the publishing of our first edition, it soon became evident that we would have to revisit our content given the rapidly changing environment and its impact on integrating dental and medical care. It has been 6 years since the publishing of the first edition, and many things have changed. For instance, at the time, the HITECH Act (Title XIII of the American Recovery and Reinvestment Act of 2009) was in full swing. As a result, we witnessed an uptake in the implementation of electronic dental records (EDRs) and electronic medical records (EMRs) as well as renewed interested in interoperability. The Centers for Medicare and Medicaid Services' Meaningful Use initiative drove the adoption through incentives for those offering Medicare/Medicaid services. It also impacted the delivery of care in other ways; for instance, by setting expectations that the general public may have regarding computerization of clinical practice ("would you go to an office that only uses paper?"). This requirement in turn changed the landscape from "if" to "when" we would achieve integration.

From the technological landscape, we can say that, for the most part, the offerings regarding EDRs and EMRs are relatively similar; however, what have evolved significantly are the environments where such technologies operate. App stores, subscription services, and mobile technology are on the rise and are now perfectly cemented mechanisms that further drive innovation. Cloud-based approaches to delivering services continue to evolve, and healthcare systems are getting more comfortable with using services beyond their usual on-premise model. All these changes are transforming the way we use technology. In these chapters, however, we made a conscious effort not to name specific technologies by brand and focused more on the principles behind their services given that, as any good technical writer knows, obsolescence is just around the corner for the written word if not done properly.

Clinically, there is still work that needs to be done, as we will review in the chapters herein. In this edition, we also aimed at bringing attention to informatics elements that are either necessary for integration or are more relevant given the aforementioned changes in the clinical care landscape. We also revisited content based on the readers' responses to the first edition and highlighted points that warranted further attention, for instance, the clinical contact points is now a whole chapter which summarizes the several connections between the oral and system conditions. This contact point chapter serves as an introduction to Section II chapters which further discuss in depth some of the key contact point areas. We also provide an update on the economic factors that play a role in integration. Optimistically, this can help facilitate discussions among those making decisions whether clinically, technologically, or in policy on why integration is beneficial as a whole. We also touched on aspects we did not work on in the previous version, and we also left elements that remain highly relevant not only clinically but also technically.

To establish continuity with initiatives which have preceded our effort in this edition of the book, the first preface by Dr. Bruce Donoff addresses the importance of integrating medical and oral healthcare and the need to eliminating the existing medical dental divide, while the second preface, by Dr. Titus K. Schleyer and Ms. Heather L. Taylor, highlights the role of biomedical and health informatics discipline in addressing the challenges that persist in the medical and dental data and care integration.

In order to help assure the appropriate interdisciplinary mix of input, we solicited contributions of varying lengths, knowing that being flexible on length would help attract contributors whose practice demands, administrative roles, and research schedules would otherwise not permit them to participate in this volume. Finally, we wanted to make sure that the two versions could be read as a continuation of our efforts. In that sense, the editions are complementary, and the reader of the earlier version will gain a better grasp of the field of dental and medical integration with this second edition. Notwithstanding, those encountering this book for the first time do not need to worry since we made sure it stands on its own and provides well self-contained content necessary to embark in the enterprise of improving dental and medical integration. Brief outlines of the coverage of the chapters are provided below:

- Chapter 1 addresses the rationale for integrating medical and dental care and patient records.
- Chapter 2 focuses on achieving the triple aim in healthcare with oral health in the equation.
- Chapter 3 provides an overview of the relationship between oral and systemic health and disease. It also presents a list of contact points between oral and systemic conditions.
- Chapters 4–10 provide an outline of the prevalence, systemic and oral manifestations, technological implications, existing risk assessment tools, care plans, and few other key topics that can serve as a guide to improve the health of patients with some of the systemic conditions and oral health.
- Chapter 11 addresses the key health information technology considerations of medical and dental data integration.
- Chapter 12 explores possible scenarios/use cases where dentists can use electronic dental record technology to increase the accuracy, coverage, and timeliness of existing public health surveillance efforts.

- Chapter 13 introduces the reader to many of the factors influencing knowledge management and representation as well as gain a better understanding of the technical aspects that can support or impede clinical integration.
- Chapter 14 provides a high-level overview of American national standards for health data integration and the social-technical issues in including oral health in national standards.
- Chapter 15 discusses dental insurance, its coverage, and its relationship to overall health status of the population in the United States and is mostly updated information from the first edition on this topic.
- Chapter 16 focuses on the need for interprofessional medical-dental education and is also an updated topic from the first edition of this book.
- Chapter 17 provides a case study of a large regional healthcare system in the United States on how integrated care delivery was achieved and supported through multifaceted approaches including development and training of integrated medical-dental healthcare delivery teams, interprofessional training, and practice implementation.
- Chapter 18 is the conclusion and focuses on reviewing models of integration in relation to academic, governmental, and private initiatives. The chapter discusses outstanding challenges and how emerging technologies may play a role in fostering dental and medical integration.
- The first two appendices present forms and material from two sources which have explicitly addressed integration of care: the University of Detroit Mercy School of Dentistry (Appendix A) and the Wisconsin Diabetes Mellitus Advisory Group (Appendix B).
- Appendix C provides the professional biography of the editorial team and the contributing authors in this edition.

Marshfield, WI, USA — Amit Acharya
Moon, PA, USA — Valerie Powell
Atlanta, GA, USA — Miguel H. Torres-Urquidy
Lubbock, TX, USA — Robert H. Posteraro
Indianapolis, IN, USA — Thankam Paul Thyvalikakath

Acknowledgments

I would like to take this opportunity to express my sincere gratitude to my mentors Mr. Greg Nycz and Dr. Susan Turney for their unparalleled support, encouragement, and guidance in shaping my career. They have provided me with several opportunities through the last decade to make a positive impact in the lives of people that Marshfield Clinic Health System serves and to bridge the chasm between medicine and dentistry. With their vision and leadership, thousands of underserved people and communities across rural Wisconsin and surrounding regions have been able to access high-quality oral healthcare within an integrated regional healthcare system, where they routinely seek medical care. I also want to thank my good friend and mentor, Dr. Murali Narayana, for his invaluable support and advice in shaping me to be a better leader and an effective healthcare/research administrator, which has been paramount for my career growth. It is heartwarming to witness and be a key part of this "Marshfield Clinic Health System" initiative under their leadership. I would also like to thank Dr. Justin Starren and Dr. Titus Schleyer for identifying the importance of dental informatics to improve oral and systemic health and providing a unique opportunity for me to pursue this field of research. I am very grateful for the support that I have received from my colleagues at the Center for Oral and Systemic Health, who are working tirelessly in making a positive difference in this important field. I would also like to thank all the authors, experts, and reviewers for their significant contributions to this book. I want to express my gratitude to my co-editors Dr. Valerie Powell who has been an inspiration to me, Dr. Miguel H. Torres-Urquidy for his camaraderie and support, Dr. Robert Posteraro for his ever-readiness to collaborate and the wealth of medical knowledge that he brought to this edition, and Dr. Thankam Thyvalikakath for keeping us focused. I am grateful for their invaluable support, enthusiasm, and perseverance in this undertaking. Finally, I would like to thank my better half, mother of my two beautiful daughters and my best friend, Rohini, who has stood by me like a guiding start, taught me never to give up when things got tough, taught me to get back up every time I fell down, and celebrated every success in my life. I could not have made it without her unwavering support and encouragement. I also want to thank my daughters, Anoushka (7 years) and Mihira (3 years), for their patience, support, and all the inquisitive questions regarding this book during its development.

> The best scientific thought is agreed that dentistry is a field of medicine. There is no logical right whatever to isolate [the oral cavity] from the rest of the body as if it were made up of ivory pegs in stone sockets." – Dr. Alfred Owre [Dean of Dentistry, University of Minnesota, 1905-27 and Columbia University, 1927-33]

Amit Acharya

I greatly appreciate the efforts of the many individuals that made the publishing of this second edition possible. First, I would like to acknowledge Grant Weston from Springer UK for his infinite patience and wisdom to support our efforts. Second, I want to thank my colleagues at CDC for supporting and allowing me to continue with this work. I especially would like to thank Barbara Nichols, Mark Berndt, Mark Frank, Emory Meeks, and Dr. Paula Yoon. I also want to thank the members of my team, Marian Dougherty, Benjamin Erickson, Guy Faler, Kathryn Harper, Emil Hristov, Susan Hughes, Marcus Kubota, and Caroline Westnedge. Additionally, I wish to thank Toby Crafton and Enrique Nieves who have always shared their wisdom, time, and, most of all, insightful conversations. Third, I want to thank all of the co-authors and co-editors whose dedication and insights made not only one but two editions of this book a reality. Especially I want to mention Valerie Powell for her unquestionable passion for this topic. It goes without saying that without her commitment, this edition would not have come to fruition. Finally, I want to thank and dedicate this book to my family, my wife Cristina, Alice, and Eva, for being so patient and letting daddy take time away to make this happen. I hope this book will serve as future inspiration when the time arrives.

Miguel H. Torres-Urquidy

First, I would like to thank my late father, Anthony F. Posteraro, AB, DDS, FACD, who instilled in me the truism that physicians and dentists are professional equals, and my late mother, Lygia P. Posteraro, for instilling in me a love of language and an understanding of grammar, punctuation, syntax, and spelling, which I only came to appreciate later in life. Next, I wish to especially acknowledge Valerie Powell for her intellectual curiosity, profound insight, and zeal in taking the lead in the struggle to integrate medical and dental healthcare records and for gathering us co-editors under her wing to help bring the message to a wider audience. She is truly one who asks not "Why?", but "Why not?". Grant Weston, from Springer UK, has been extremely patient as the second edition took shape and has also been a prime mover in getting us to bring it to fruition. Thank you, Grant! I wish to thank my fellow co-editors, Valerie Powell, who initiated the project; Amit Acharya, who stepped up to the plate when Valerie had more pressing issues to attend to and who set us on the course to completion; Miguel H. Torres-Urquidy, whose insights and suggestions were very helpful to me; and Thankam Thyvalikakath, who also offered well-appreciated insights and suggestions and was my co-reviewer and co-proofreader. Other than Valerie, I have not had the pleasure of meeting my other co-editors, face-to-face, but I feel that I have come to know them "virtually" and I hold them all in highest regard and thank them for welcoming me into their fold. I'd like to thank my program director, Sharon Hunt, and my chairman, Ryan Schmidt, who have been very understanding of the time I have had to work on this project. Finally, thank you, Elaine, for your support and patience, for listening calmly and offering encouragement when things got hectic, and for more things than I can list in this limited space.

Robert H. Posteraro

I would like to acknowledge Dr. Valerie Powell for convincing me to be co-editor of the second edition and my colleagues, Dr. Amit Acharya, Dr. Robert Posteraro, and Dr. Miguel H. Torres-Urquidy for their support. At this time, I am grateful to my professors from predoctoral and residency years who taught me the importance of oral-systemic disease connection. I would also like to acknowledge Dr. Titus Schleyer and Dr. Wishwa Kapoor for their support and guidance, especially during the early stages of my career in biomedical informatics. My colleagues and students have played a major role in enhancing my knowledge in dentistry and informatics, and I will always be indebted to them. Finally, I am thankful to my dear husband, Dr. Biju Cheriyan, who has been my source of strength and inspiration and my children, Ashok and Ashwin, who have been very understanding when I am away from them working.

Thankam Paul Thyvalikakath

Abbreviations

3D	3 Dimensional
AAMC	Association of American Medical Colleges
AAP	Aspiration-associated pneumonia
ACA	Affordable Care Act
ACC	American College of Cardiology
ACEI	Angiotensin converting enzyme inhibitor
ACGT	Advancing Clinico-Genomic Trial
ACO	Accountable Care Organization
AD	Autoimmune disease
ADA	American Dental Association
ADA	American Diabetes Association
ADEA	American Dental Education Association
AGE	Advanced glycosylation end products
AEGD	Advanced education general dentistry
AHA	American Heart Association
AHRQ	Agency for Healthcare Research and Quality
AI	Artificial intelligence
AIDS	Acquired immunodeficiency syndrome
AMI	Acute myocardial infarction
AMP	Anterior mandibular positioning
ANSI	American National Standards Institute
AP	Antibiotic prophylaxis
APACHE II	Acute physiology and chronic health evaluation II
ARRA	American Recovery and Reinvestment Act
ASCP	American Society of Clinical Pathologists
ASTHO	Association of State and Territorial Health Officials
ATS	American Thoracic Society
BBS	Bardet-Biedl syndrome
BDS	Bachelor of Dental Surgery
BMI	Body Mass Index
BON	Bisphosphonate-associated osteonecrosis

BTH	Brown tumor of hyperparathyroidism
CAD	Coronary artery disease
CAHPS	Consumer assessment of healthcare providers and systems
CAMBRA	Caries management by risk assessment
CAP	College of American Pathologists
CAP	Community acquired pneumonia
CBP	Complete blood picture
CBT	Computer based testing
CBT	Computer based training
CCHIT	Certification Commission for Health Information Technology
CDA	California Dental Association
CDA	Canadian Dental Association
CDC	Centers for Disease Control and Prevention
CDS	Clinical decision support
CDT	Current dental terminology
CE	Continuing education
CeVD	Cerebrovascular disease
cGVHD	Chronic graft-versus-host disease
CHC	Community Health Center
CHD	Coronary heart disease
CIED	Cardiovascular implantable electronic device
CKD	Chronic kidney disease
CKD-MBD	Chronic kidney disease—mineral and bone disorder
CMS	Centers for Medicare and Medicaid Services
CMS	Clinical Management System
CODA	Commission on Dental Accreditation
COHR	Computer-Based Oral Health Record
COSH	Center for Oral and Systemic Health
COTS	Commercial off-the-shelf
COPD	Chronic obstructive pulmonary disease
CPOE	Computerized physician order entry
CRP	C-Reactive protein
CSA	Cross-subspace analysis
CT	Computed tomography
CTSC	Cathepsin C gene
CVDs	Cardiovascular diseases
DART	Diagnostic Aid Resource Tool
DDS	Dental Diagnostic System
DDS	Doctor of Dental Surgery
DICOM	Digital imaging and communications in medicine
DKA	Diabetic ketoacidosis
DL	Description logics
DM	Diabetes mellitus
DMD	Doctor of Dental Medicine
DNM	Descending necrotizing mediastinitis

DOQ	Doctor's office quality
E&M	Evaluation and management
EBICP	Evidence-based integrated care plan
EDR	Electronic Dental Record
eGFR	Estimated glomerular filtration rate
EHR	Electronic Health Record
EHT	Electronic health technologies
EMR	Electronic Medical Record
ENT	Ear, nose and throat
EP	Eligible professional
ER	Emergency room
ESC	European Society of Cardiology
ESRD	End stage renal disease
FFS	Fee for service
FHC	Family Health Center
FQHC	Federally Qualified Health Center
GCF	Gingival crevicular fluid
GDP	Gross domestic product
GFR	Glomerular filtration rate
GH	Group health
GMP	General medical practitioner
GO	Gene ontology
GPRO	Group practice reporting option
GVHD	Graft-versus-host disease
GWAS	Genome Wide Association studies
HAART	Highly active anti-retroviral therapy
HAP	Hospital-acquired pneumonia
HCAP	Health care acquired pneumonia
HCP	Healthcare provider
HCT	Hematocrit
HCT	Hematologic stem cell transplant
HDL-C	High density lipoprotein-cholesterol
HHS	Health & Human Services
HIE	Health Information Exchange
HIO	Health Information Organization
HIPAA	Health Insurance Portability and Accountability Act
HIT	Health Information Technology
HITECH	Health Information Technology for Economic and Clinical Health
HIV	Human immunodeficiency virus
HMO	Health Maintenance Organization
HONK	Hyperosmolar hyperglycemic non-ketotic
HPO	Human phenotype ontology
HPT	Hyperthyroidism
HRSA	Health Resources and Services Administration
hsCRP	High sensitivity C-reactive protein

HSDM	Harvard School of Dental Medicine
HTC	Hemophilia Treatment Centre
Hx	History
ICD	Implantable cardioverter-defibrillator
ICD	International Classification of Diseases
ICD-10	International Classification of Diseases, Tenth Revision
ICD-10 CM	International Classification of Diseases, Tenth Revision, Clinical Modification
ICD-9	International Classification of Diseases, Ninth Revision
ICD-9 CM	International Classification of Diseases, Ninth Revision, Clinical Modification
ICU	Intensive care unit
IDSA	Infectious Diseases Society of America
IE	Infective endocarditis
iEHR	Integrated Electronic Health Record
iEDW	Integrated Enterprise Data Warehouse
IHI	Institute of Healthcare Improvement
INR	International Normalized Ratio
IOM	Institute of Medicine
IOTF	International Obesity Task Force
IT	Information Technology
JNC	Joint National Committee
KBTA	Knowledge based temporal abstraction
KDIGO	Kidney disease: improving global outcomes
LBW	Low birth weight
LDL	Low density lipoprotein
LIS	Laboratory Information System
LOP	Late onset pneumonia
LPS	Lipopolysaccharide
MA	Moving average
mBTS	Modified British Thoracic Society
MC	Marshfield clinic
MCEF	Marshfield Clinic Education Foundation
MCHS	Marshfield Clinic Health System
MCRI	Marshfield Clinic Research Institute
MCIS	Marshfield Clinic Information system
MD	Doctor of Medicine
MDPP	Medicare Diabetes Prevention Program
MEF	Mean etiologic fraction
MESA	Marshfield Epidemiologic Study Area
MetS	Metabolic syndrome
MGED	Microarray Gene Expression Data
MHD	Medical History for Dentists
MI	Myocardial infarction
MLR	Minimum loss rate

MOL	Maximum owed losses
MRI	Magnetic resonance imaging
MRSA	Methicillin-resistant *Staphylococcus aureus*
MSR	Minimum Savings Rate
MSS	Maximum Shared Savings
MSSP	Medicare Shared Savings Program
MU	Meaningful use
MVP	Mitral valve prolapse
NADP	National Association of Dental Plans
NCQA	National Committee for Quality Assurance
NHANES	National Health and Nutrition Examination Survey
NHE	National Health Expenditure
NHLBI	National Heart, Lung and Blood Institute
NIDDK	National Institute of Diabetes and Digestive and Kidney Diseases
NIH	National Institutes of Health
NIS	Nationwide inpatient sample
NJDOH	New Jersey Department of Health
NJDDCS	New Jersey Discharge Data Collection System
NK	Natural killer
NLP	Natural language processing
NPC	Nasopharyngeal carcinoma
NSACO	National Survey of Accountable Care Organizations
OF-RO	Osteitis fibrosa/renal osteodystrophy
OMS	Odontogenic maxillary sinusitis
ONCHIT	Office of the National Coordinator for Health Information Technology
OPG	Orthopantomogram
ORN	Osteoradionecrosis
OWL	Ontology Web Language
PCI	Percutaneous Coronary Intervention
PCMH	Patient Centered Medical Home
PD	Periodontitis
PD	Periodontal disease
PDQ	Physician Data Query
PGP	Physician group practice
PHI	Protected Health Information
PHR	Personal Health Record
PLS	Papillon-Lefèvre syndrome
PQRI	Physician quality reporting initiative
PPM	Permanent pacemaker
PSF	Privacy and Security Framework
PSI	Pneumonia Severity Index
PVD	Peripheral vascular disease
PY	Performance year
RDW	Research Data Warehouse

RECIN	Registry for Effectively Communicating Immunization Needs
RMED	Rural Medical Education
RODS	Real-Time Outbreak and Disease Surveillance Laboratory
RSV	Respiratory syncytial virus
SAPS	Simplified Acute Physiology Score
SARS	Severe acute respiratory syndrome
SCORE	Systematic coronary risk evaluation
SDOs	Standards Development Organizations
SHEA	Society for Healthcare Epidemiology of America
SLE	Systemic lupus erythematosus
SNODENT	Systematized Nomenclature of Dentistry
SNOMED CT	Systematized Nomenclature of Medicine—Clinical Terms
SS	Sjögren syndrome
SSN	Social Security Number
TNFα	Tumor necrosis factor-alpha
UAE	Urinary albumin excretion
UI	User interface
US	United States
USA	United States of America
USDHHS	US Department of Health & Human Services
USAMRIID	US Army Medical Research Institute of Infectious Disease
USRDS	United States Renal Data System
UWSMPH	University of Wisconsin School of Medicine and Public Health
VA	Veterans Administration
VATS	Video-assisted thoracoscopic surgery
VAP	Ventilator acquired pneumonia
VSD	Vaccine Safety Datalink
WARM	Wisconsin Academy for Rural Medicine
WBC	White blood cell
WDS	Washington Dental Service
ZIP	Zone Improvement Plan

Contents

Contributors

Amit Acharya, B.D.S., M.S., Ph.D. Center for Oral and Systemic Health, Marshfield Clinic Research Institute, Marshfield, WI, USA

Mureen Allen, M.D., M.S., M.A., F.A.C.P. UnitedHealth Group, New York City, NY, USA

Jordan L. Ashton, D.O. Marshfield Clinic-Stettin Medical Center, Stettin, WI, USA

Valerie Bertaud-Gounot, D.M.D., Ph.D. Psychiatric Hospital of Rennes, Rennes, France

Kelly Boggs, M.B.A. Network Engagement, Aspirus Network Inc., Wausau, WI, USA

Monica Chaudhari, Dr.P.H. Cancer Research and Biostatisticians, Seattle, WA, USA

Louay O. Danial, M.D. Marshfield Clinic-Park Falls Medical Center, Park Falls, WI, USA

Richard Dart, M.D. Center for Human Genetics, Marshfield Clinic Research Institute, Marshfield, WI, USA

Mark Diehl, D.D.S., M.A., M.P.H. Health Informatics Program, Misericordia University, Dallas, TX, USA

Franklin Din, D.M.D., M.A. FraudLens Inc., Arlington, VA, USA

Bruce Donoff, D.M.D., M.D. Harvard School of Dental Medicine, Boston, MA, USA

Stephen Foreman, J.D., Ph.D., M.P.A. Health Economics, Robert Morris University, Pittsburgh, PA, USA

Shin-Mey Rose Yin Geist, D.D.S., M.S. Departments of Biomedical and Diagnostic Sciences and Patient Management, University of Detroit Mercy School of Dentistry, Detroit, MI, USA

Ingrid Glurich, Ph.D. Center for Oral and Systemic Health, Marshfield Clinic Research Institute, Marshfield, WI, USA

Casey Hein, B.S.D.H., R.D.H., M.B.A. International Center for Oral-Systemic Health, College of Dentistry, University of Manitoba, Winnipeg, MB, Canada

Rady Faculty of Health Sciences, University of Manitoba, Winnipeg, MB, Canada

Mark Jurkovich, D.D.S., M.H.A. HealthPartners Institute, Minneapolis, MN, USA

Joseph Kilsdonk, Au.D. Office of Medical Education, Aspirus Healthcare Systems, Wausau, WI, USA

Ted Klein, M.S. Klein Consulting Informatics, LLC, Star Valley Ranch, WY, USA

Kori Krueger, M.D., M.B.A. Institute for Quality Innovation and Patient Safety, Marshfield Clinic, Marshfield, WI, USA

Jayanth Kumar Medam, B.D.S. Dental Informatics Core, Department of Cariology, Operative Dentistry and Dental Public Health, Indiana University School of Dentistry, IUPUI, Indianapolis, IN, USA

School of Informatics and Computing, IUPUI, Indianapolis, IN, USA

William Melms, M.D. Marshfield Clinic-Minocqua Medical Center, Minocqua, WI, USA

Sushma Mishra, Ph.D. Robert Morris University, Pittsburgh, PA, USA

John O'Brien, D.D.S. Family Health Center Inc., Marshfield, WI, USA

Aloksagar Panny, B.D.S., M.S. Center for Oral and Systemic Health, Marshfield Clinic Research Institute, Marshfield, WI, USA

Ram Pathak, M.D., F.A.C.P., F.A.C.E. Department of Endocrinology, Marshfield Clinic, Marshfield, WI, USA

Robert H. Posteraro, M.D., M.B.I. Department of Healthcare Management and Leadership, Texas Tech University Health Sciences Center School of Health Professions, Lubbock, TX, USA

Valerie Powell, Ph.D., M.S., R.T.(R). Robert Morris University, Moon Township, PA, USA

Frank Scannapieco, D.M.D., Ph.D. Department of Oral Biology, School of Dental Medicine, State University of New York at Buffalo, Buffalo, NY, USA

Titus K. Schleyer, D.M.D., Ph.D. Center for Biomedical Informatics, Research Scientist, Regenstrief Institute, Inc., Indianapolis, IN, USA

Department of Medicine, Indiana University School of Medicine, Indianapolis, IN, USA

Neel Shimpi, B.D.S., M.M., Ph.D. Center for Oral and Systemic Health, Marshfield Clinic Research Institute, Marshfield, WI, USA

Cynthia A. Sorenson, F.N.P. Marshfield Clinic Stettin Medical Center, Stettin, WI, USA

Heather L. Taylor, M.P.H., L.D.H. PhD Student, IUPUI School of Public Health, Indianapolis, IN, USA

Thankam Paul Thyvalikakath, D.M.D., Ph.D. Dental Informatics Core, Department of Cariology, Operative Dentistry and Dental Public Health, Indiana University School of Dentistry, IUPUI, Indianapolis, IN, USA

School of Informatics and Computing, IUPUI, Indianapolis, IN, USA

Centre for Biomedical Informatics, Regenstrief Institute, Indianapolis, IN, USA

Miguel H. Torres-Urquidy, D.D.S., M.S., Ph.D. (candidate) Centers for Disease Control and Prevention, Atlanta, GA, USA

Peter Umukoro, M.D., M.P.H., Sc.D. Department of Internal Medicine, Marshfield Clinic, Marshfield, WI, USA

Jayanth Vedre, MD, M.P.H. Medical Intensive Care Unit, Marshfield Clinic, Marshfield, WI, USA

About the Editors

Amit Acharya B.D.S., M.S., Ph.D., is the executive director of the Marshfield Clinic Research Institute (MCRI) at Marshfield Clinic Health System (MCHS) in Wisconsin, USA. Dr. Acharya provides leadership and direction to support the mission and vision of the Institute, and he is responsible for the oversight of the research operations. He subsequently serves as the chief dental informatics officer (CDIO) of the Family Health Center (FHC) at MCHS. FHC provides care to low-income, Medicaid, and uninsured populations at 19 medical and 10 dental FQHC sites (44 general dentists, 2 oral surgeons, and 44 hygienists) in partnership with Marshfield Clinic. As the CDIO, Dr. Acharya is responsible for developing strategic road map and advising specific implementation groups of key informatics and information technology best practices to support patient care, research, and educational activities. He is actively involved in development and implementation of effective clinical systems and applications that brings the practice of medicine and dentistry at MCHS closer, contributing to cost reduction and helping streamline the process of delivering healthcare.

Dr. Acharya is also a tenured research scientist at the Center for Oral and Systemic Health at MCRI. Dr. Acharya has been a leading researcher and is well-regarded throughout the United States on his expertise in biomedical and dental informatics. As a general dental surgeon and a computer scientist with expertise in the field of biomedical informatics, Dr. Acharya's research focus has been in the area of applied clinical informatics focusing on integration of medical and dental data, clinical and research information systems, and design and architecture of electronic health records; developing clinical decision supports; and investigating the oral-systemic relationship between periodontal and systemic disease, such as diabetes, and cardiovascular and respiratory diseases. Dr. Acharya's desire to pursue the field of health information technology and informatics developed due to a desire to bridge the gap between medical and dental care.

Dr. Acharya has been instrumental in the founding of the Center for Oral and Systemic Health (COSH) (formerly known as the Institute for Oral and Systemic Health) which is one of the six research centers at MCRI, the integration of

Marshfield Clinic's electronic dental record with its propriety electronic medical record, and the establishment of one of the very few oral health informatics postdoctoral fellowship programs in the nation. Dr. Acharya places a strong emphasis on education and the development of the future research workforce. He served as the program director of this NLM-/NIDCR-funded Oral Health Informatics postdoctoral fellowship program at MCRF (in collaboration with the University of Wisconsin-Madison) from 2012 to 2017. He also served on the management committee of UW-Madison's Computational and Informatics in Biology and Medicine program and has mentored several graduate students and postdoctoral fellows as part of this program. Marshfield Clinic along with UW-Madison is one of the only three institutions in the nation to offer postdoctoral training in dental informatics training.

Dr. Acharya completed his Bachelor of Dental Surgery from Bangalore University, India, in 2000 after which he practiced clinical dentistry as a house surgeon and a dental officer for few years. He then completed his master's in computer science from Western Kentucky University, KY, in 2004 moving on to completing his doctoral in biomedical informatics from University of Medicine and Dentistry in New Jersey, NJ, in 2010. He also pursued additional training in leadership strategies for information technology in healthcare from Harvard School of Public Health, Boston. Before moving to Marshfield Clinic in 2010, Dr. Acharya served as a visiting scholar at the Center of Dental Informatics, University of Pittsburgh.

Dr. Acharya has published over 100 scientific abstracts and manuscripts in national and international peer-reviewed journals. He was also one of the original editors on the first edition of this book, *Integration of Medical and Dental Care and Patient Data* which was published by Springer. He was invited to serve on the 2012 American Medical Informatics Association (AMIA) Scientific Programming Committee (SPC). He has received multiple grant funding dedicated to bridging the medical and dental divide throughout the course of his career.

Dr. Acharya has held several national leadership roles including secretary, chair-elect, and chair of the American Dental Education Association's Dental Informatics Section and co-chair-elect and co-chair of the American Medical Informatics Association's Dental Informatics Work Group. He had served as the chairman of the clinical informatics subcommittee of the American Dental Associations' (ADA) Standards Committee for Dental Informatics and the ADA representative to the Health Level Seven (HL7) in the past. He has also served on national HIT expert panels coordinated by entities like Agency for Healthcare Research and Quality (AHRQ), Office of the National Coordinator (ONC) for Health Information Technology, and National Quality Forum (NQF). Dr. Acharya currently serves as a member on the advisory board of the National Center for Community Health Research and ADA Dental Quality Alliance's Implementation and Evaluation Committee.

He is a strong advocate for child health and volunteers with the Children International Organization, which is dedicated to fighting poverty and supporting children in need in poor and developing countries.

Valerie Powell Ph.D., M.S., R.T.(R)., a native of Racine, Wisconsin, USA, first studied humanities, with a focus on languages, philosophy, and linguistics, then computer science and information systems, and finally radiologic technology. Her undergraduate studies in German and philosophy at Wabash College in Indiana included a year of studies of philosophy and linguistics at the Albert-Ludwigs-Universität, Freiburg im Breisgau, Germany. She then earned a master's degree and a PhD at the University of Texas at Austin. Her postdoctoral master's degree in computer science was completed at Texas A&M University in Commerce, Texas. She started teaching at the University of Texas at Austin in the fall of 1959 and has been teaching for over 50 years. She spent a sabbatical semester as a visiting scientist in dynamic systems at the Software Engineering Institute of Carnegie Mellon University, where the focus of her work was formal modeling of resectorization in the FAA Air Traffic Control System. Dr. Powell's studies in philosophy sensitized her to the properties of classification systems. She feels this foundation helped her question the routine sense of medical care that omitted attention to the stomatognathic system in certain critical respects.

When she began to work with and teach MUMPS (Massachusetts General Hospital Utility Multi-Programming System) in computer science in the early 1980s, she was soon invited to work with the US Department of Veterans Affairs (VA). Her first publications in the field of hospital information systems appeared in the mid-1980s. She taught databases, including clinical databases, for a number of decades (both relational SQL technology and the MUMPS-based VA FileMan database technology of the US Department of Veterans Affairs. She was admitted to the Sigma Xi science research honor society for research leading to a paper presented in Nagoya, Japan, in 1988: "Implications of Non-1NF Extensions to the Relational Database Model for the MUMPS Standard and MUMPS Databases." From 1988 through 1996, she served as a consulting scholar in medical computing for IBM Corporation. Dr. Powell carried out a number of projects for the VA (and also for the Indian Health Service (IHS)) over the years through 1999. From 1988 through 1992, she worked with Trident Technical College in Charleston, SC, to add an electronic dental record for patients served by their oral health education programs (dental hygiene and dental assisting).

During this period, she also served on software standards committees: X3/DBSSG (Database Systems Study Group), X11 (MUMPS Users Group), NCITS/T3 (OSI Telecommunications), and as chair of NCITS/J21 (model-based formal specification systems), a committee with US technical advisory group (TAG) responsibilities for the Z and VDM international standards. Dr. Powell learned health informatics through collaboration with Dr. Charles J. Austin, author of textbooks on hospital information systems, and Dr. med. Wolfgang Giere, Director, Zentrum für medizinische Informatik, Goethe University, Frankfurt am Main, Germany, and through almost 20 years of experience assisting the US Veterans Health Administration and working with its DHCP (later VistA) electronic health record (EHR) technology. In 1999, she gave invited lectures on health informatics and Year 2000 concerns at the Zentrum für Medizinische Informatik, Goethe University, Frankfurt am Main, Germany. She also lectured on Year 2000 issues at the Brandenburg Technische Hochschule in Cottbus. These lectures were sponsored by the US Embassy in Berlin.

In 2000, she felt she needed clinical experience to do the kind of work in healthcare informatics she wished to do and completed the prerequisites for a degree in radiologic technology and then the degree itself, passing the ARRT registry exam in 2002. She found this clinical experience valuable in her informatics work. She chose imaging as it would (and did) give her contact with many subspecialties of medical care as well as first-hand experience in the emergency department and with a variety of surgical procedures in the operating room environment. It gave her experience with the workflow of the care setting and the necessary sense of delivering care to an individual patient for which one is responsible and not just for patient data. Since 1999, Dr. Powell has worked with WorldVistA, a nonprofit organization making open-source VA VistA EHR technology available domestically and internationally. In 2007, she was invited by the Mexican government agency Instituto Mexicano del Seguro Social (IMSS) to provide technical advice on health information technology (HIT) in Mexico City. She taught healthcare informatics at Robert Morris University.

In 2007, Pennsylvania Gov. Ed Rendell appointed Dr. Powell to the Governor's Commission on Chronic Care Management, Reimbursement, and Cost Reduction, because of her extensive work with health information technology. With this assignment and facing the question as to whether performance measures proposed for the Commission's strategic plan were adequate, she noticed the omission of "dental referral" from the set of diabetes performance measures. She sought advice from the American Academy of Periodontology research staff in Chicago to learn what she needed to know to evaluate diabetes performance measures. She set about bringing her evaluation to the attention of the American Diabetes Association (ADA) and encouraged the ADA to add "dental referral" to its standards of care (SoC) for diabetes. This was done in 2007–2008. In 2008, she started giving lectures on and writing on the need to integrate medical and dental care and patient data. In 2018, Dr. Powell was named to the Board of Directors, Metro Community Health Center, South Braddock Ave., Pittsburgh, PA. She holds an appointment as university professor of computer and information systems emerita at Robert Morris University, Moon Township, Pennsylvania, where she has taught for 20 years.

Miguel H. Torres-Urquidy D.D.S., M.S., Ph.D. (candidate), is a Senior Service Fellow with the Division of Health Informatics and Surveillance of US Centers for Disease Control and Prevention. Because of his clinical and informatics expertise, he has served in multiple roles and projects within CDC. He currently supports the Medical Countermeasure Tracking System (CTS). Elements of CTS are used to distribute medications and medical supplies to the general population during national and regional public health emergencies. Previously he managed the public web release of information for the National Notifiable Disease Surveillance System (NNDSS) used by all US public health departments to report notifiable conditions. He served as lead for the Public Health Informatics Fellowship Program and also as former acting program manager for BioSense (now the National Syndromic Surveillance Program).

As part of the National Syndromic Surveillance Program, he oversaw the Influenza-Like Illness, Hepatitis and Opioid-Overdose Pilot Projects. As Ebola responder, he served as senior informatics advisor for the CDC's Domestic Clinical Inquiries Team supporting US hospitals and clinics, as well as public health departments when handling confirmed and suspected Ebola cases in the United States.

He first joined CDC as informatics fellow for CDC's Influenza Division. During his tenure, he worked on facilitating access to CDC data to the general public by creating several visualization systems of influenza information (FluView Interactive). In addition, he developed two iPhone/iPad applications, one that provides data on national influenza activity and another that assists triaging patients with flu-like symptoms. He also supported the Idaho Department of Health and Welfare in improving the matching of Vehicle Accident Data with other information sources. Internationally, he aided the Influenza Division in assessing influenza surveillance capabilities in Central America. His work earned him the Best Poster Award at the International Society for Disease Surveillance Conference in 2010. He and his colleagues also received the 2013 National Center for Immunization and Respiratory Diseases (NCIRD) Honor Award for "Excellence in Domestic Epidemiology" for their work in FluView.

Before joining CDC, he worked as postdoctoral associate at the Center for Dental Informatics at the University of Pittsburgh where he conducted NIH-funded research focused on diagnostic terminologies. Dr. Torres-Urquidy was trained as a dentist at the National Autonomous University of Mexico and continued his education with a master's degree in biomedical informatics from the School of Medicine at the University of Pittsburgh where he also pursued his doctoral studies. He also rotated with the NIH's National Library of Medicine in the summer of 2004. During his rotation, he conducted analyses on US public policy related to the establishment of the National Health Information Infrastructure. Previously, in 1996 and 1999, he collaborated with the Department of Dental Informatics at Temple University conducting and publishing studies in the adoption of information technology and use of Internet by clinicians.

He is past chair of the Dental Informatics Working Group at the American Medical Informatics Association. He has published and currently serves as reviewer in several grant and contract review panels, scientific journals, and conferences.

Robert H. Posteraro M.D., M.B.I., F.A.C.R., is a professor and assistant program director in the Master of Science in Healthcare Administration (MSHA) program at Texas Tech University Health Sciences Center—School of Health Professions. Dr. Posteraro graduated Phi Beta Kappa, magna cum laude, in cursu honorum, with a Bachelor of Science degree from Fordham College and earned his MD degree from Yale University School of Medicine. He did a fellowship in chest radiology at Yale and a fellowship in magnetic resonance imaging at Duke. He earned his Master of Biomedical Informatics degree from Oregon Health & Science University. Prior to joining the MSHA faculty, Dr. Posteraro practiced radiology in both academic and private practice settings. He was chairman of the Department of Radiology at Texas Tech University HSC School of Medicine. He continues to stay current in radiology and teaches radiation biology, radiation protection, and digital imaging, on a voluntary basis, at the Covenant School of Radiography, in Lubbock, TX.

Dr. Posteraro has numerous publications, presentations, and guest lectures to his credit. He has been named Outstanding Faculty Member seven times, by the students in the MSHA program. He is a peer reviewer for three journals and is a member of the American Medical Informatics Association and the Society for Imaging Informatics in Medicine. His current work is on the use and effects of informatics in distance education and the development of critical thinking skills in students.

Thankam Paul Thyvalikakath D.M.D., M.D.S., Ph.D., is the director of dental informatics core at the Indiana University School of Dentistry as well as a research scientist at the Center for Biomedical Informatics, Regenstrief Institute, Indianapolis, IN. As core director, she has established a program to enhance patient care through improved data capture and retrieval to assess treatment outcomes. Dr. Thyvalikakath earned her PhD degree in biomedical informatics in 2012 from the University of Pittsburgh School of Medicine. She also holds a dental degree and certificate in clinical research from the University of Pittsburgh as well as a dental degree from the University of Kerala, India, and a master's degree in oral and maxillofacial surgery from the University of Calicut, India.

Dr. Thyvalikakath has served as principal investigator, co-investigator, or consultant on numerous National Institute of Health grants. Her research established foundational knowledge on applying user-centered design and cognitive engineering methods to design and evaluate clinical systems in dentistry. Currently, she is leading a study supported through the National Dental Practice-based Research Network of the NIDCR to explore the feasibility of mining electronic dental record data from network practices to assess treatment outcomes. In addition, she is co-investigator on a recent NIDCR-funded study to implement clinical decision support for tobacco cessation in dental practices. Dr. Thyvalikakath also participates in clinical teaching and practice at the IU School of Dentistry. She has several publications, presentations, and guest lectures to her credit and is a peer reviewer for five journals. She was a member of the American Medical Informatics Association (AMIA) Task Force to develop eligibility requirements for the Advance Health Informatics Certification (AHIC). She is also a past chair of the Dental Informatics Work Group at AMIA and Dental Informatics Section at American Dental Educators Association (ADEA).

About the Authors

Mureen Allen M.D., M.S., M.A., F.A.C.P., has held several positions involving health information technology (IT) and data analytics. She has worked on a variety of initiatives involving the acquisition and aggregation of clinical data with administrative data to identify signals that drive variation in clinical care. Dr. Allen is committed to the development of solutions that improve the delivery of healthcare. Her interests include clinical decision support, quality measurement, systems interoperability, usability, and the patient-centered medical home. Dr. Allen was the senior associate for informatics and practice improvement at the American College of Physicians (ACP), providing support for health IT public policy initiatives. Dr. Allen served as a co-chair of the Health Information Technology Standards Panel. As a co-chair, she was active in identifying the appropriate standards to support consumer empowerment while using a personal health record, and she supported the identification of standards for consumers to express their preferences for sharing data. Dr. Allen is board-certified in internal medicine. Beyond her recognition as a fellow of the American College of Physicians, she is a member of the American Medical Association and the American Medical Informatics Association. Dr. Allen holds master's degrees in biomedical informatics and in technology management.

Jordan Ashton D.O., practices family medicine in a holistic manner, which incorporates all aspects of medicine, including oral health. As a clinical oral health champion, she has been engaged in a pilot study incorporating oral healthcare for her diabetic patients. Her passion for the integration of oral-systemic health has led to national recognition of her efforts, including speaking on behalf of Marshfield Clinic at the National Interprofessional Initiative on Oral Health (NIIOH) Symposium and creating a webinar for the American Diabetic Association (ADA). She received her Bachelor of Science from the University of Wisconsin-Madison and attended medical school at Michigan State University College of Osteopathic Medicine. Dr. Ashton completed her family medicine residency at Botsford Hospital in Farmington Hills, Michigan. Now in her fifth year of practice with Marshfield Clinic, she is putting her values of integrated healthcare into fruition. As a Wisconsin native, Dr. Ashton understands the importance of giving back to her community, as she is also actively engaged in medical education for students.

Valerie Bertaud-Gounot Ph.D., is full professor and hospital practitioner at the Health Big Data Department of the University of Rennes, France. She obtained her bachelor's degree in computer engineering and subsequently her dental degree. She later obtained a PhD in biomedical informatics followed by a master's in statistics. She teaches preventive medicine, biostatistics, evidence-based medicine, and dental informatics. In addition, she continues her clinical activities providing care for patients at the dental emergency facility of the University Hospital and the Dental Office of the Psychiatric Hospital of Rennes.

Kelly A. Boggs B.S., M.B.A., achieved her undergraduate degree in political science and public administration from UW-Stevens Point in 2001. After college, Kelly spent 7 years in the mortgage industry before going back to school for an MBA with a healthcare focus in 2006 and graduating in 2008. Kelly completed a 2-year Academic Administrative Fellowship at Marshfield Clinic. Her capstone project of her fellowship involved of the completion of an application to the Commission on Dental Accreditation for a dental residency program, which was ultimately approved. In 2012, Kelly joined Ministry Health Care as an account executive working on dual programs for cardiology and oncology with Marshfield Clinic. In the next 5 years, she progressed from an account executive to the director of physician relations. Kelly completed a Leadership Development Program with American College of Healthcare Executives and has been a member of the Medical College of Wisconsin's Regional Advisory Admissions Committee (RAAC) since the inaugural class in 2015. In 2018, she accepted a director of network engagement position with Aspirus Network, Inc., a clinically integrated network. Kelly lives in Stevens Point, WI, with her husband, Dan, and sons, Harrison and Griffin.

Monica Chaudhari Dr.P.H., is a doctoral biostatistician providing methodological, analytical, and statistical support in the field of healthcare research. She began her career at WDS (2006–2011) after attaining a master's degree in biostatistics from the University of Washington. Her functional areas at WDS included facilitation of medical-dental collaborative research, multicenter provider profiling, dental utilization and cost analysis, and dental treatments and outcomes assessment. During her tenure, Dr. Chaudhari and Group Health investigators examined association between diabetes mellitus and periodontal disease in health outcomes and medical costs. They also looked at implications of diabetes in use of dental services and costs.

Since then, she has had experience in multiple therapeutic areas (clinical phase-II/phase-III or observational studies) including immunology, diabetes type-I/type-II, post-traumatic stress disorder (PTSD), gynecology, and oncology. Her statistical work has focused on methodologies for precision medicine and other modeling techniques including, but not limited to, stochastic/mixed effect, survival/longitudinal, Bayesian, skewed/overdispersed/missing data, causal inference, multistate disease progression, and high-dimensional supervised and unsupervised learning. She has contributed significant independent scientific insights and has demonstrated the ability to develop and apply new methods to studies of a relatively new field of inquiry.

Dr. Chaudhari serves as a journal referee and belongs to professional organizations including the International Biometric Society and the American Statistical Association (ASA).

Louay Danial M.D., is a family medicine practitioner at the Marshfield Clinic Park Falls Center and Marshfield Clinic Phillips Center. He has more than 20 years of clinical experience. He completed his residency in family medicine from Swedish Covenant Hospital, Chicago, in 2005. His interests include primary care including OB/GYN, pediatric medicine, and geriatric medicine.

Richard Dart M.D., M.A.C.P., F.C.C.P., F.A.H.A., F.A.S.N., F.A.S.H., is a Marshfield Clinic Emeritus Research Clinician. Dr. Dart has been actively engaged in the research process to varying degrees throughout his nearly 50-year career as a physician. During special fellowship training in the research division of the Cleveland Clinic Foundation, he was engaged in a study of total body sodium under the tutelage of Harriet P. Dustan, MD. Upon entering clinical practice in the Department of Hypertension and Nephrology at Marshfield Clinic in 1973, he participated in clinical studies as well as collaborative research with basic scientist Duane Tewksbury, PhD, in the Marshfield Clinic Research Foundation on a study exploring high molecular weight angiotensinogen in pregnancy-induced hypertension. Later collaborative work resulted in characterization of the placental location of an angiotensinogen receptor in the human placenta.

In addition to this collaborative work, he has also participated in numerous clinical trials, including a phase three trial of Capoten, one of the first oral angiotensin-converting enzyme inhibitors, and the membranous glomerulonephritis/nephrotic syndrome Prednisone trial. In addition, Dr. Dart served as site PI for a number of multi-institutional initiatives, including the IgA Nephropathy/Fish Oil trial, the National Heart, Lung, and Blood Institute's Antihypertensive, Lipid Lowering, Heart Attack Prevention Trial (ALLHAT), and the Focal Sclerosing Glomerulonephritis Genetics Trial. More recently, Dr. Dart's efforts have been focused on genetic-based studies, including an investigation of the genetic variation in 25-hydroxyvitamin D 1 alpha hydroxylase (CYP27B1) in congestive heart failure patients with hypertension and additional studies related to the relationship between single nucleotide polymorphisms and high-sensitivity C-reactive protein and other covariables (1–3).

Outside the clinical research environment, he has also been involved in several educational and bioethical projects serving as a contributing member and co-author for several writing committees.

Mark Diehl D.D.S., was the director of the Health Informatics Program at Misericordia University, Dallas, PA, where he built a comprehensive undergraduate, graduate, and continuing education program. His research interests included data architecture and modeling, information governance, and the human-system interaction.

Dr. Diehl was member of the US Technical Advisory Group of the International Standards Organization Technical Committee 215 on Health Informatics, chair of the American Dental Association Standards Committee on Dental Informatics Subcommittee 11 on Clinical Informatics, and co-chair of the ASTM subcommittee E31.25 on Healthcare Data Management, Security, Confidentiality, and Privacy. He is the principal author of several health informatics standards such as the ANSI/ADA Specifications 1000, 1027, and 1039 and ASTM standards E2145 and E2436.

He also contributed to standards work in Health Level Seven, serving as the HL7 liaison to the American Dental Association, and worked on standards activities in the ANSI Health Information Technology Standards Panel and the National Council for Prescription Drug Programs.

Among his degrees, Dr. Diehl received a DDS from Temple University, an MA in computer data management and health systems management from Webster University and an MPH in Health Services Administration from the Uniformed Services University.

Franklin M. Din D.M.D., M.A., is currently the chief medical information officer for FraudLens Inc. Previously he was a solution architect for Transactions, Code Sets & Informatics, HP Enterprise Services, Global Healthcare, and is responsible for providing medical informatics, terminology, and other healthcare data standards expertise improve healthcare delivery, costs, outcomes, and future trends. Standardization of data is essential to the informatics goal of turning massive amounts of data into useful and actionable knowledge.

Frank worked at HP from 2009 until 2012. In July 2009, he led the Medical Informatics Center of Excellence (MICOE) team successfully partnered with a Title XIX Account to seamlessly in-source business analytic work that was previously outsourced at a cost of millions of dollars. In March 2010, he led the MICOE team that successfully delivered an HP proprietary, Medicaid-specific predictive model for diabetes. In November of 2010, Frank successfully designed, prototyped, and demonstrated an approach to perform medical term standardization, natural language processing, and ontology development, all in Mandarin, for a Nationwide Medical Records Project in China.

Before joining HP, Frank was a senior informatics consultant for Apelon, Inc. He was involved with data standardization for two rounds of the National Health Information Network (NHIN); he led the team that produced a strategy to cross map discrete medication data streams which resulted in simplified analytics for an academic medical center; he devised a plan to bring SNODENT terminology into compliance with SNOMED CT; he worked on the improvement to the National Cancer Institute's NCI Thesaurus that resulted in the new BioMed GT terminology while simultaneously creating the prototype of a collaborative semantic media wiki that permits remote collaboration on BioMed GT. While working for the VHA in the Salt Lake City Office of Information, Frank created a tool to map concepts in VistA with SNOMED CT for the LDSI (Lab Data Sharing Initiative) which links the VHA and the Department of Defense lab systems; he created an MS Excel mapping tool to convert the Kaiser Permanente ICD-9-based problem list into a SNOMED CT-based list. This work became the basis of the FDA's SPL problem list.

Prior to his specialization in biomedical informatics, Frank was a practicing dentist, assistant clinical professor of dentistry at NYU Dental School, and course director for forensics dentistry at Columbia University School of Dental and Oral Surgery. He currently serves as a member of DMORT (Disaster Mortuary Operational Response Team) to perform forensic dental services at mass disaster sites, with previous deployments to the World Trade Center and Hurricane Katrina.

Frank has active memberships in AMIA (American Medical Informatics Association) and HIMSS (Healthcare Information Management Systems Society). He was a member of HITSP and co-chaired the subcommittee on planning and internal communications for HITSP's Education, Communication, and Outreach (ECO) Committee.

Frank received a BS in biology from Lehigh University and a DMD from Fairleigh Dickinson University and completed an NLM (National Library of Medicine) postdoctoral fellowship in Biomedical Informatics with an MA from Columbia University.

Stephen Foreman J.D., Ph.D., M.P.A., is professor of health economics at Robert Morris University, Pittsburgh, PA, where he teaches health economics, health policy, statistics, and health law and ethics in the University's graduate programs. Steve has been a Fulbright scholar at the Crimea State Medical University, Simferopol, Crimea, where he lectured and conducted research in comparative international health policy. Dr. Foreman's research focuses on structure, performance, and strategy in health insurance, hospital and physician markets, and health insurance data. His work includes the international economics of aging, economic mechanisms as they relate to corruption, and the economics of human trafficking. Professor Foreman holds a PhD in health economics from the University of California, Berkeley, a JD with honors from the University of North Carolina and a Master in Public Administration from Harvard's Kennedy School of Government where he was a Littauer fellow.

Shin-Mey Rose Yin Geist D.D.S., M.S., is an associate professor in the Departments of Biomedical and Diagnostic Sciences and Patient Management at the University of Detroit Mercy School of Dentistry. Born and raised in Taiwan, Republic of China, Dr. Geist graduated from Dental School in Taiwan in 1974. She specialized in oral surgery and was teaching in the University Hospital when she found her passion for oral medicine. She completed her master's degree in oral diagnosis/oral medicine at the Indiana University School of Dentistry in 1985 and then studied and worked in molecular biology and DNA cloning research at the medical schools at Indiana University and Wayne State University. Dr. Geist received her DDS degree in 1990 from the University of Detroit and has been teaching oral diagnosis and oral medicine at UDM since that time. She has been course director of the advanced oral medicine course for graduate students in periodontics and advanced general dentistry. Dr. Geist served as chair of the oral diagnosis and oral medicine section of the American Dental Education Association (ADEA) and is presently serving on the editorial review board of the *Journal of Dental Education*, the official journal of ADEA. She was recently appointed as a member of the content analysis working group of MedEdPORTAL Oral Health in Medicine Model Curriculum. *MedEdPORTAL* is a peer-reviewed online publication of the Association of American Medical Colleges (AAMC), partnered with ADEA.

Dr. Geist has held a diplomate of the American Board of Oral Medicine since 1992 and has special interest in medically complex dental patient management. She is committed to improving the interface between medical and oral healthcare. Her research interests include the efficiency in teaching and service in providing comprehensive coordinated care.

Casey Hein In July 2018, Casey Hein, B.S.D.H., R.D.H., M.B.A., retired from her decade-long appointments at the University of Manitoba, where she was an assistant clinical professor in the Department of Periodontics, director of education of the International Centre for Oral-Systemic Health in the College of Dentistry, and the director of continuing professional development for dentistry and dental hygiene in the Rady Faculty of Health Sciences at the University of Manitoba (Canada). One of her responsibilities at the University of Manitoba was to lead a team in the development of her vision for the first comprehensive curriculum about oral health for physicians, nurses, and other non-dental healthcare providers (Oral-Systemic Health Education for Non-Dental Healthcare Providers), which won for the University of Manitoba the prestigious William J. Gies Award for Outstanding Innovation in 2015. She maintains a faculty appointment as an assistant professor in the University's School of Dental Hygiene and writes and lectures on the topic of dental-medical collaboration in caring for people at risk for oral-systemic diseases and conditions. She has developed two educational websites that provide resources for implementation of periodontal-systemic science (www.caseyhein.com) and online courses related to oral-systemic health for both the dental and medical communities (www.oralhealthed.com).

Glurich Ingrid Ph.D., earned her degree in microbiology and microbial pathogenesis with a special emphasis on autoimmunity and immunopathology from the State University of New York at Buffalo. Dr. Glurich has been involved in research for over 30 years and is currently a project scientist in the Center for Oral and Systemic Health at Marshfield Clinic Research Institute in Marshfield, Wisconsin. Her basic and clinical research has focused on oral-systemic health connections and has included studies surrounding immune and inflammatory mechanisms and the role of host response to microbial pathogens. Her current research activities include advancing integrated care delivery models for oral and medical management of patients with diabetes, defining a potential role for immune and inflammatory response to oral pathogens in exacerbation of renal disease, characterizing the role of oral health status in patients with emergent pneumonia, and translating precision medicine into the oral healthcare delivery arena. To date, Dr. Glurich has authored/co-authored over 60 manuscripts and book chapters.

Mark W. Jurkovich D.D.S., M.B.A., M.H.I., is a senior fellow at the HealthPartners Institute in Bloomington, MN, and is a graduate of the University of Minnesota School of Dentistry, the Carlson School of Business, and the Institute of Health Informatics at the University of Minnesota. He provided direct patient care in a variety of private practice formats for 38 years. He currently works in the areas of research, terminology development, and data analytics, with a focus on the dental field. He currently serves on the American Dental Association's (ADA) oversight committee of the Standards Committee on Dental Informatics, on the State of Minnesota e-Health Advisory Committee, and on the Information Exchange oversight committee. He is chair of the

ANSI SNODENT Maintenance Committee and lead for the SNOMED International Dental CRG. He has provided numerous presentations throughout the country on dental topics involving electronic dental record systems and terminologies.

Joseph Kilsdonk Au.D., has served as the administrator for Marshfield Clinic's Education Division since 2004. The Division oversees the largest community health center-based training programs in the State of Wisconsin. Prior to that, he served as an associate dean overseeing health careers for a public college, served as an executive for a national ancillary healthcare service corporation, served on the management team of a multispecialty physician group practice and a community hospital, taught as an assistant professor, and founded and managed hospital and community-based outreach practices.

Dr. Kilsdonk was the lead author on the Clinic's dental education feasibility study leading to its current efforts in dental education resulting in a public-private partnership for rural dental education expansion. He has presented locally, regionally, and nationally on a number of healthcare and practice management topics. Most recently, he has presented to the "National Health Policy Forum on Oral Health; 10 Years after the Surgeons General's Report" in Washington, DC. He has served on Wisconsin's Dental Education Feasibility Study Advisory Committee and presently serves on the Advisory Committee for the Wisconsin Academy for Rural Medicine, the Committee for the Wisconsin Rural Physician Residency Assistance Program, and the Chancellor's Advisory Committee for University of Wisconsin at Stevens Point. He has been a manuscript reviewer for the *Journal of Dental Education* since 2009.

Dr. Kilsdonk received his doctorate in audiology for the Arizona School of Health Sciences, a master's degree from the University of Wisconsin, Oshkosh, and his undergraduate degree in communicative disorders from the University of Wisconsin, Stevens Point.

Ted Klein M.S., Klein Consulting, Inc. Vocabulary Co-chair, HL7 International.

Kori Krueger M.D., M.B.A., is the medical director of the Institute of Quality, Innovation, and Patient Safety at Marshfield Clinic, Marshfield, Wisconsin. Dr. Krueger attended medical school at the University of Wisconsin Medical School in Madison and completed his residency at Marshfield Clinic in Marshfield, Wisconsin. He is board-certified in internal medicine and pediatrics. He is involved in medical education and works as a primary care provider in pediatrics and internal medicine at Marshfield Clinic, Stratford Center. Dr. Krueger completed his medical MBA degree at the University of St. Thomas in Minneapolis, Minnesota, in 2013. Dr. Krueger is also the medical director of the Marshfield Clinic ACO.

Jayanth Kumar Medam B.D.S., is currently pursuing MS in health informatics at the School of Informatics and Computing, Indiana University. He holds a bachelor's in dental surgery from Dr. NTR University of Health Sciences, India. Following dental residency in India, Jayanth Kumar worked with multiple IT organizations and served in different roles such as medical content developer, subject matter expert in revenue cycle, and clinical analyst. This experiential learning inspired him to pursue a career focused in the application of information technology in healthcare to improve healthcare outcomes. This eventually stimulated him to pursue an advanced degree in health informatics.

Jayanth Kumar Medam is a graduate research assistant at the Dental Informatics Core directed by Dr. Thankam Paul Thyvalikakath, Indiana University School of Dentistry. He is presently working on his master's thesis under her valuable guidance. This explorative study would address some of the existing communication gaps between medical and dental providers. His ultimate goal is to be a clinical informatics professional and contribute significantly to this domain.

William Melms M.D., is the Northeast Regional Primary Care Medical Director at Minocqua Center of Marshfield Clinic. Dr. Melms has more than 20 years of clinical experience in urgent care and family medicine. He has authored/co-authored research papers. He pursued his MD from the University of Wisconsin School of Medicine and Public Health in 1986 and completed his residency in family medicine from Medical College of Wisconsin Affiliated Hospitals in 1989. Dr. Melms interests include general family medicine.

Sushma Mishra M.B.A., Ph.D., is an associate professor of computer information systems at Robert Morris University. She is the director of doctor of science (DSc) program at RMU. She has an MBA degree from India and a PhD in information systems from Virginia Commonwealth University. Dr. Mishra's research interests include information security, information assurance issues in healthcare information systems, systems auditing, and systems development methodologies. Dr. Mishra has published in several conference proceedings, book chapters, and journal articles on these topics. She teaches information security and decision support systems.

John O'Brien D.D.S., is the clinical dental director of the Family Health Center Dental Clinics and is a practicing dentist. He pursued his DDS from the State University of New York at Buffalo School of Dental Medicine. He has been involved in various research studies.

Aloksagar Panny B.D.S., M.S., is the research specialist at the Center for Oral and Systemic Health, Marshfield Clinic, Marshfield, Wisconsin. In March 2013, he obtained his Bachelor of Dental Surgery (BDS) from Dr. NTR University of Health Sciences, India. In May 2016, he earned a Master of Science in medical informatics and a graduate certificate in healthcare data analytics—both from George Mason University, Fairfax, VA. He is also a SAS-certified programmer. Mr. Panny was an intern at the National Institutes of Health where his work was focused on using a range of informatics and natural language processing (NLP) techniques to analyze clinical research documents of both active and terminated clinical trials. Mr. Panny has a strong clinical background. His research interests include oral-systemic connections, clinical decision support systems, and dental informatics.

Ram Pathak M.D., F.A.C.P., is a consultant in the Department of Endocrinology at Marshfield Clinic in Wisconsin. He also serves as the director of Diabetes Education Program across the Marshfield Clinic Health System. He has more than two decades of experience caring for patients with diabetes and formerly served as the chair of the Department of Endocrinology.

Dr. Pathak has been a principal investigator for various studies in the diabetes field and has published more than two dozen manuscripts in national and international journals. He served as a member of the research committee for 6 years and as a trustee for the Marshfield Clinic Research Foundation from 2011 to 2014. Currently, Dr. Pathak is active in patient care, medical teaching, and clinical research.

Frank Scannapieco D.M.D., Ph.D., professor and chair of the Department of Oral Biology and associate dean for faculty and professional development, School of Dental Medicine, State University of New York at Buffalo, is a periodontist and investigator with over 25 years of research experience. He studies oral microbiology, molecular mechanisms of bacterial colonization, and the interface between oral and systemic health, especially the role of oral conditions in the process of respiratory infection. He received the DMD from the University of Connecticut and the PhD in oral biology and certificate in periodontology from the University at Buffalo.

Dr. Scannapieco is a past associate editor of the *Journal of Periodontology*, has edited an issue of *Dental Clinics of North America*, has served on the editorial board of the *Journal of Dental Research*, and as a referee for over 40 medical, dental, and scientific journals. He has received substantial funding from NIH to support his research and has authored or co-authored over 150 peer-reviewed papers and abstracts.

Neel Shimpi B.D.S., M.M., Ph.D., is currently working as a tenure-track associate research scientist at the Center for Oral and Systemic Health at Marshfield Clinic Research Institute at Marshfield, Wisconsin, USA. Dr. Shimpi was trained as a general dental surgeon and received her PhD in the field of biomedical and health informatics. Additionally she has master's degree in healthcare management from Cambridge, Massachusetts, and diplomas and certificates in hospital administration and clinical research. Dr. Shimpi has been involved in research for over 5 years, applying her expertise to research focused on applying informatics to projects involving artificial intelligence, educational curriculum development, natural language processing, and clinical and oral-systemic health research, among other applications. She has published in many national journals and presented at national and international conferences. Her work on assessment of oral cancer knowledgeability among healthcare providers was highlighted by the Oral Cancer Foundation in 2016. She has also been involved in conducting quantitative studies surrounding oral cancer, mixed methods approaches for conducting oral-systemic health research, and data-driven and exploratory analysis of quantitative health informatics data to develop and evaluate various clinical decision support tools at point of care. She has co-mentored and mentored many summer interns and dental residents in the conduct of research studies. Dr. Shimpi's research interests include medical and dental informatics, developing clinical decision supports and expert systems, educational toolkits for healthcare providers, ontologies and terminologies, principles of evidence-based practices, and investigating the oral-systemic relationships with high potential for translation into clinical practice.

Cindy Sorenson F.N.P., graduated from Viterbo University in 1983 with bachelor's in nursing. Her nursing career started in the intensive care unit and the emergency department at Marshfield Clinic. Due to her keen interest in family practice, she went back to school and pursued a master's degree in nursing with an emphasis in family practice in 1955. She has been working for 22 years at the Marshfield Clinic Stettin Center. She played a key role in a pilot study surrounding integration of oral healthcare in diabetic patients.

Peter Umukoro M.D., M.P.H., Sc.D., is a physician and researcher with extensive cardiovascular experience. While at Harvard, his research focused on elucidating the determinants of ischemic heart disease and autonomic cardiac disease among occupational groups with peculiar exposures at work such as nurses, construction workers, and welders.

His research work spans cardiac autonomic function, physical activity determinants of nurses and construction workers, ergonomic intervention assessments among construction workers, and key determinants of ischemic heart disease risk in welders. His research with the Harvard Center for Work, Health, and Well-being has publications that have linked trunk bending to physical activity of nurses and described associations between occupational and leisure time physical activity. He has authored/co-authored original publications from his work with Harvard including a landmark publication in the *British Medical Journal* which describes associations between particulate exposure and decreases in cardiac acceleration and deceleration capacities.

He is currently a resident physician at the Marshfield Medical Center, an investigator with the Marshfield Clinic Research Foundation, and a member of the American Public Health Association, American College of Physicians, and American College of Cardiology.

Jayanth Vedre M.D., M.P.H., is a pulmonologist and intensivist licensed in Wisconsin and Minnesota, with board certification in critical care medicine, neurocritical care medicine, and internal medicine with over 12 years of experience in medical practice. Dr. Vedre is currently the director of the medical intensive care unit and intensivist at Marshfield Clinic Health Systems in Marshfield Wisconsin. Dr. Vedre was engaged in research in the critical care medicine during his tenure as a research fellow in the Mayo Clinic Epidemiology and Translational Research in Intensive Care (METRIC) at Mayo Clinic in Rochester, MN. His research interests include intensive care quality improvement projects, pneumonia management, critical care bedside ultrasound development, and extracorporeal membrane oxygenation. Dr. Vedre has 4 published abstracts and has authored/co-authored 17 additional abstracts/posters to date at national/state conferences. Dr. Vedre also holds an MPH in public health education from Western Kentucky University in Bowling Green, KY, and proactively engages in medical education of residents. He has received two excellence-in-teaching awards.

Chapter 1
Mouth: The Gateway to the Body and the Importance of Medical and Dental Data Integration

Miguel H. Torres-Urquidy and Valerie Powell

1.1 Introduction

This book starts from a simple premise "the oral cavity and related clinical conditions" still remain part of the rest of the body. Although this may seem obvious, administratively, clinically, historically, and technologically this may not be the case when a patient seeks care. Dentists and physicians have operated (literally and figuratively) separately, making the care of patients challenging, given that both perform treatments, prescribe medications, and even bill through different mechanisms.

This book gets to the root of this divide by characterizing how such a gap evolved and what can, could, and should be done to close it. Our book starts by describing how clinical information is used in this two-tier system (dental and medical). We provide examples on how this can impact health of the patients and also provide the perspectives of those having to deal with the complexities of living in these two tiers (patient and provider perspective).

We then explore how there are a variety of Clinical Contact Points, instances where there is a clear need of integration as well as supportive clinical evidence suggesting that dentists and physicians need to operate in a fully integrated fashion. The reader will be exposed to the consequences created by having limited integration (for instance, poor oral health can lead to physiological issues—by virtue of being unable to eat properly—which in turn lead to extreme cases of malnutrition in elderly or disabled patients). Unfortunately, these cases occur in isolation, making

M. H. Torres-Urquidy (✉)
Centers for Disease Control and Prevention, Atlanta, GA, USA
e-mail: miguel@forwardthinkingconcepts.org

V. Powell
Robert Morris University, Pittsburgh, PA, USA
e-mail: powell@rmu.edu

A. Acharya et al. (eds.), *Integration of Medical and Dental Care and Patient Data*, Health Informatics, https://doi.org/10.1007/978-3-319-98298-4_1

them difficult to assess or being dismissed by the single caretaker. In reality, a pattern may exist that should be comprehensively addressed.

We also evaluate how health systems have different or (most likely) similar approaches. We also discuss how different technological solutions at different points of care can address closing that divide between dental and medical care. From the public health perspective, we can also describe how not having a fully integrated approach can limit the effect of interventions. On the other hand, integrated approaches are already in place and we describe cases where public health has made inroads in this regard. We also discuss how education fits the integration agenda. It makes sense that integration between dental and medical care should start when we train dentists and physicians; yet, this still remains a moving target. Thus we highlight how different models are being created to increase this integration.

In terms of patient care, we illustrate how different practical aspects of care, such as the use of guidelines, patient engagement, personalized care, and risk assessment can be supportive of a new, integrated way, of caring for patients. On the other hand, the book also not only pinpoints the separation of care but also provides an extensive description of informatics methods that can support and ultimately achieve the integration of dental and medical care.

The book then provides information on the different outcomes that should be expected from having such integration, whether better health outcomes or economic benefits, and we establish a clear description of what would be gained by achieving integration.

Finally, we embark on describing what the future research agenda should be that hopefully provides a strategy on how to tackle the most immediate as well as the long term problems of the dental and medical integration of patient care.

1.2 Separation of Care: How Did We Get Here?

There are several ways in which it is possible to see why dental care, although a fully recognized medical sub-specialty is taught, practiced, billed, and managed separately from the rest of the medical realm. For this book we believe it is important that the reader becomes fully aware of the historical, economical, and empirical reasons why such separation occurred.

In the beginnings of medicine, independent of culture, the managing of oral and systemic diseases did not appear separately. As pointed by Ring (1992) in his now classic book "Dentistry An Illustrated History", early civilizations treated oral conditions as part of other systemic conditions.

In Mesopotamia (Ring 1992, p. 27) physicians started treating disease and laws were drawn up during the time of Hammurabi (1792–1750 B.C.) to characterize the punishments and rewards as a result of treatments. In here we can find that both dental and medical treatments are listed side by side.

Among the Greeks, it is with Hippocrates' writings (B. 460 B.C.–D. 377–359 B.C.) that we can find references to issues of dentition and dental disease, as well as treatment. As the father of medicine, Hippocrates included oral issues as part of what is the Hippocratic Corpus (Ring 1992, p. 40). Aristotle's (B. 384 B.C.–D. 322 B.C.) work in comparative anatomy included dental anatomy as well.

In the Roman empire Ring (1992, p. 46) states that "There is no separate word for dentist in the early Latin language, for dentistry as a separate profession did not exist among the Romans but was included as part of medical practice, and Roman physicians made no distinction between diseases affecting the mouth and those affecting other parts of the body. Nor did nonprofessionals specialize in dentistry, although we have extensive knowledge of the services performed by Roman barbers, no mention is ever made of their extracting teeth."

In China, in 659 A.D. Su Kung (Ring 1992, p. 81), with 23 other scholars wrote how "Silver Paste" can be used for fillings as part of the first medical pharmacopoeia, which included 54 chapters and 850 remedies.

During the seventh Century, the expansion of the Islamic World beyond the Arabian Peninsula included the Middle East, North Africa, and significant portions of Spain. During the next centuries, translations of classical Greek writings would lead to establishing the foundation of later modern medical texts (Ring 1992, p. 63). In the case of Islamic medical texts there is little devoted primarily to dentistry, usually embedding information of one within the other. Ali Abbas's (Ali ibn'l-Abbas al-Majusi) Royal Book, Albucasis's (Abul Kassim) Al-Tasrif (The Method), Aviccenna's (abu-'Ali al-Husayn ibn-Sina) Al-Qanun (The Canon) and Rhazes's (Abu-Bakr Muhammad ibn-Zakariya al-Razi) Kitab al-Hawi (Compilation) all provide chapters dedicated to dentistry as part of broader medical treaties of that time. Again, dental care was seen as an integral part of medical care.

A notable exception may be the Egyptians, who established early professing of specialized medicine, where physicians would specialize on certain parts of the body or diseases, as described by Herodotus of practices 2000 earlier in Egypt (Ring 1992, p. 33). Yet it is worth mentioning that physicians were responsible for healthcare (and not a separated professional entity) and it was the clinical conditions (and understanding) of the time that dictated specialization. This last point provides a good segue to a key element that is necessary to highlight which is: within given conditions, it is important to retain a separation of practices, if it allows for gains in efficiency of care. Given the state of knowledge at the time, Egyptian physicians naturally evolved to such a specialized state.

Fast forward several centuries and the modern western practice of dentistry had, from the beginning, a divergent origin from medical care. Well known is how dentistry had its humble beginnings among barbers around the Middle Ages. While physicians were practicing earlier forms of medicine, proto-dentists (barbers) fulfilled a function, which was mandated primarily for what are anatomical and physical reasons. Although obvious today, such factors are worth mentioning. Barber-surgeons (Ring 1992, p. 109) had the physical equipment necessary to perform procedures in proximity to the craniofacial structures. Per their profession, they would handle instruments and conduct activities that would "prepare them" to just "extend" their area of work inside and around the oral cavity. In addition, simplicity of access to the oral anatomical structures made it consequential for them to expand the repertory of services they could offer (besides "bleeding, cupping, giving enemas, leeching and extracting teeth") (Ring 1992, p. 109). Additionally, their tools of the trade would easily support functions of barber and dentist (dental chairs make a good example). Another element which comes into play is the philosophy of their activities: in the abstract, cutting hair and extracting teeth both refer to the notion of removing human body elements which are no longer performing as intended. Hence, in the case of early barbers, it did not require them to have distinct work philosophies to fulfill these enhanced roles.

In the seventeenth century western physicians, surgeons, and dentists could now be found operating as separate guilds (Ring 1992, p. 147). Physicians would practice based on prior "Classical and Arabic writings" taking limited input from more recent scientific discoveries. The surgeons were tied to militaries and would conduct not only medical treatments but also barber functions. As such they would perform dental treatments and/or cure medical maladies using dental procedures. Dentists/barbers, now would publicize their ability to perform extractions usually in marketplaces. It wasn't until the eighteenth century that dentistry formalized through ongoing trial-and-error. Yet advances were significant and led to formal recognition in the form of regulating the practice and requiring formal examinations by a committee of surgeons in order to be allowed to practice (France, Germany) (Ring 1992, p. 157). From this point forward we can see the early foundations of what are now the separated realms for care between dentistry and medicine.

Both the dental and medical professions organically established separated paths as a result of their origins but also of their evolution. The ability to apply emerging scientific findings, to secure professional sovereignty, and to establish within society at large their professional authority beyond the clinical realm, at least in the United States, has granted dentistry and medicine as professions, access to higher social status, economic privilege, and political influence (Starr 2017). Although in their modern beginnings both professions were not highly regarded, both evolved in parallel to attain such high status. The establishment of educational requirements and respective accreditation boards provided a natural way to set higher standards of care, as well as formalizing educational processes while establishing separate schools and curriculums. This, tied to the adoption of scientifically backed findings, naturally led to actual improvements in results obtained in actual clinical care.

Here it is important to distinguish that this parallel evolution of separate guilds, boards, schools, etc. led to the proliferation of different facilities in which to provide care (hospitals vs. dental clinics), insurance models, and regulatory frameworks among other long term disintegrated elements. Obviously, there are exceptions to this; for instance, in large integrated healthcare systems (e.g., the US Veterans Affairs (VA), US Military (MHS), and Indian Health Service (IHS) health systems) and hospital dentistry. Yet, the patient remains the single unit under which such separate, parallel, professions need to operate. As a result, patients now carry the burden of visiting different places for care, having to record information multiple times, keeping separate insurance cards, and carrying their information between points of care through a "Sneakernet" as described by Powell and Din (2012, p. 19) in the previous edition of this book. Furthermore, we have in the electronic realm, well-defined separate classes of information recording systems in the form of both Electronic Dental Records (EDRs) and Electronic Medical Records (EMRs).

1.3 Addressing Dental-Medical Records Discrepancies

As stated, having multiple health data repositories (EDRs and EMRs) evolved as a natural result of the respective professional emergence of dentists and physicians. These record systems also reflect the practical realities of their respective owners. Dentists have specialized sections for recording dentition and craniofacial anatomical features. Physicians' EMRs as well have the ability to store information that is highly relevant to general medical practice, which may be less required during day-to-day dental practice. For instance, laboratory results or immunization status can be found more prominently on an EMR than an EDR. On the other hand, both types of systems still have a large amount of overlap in terms of information needed to support clinical operations (patient demographics, vital signs, health history, etc.) As a result, during ongoing clinical practice we can find different locations where clinical information is first captured/generated, maintained, and stored. This separation has led to multiple places where information resides creating an uncoordinated reality of keeping the patient's health information.

It is well known in computer science that discrepancies arise in the maintenance of a database either by a failure to correctly record information in a repository external to the database, or by maintaining more than one copy of the database (or a part of it) and failing to adequately synchronize the copies. In each case, there is more than one copy of the data, and the copies don't agree in what each communicates.

The process of getting medical history from the medical or dental patient's recollections onto a paper chart or into an electronic record system faces challenges from the outset.

As one might easily imagine from Fig. 1.1, there are two classes of opportunities for inaccuracies to arise in a patient record system: (1) some of the information in the patient record might be inaccurate because the patient's memories are inaccurate, because the patient made errors in filing out a medical history form, because the person taking a patient's medical history (in the process called anamnesis or Hx) may have misinterpreted a response or may have incorrectly transcribed information or (2) the multiple copies of the patient's Hx may not agree with each other, especially if there are structured formats rather than a direct transcription of a narrative, due to a process sometimes called *information refraction* that can affect the reformulation of information when it crosses the boundary from human representa-

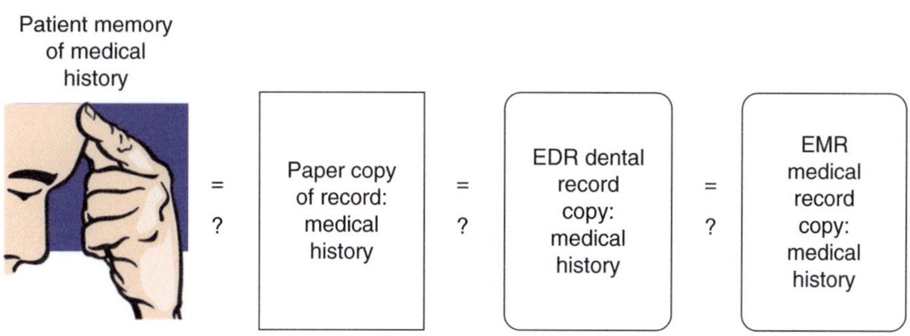

Fig. 1.1 Multiple copies of medical history

tion to machine representation or from representation in one automated system to another automated system, or even in transmission by speech and interpretation from one human to another, as occurs in anamnesis, in spite of the professional training of the individuals who carry out anamnesis in health care organizations.

Computer science documents the occurrence of discrepancies under two conditions in database technologies where there is more than one copy of a record. (1) A well-known "unstable condition of the database" occurs in database arithmetic operations while changed and unchanged copies temporarily co-exist and (2) distributed databases intentionally maintain multiple copies of data to support availability at multiple sites and thus must explicitly synchronize these copies to assure distributed accuracy to support (transparency of location.)

What evidence of discrepancy problems in patient record systems (paper or electronic) has been described? The questionable reliability of a patient's own documentation in filling out a history form has been described. A number of studies have described the occurrence of discrepancies between medical and dental records of the same patient (or more correctly, between the patient's medical record and the medical history portion of the dental record or between the patient's dental record and the dental history portion of his/her medical record) (see Fig. 1.2).

The U.S. Department of Defense has been aware since 1977 that as many of 10% of dental records of active duty personnel could have discrepancies when compared with their medical records (Lewis et al. 1977). In a group of 100 randomly selected active duty personnel at Walter Reed Medical Center, "11 discrepancies of major medical significance were found."

In 1985 Dunne and Clark reported that, "Medical histories were obtained from 130 dental outpatients by questionnaire. A total of 109 medical conditions were

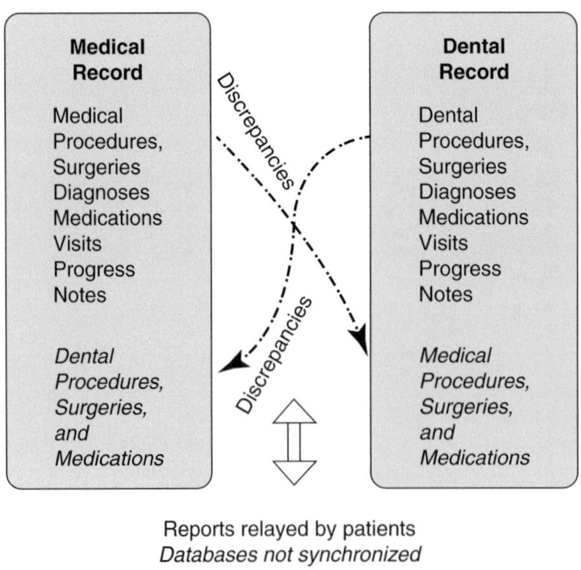

Fig. 1.2 Discrepancies in the medical and dental health record

recorded. The dental records of 50 of these patients, selected at random, were examined retrospectively and compared to the questionnaire responses. Twenty-eight omissions were found in the dental records, 11 of which were potentially serious, while 3 were potentially life threatening. These results indicate the ease by which relevant medical details can be missed in a hurried interview, and illustrates the usefulness of a simple self-answering questionnaire."

Haughney et al. (1998) reported 99 discrepancies between medical and dental records for 178 joint patients (records of about 40% of the patients). Six of these discrepancies were classified as "life-threatening." Haughney et al. (1998) recommended that "the joint use of patient record systems avoided discrepancies in patient information which would have affected the quality of patient care" and pointed out that "joint consultations reduced the need for secondary referrals."

Almas and Awartani (2003) studied 743 "medically compromised patients" referred for periodontal treatment in a teaching hospital. They reported that approximately "90% of the patients were systemically healthy. The remaining 10% of the patients were with different systemic diseases or sequelae. Diabetes mellitus, hypertension, asthma and rheumatic fever were most commonly present. Thirty-one (4.2%) of the medically compromised were diabetic. Hypertension was reported in 9 (1.2%) patients. Rheumatic fever and asthma were equally present in 7 (0.9%) patients. Periodontal diseases were equally prevalent in both male and female patients. Approximately 50% of the patients had moderate periodontitis while severe periodontitis was common among 9% of the male and female patients." They concluded that, "Diabetes and heart related conditions were most common among the specialist patients referred for periodontal treatment. Advanced periodontitis was prevalent among 9% of the patients. It is recommended that physicians are [sic] become more familiar with the systemic associations to periodontal diseases. The dental practitioners should be well versed in the interplay between oral and systemic disease. More extensive knowledge of oral and physical medicine will be needed in order to provide quality care and appropriate treatment of patients with periodontal diseases suffering with systemic conditions."

In 2016 Al Hibshi et al. reported that "75% of the patients [Al Hada Armed Forces Hospital, Taif, Saudi Arabia] who directly or indirectly accessed the dental services showed discrepancies." Al Hibshi et al. found that "Two hundred and seventy-nine (96.5%) of the 289 dental records had medical information discrepancies compared to the corresponding medical records. One hundred percent of systemic lupus erythematosus and rheumatic fever cases were not documented in the dental records followed by 93% of medications, 92% of stroke, and 88.5% of hyperlipidemia, whereas the least prevalent were cardiac disease (26%) and diabetes mellitus (22.2%)." Al Hibshi et al. cautioned that a "well-established model for efficient communication among medical and dental care providers caring for cardiac patients does not appear to exist. The absence of such a model can threaten the overall health of patients."

Discrepancies between medical and dental records are due largely to the reliance on patient reports from treatment in the other discipline, rather than on an integrated electronic record system. Selzer and McDermott reported in 1999 that "of patients who completed the same medical history questionnaire twice within a certain time period, 66% had at least 1 significant omission in their history."

According to Lutka and Threadgill (1995), "medical history questionnaires and outpatient medical records of 115 patients were compared. All patients had a medical history of at least two years in both records. The dental records were initially reviewed, and patients' responses were compiled; when these were compared with the outpatient medical records, the overall discrepancy rate was >86 percent. This overwhelming rate of error should make dentists aware that many routinely treated patients have medical conditions that are unknown to providers. Use of universal precautions, adequate medical-emergency training, and oral review of the dental health questionnaire are recommended."

Jones et al. (1999) reported that "eighty per cent of dentists had contacted a doctor and 16% of doctors had contacted a dentist in the previous three months; 87% of dentists and 68% of doctors thought an integrated medical-dental PHR would be of some use. Twenty-one per cent of dentists and 85% of doctors had practice computers. Most patients wanted to be able to see and read their own records. Twenty-four per cent of patients said there were mistakes and 30% noticed omissions in the integrated medical-dental PHR issued. Experience of having an integrated medical-dental PHR made patients more positive towards the idea of having a patient-held record and being able to check the accuracy of records."

Theis et al. (2010) report on automated record linkage as a method of solving the problem and Stilley and Berthelson report on the adequacy (2000) of patient input of health history to a hand-held computer, but don't compare this method of gaining medical history with access to a medical record in the context of an integrated health record system.

1.4 Why Then, Has integration Not Occurred?

As we have reviewed, the reasons behind the lack of integration of dental and medical care can be traced back to the early origins of both professions as well as to the way the professions have evolved and also to how specialization of care naturally requires us to provide care. Hence it is important to ask the question, what is the true impact of such lack of integration? What would integration bring given that, so far, we have health systems (dental and medical) that are parallel? Still, it is possible to argue that natural forces created this parallelism in care and it is for good (and/or practical) reasons. To address this question it is necessary to consider that, first, the human body, as a result of evolutionary forces, has become an extraordinarily resilient machine. Redundancy and self-healing combined with a highly sophisticated immune system allows humans to tolerate significant damage to their biological integrity. In the case of dentistry, it can be argued that patients (fortunately) rarely die of not only dental conditions but also as a result of dental care, up to the point where, in those unfortunate cases where dental care results in death (when compared to medical care), they become subject to national attention by media outlets (Egerton 2015). The same can be argued of dental conditions leading to fatal results (Sgobba 2017). However, this focuses only on the most extreme of possible health outcomes. There are a myriad of other less dramatic, yet highly important, examples where integration would greatly benefit both direct patient outcomes and also improve the efficiency and efficacy of care. As argued in the subsequent chapters, contact points of care are extensive and improving the overall understanding of the patients' current clinical status will naturally lead to avoiding errors, reducing costs, and maximizing outcomes for the overall health system.

Integration of dental and medical care, in order for it to be successful, has to occur while understanding the history and rationale behind the existence of such parallel health systems. Otherwise such efforts may fail to gain traction. As an example we can cite how, despite attempts by dentists to be allowed to dispense vaccines (Fox 2013), this has been met with opposition from organized medical groups (ISMS 2013). Factors listed behind the opposition include "…little to no experience with the vaccine schedule, its administration, handling and storage". In addition, "additional training is inadequate and will not protect patients, especially those who suffer from chronic illnesses, experience allergic reactions and/or those who are on other drugs that may negatively interact with an immunization." It is only under special circumstances, like the H1N1 pandemic, where dentists have been allowed to expand their scope of practice to dispense vaccines (ASTHO 2012). On the other hand, highly successful interventions such as Tobacco Cessation, diabetes control, and hypertension programs can be seen as well integrated efforts between medicine and dentistry to improve health care outcomes.

1.5 Conclusion

In closing, it is ethically imperative to seek integration of dental and medical care. It is the responsibility of health care providers to be comprehensively aware of the health status of the patient. Medical and oral conditions, medications, problem lists, social factors, etc. should be available at the point of care, at the time of planning and rendering care. We anticipate that this volume will help achieve such integration in tangible ways by providing those interested in making it happen, clarity on what, why, and how to achieve it.

Disclaimer The views presented in this chapter are solely of the authors and do not necessarily represent the views of the US Government, Department of Health and Human Services and/or the Centers for Disease Control and Prevention.

References

Al Hibshi SM, Al-Raddadi RM, Assery MK. Discrepancies between dental and medical records of cardiac patients in AlHada Armed Forces Hospital, Taif, Saudi Arabia. J Int Soc Prev Community Dent. 2016;6(6):568–74.

Almas K, Awartani FA. Prevalence of medically compromised patients referred for periodontal treatment to a teaching hospital in Central Saudi Arabia. Saudi Med J. 2003;24(11):1242–5.

Association of State and Territorial Health Officials (ASTHO). Modified scope of practice used by states in the 2009 H1N1 influenza pandemic, Fact sheet. Astho legal preparedness series scope of practice toolkit. 2012. http://www.astho.org/Programs/Preparedness/Public-Health-Emergency-Law/Scope-of-Practice-Toolkit/Modified-Scope-of-Practice-Used-by-States-in-the-2009-H1N1-Influenza-Pandemic-Fact-Sheet/. Accessed 10 June 2018.

Dunne SM, Clark CG. The identification of the medically compromised patient in dental practice. J Dent. 1985;13(1):45–51. https://doi.org/10.1016/0300-5712(85)90062-4.

Egerton B. Elusive numbers. We asked for death totals, but most states weren't counting. The Dallas Morning News. 2015. http://interactives.dallasnews.com/2015/deadly-dentistry/part2.html. Accessed 10 June 2018.

Fox K. Who calls the shots? Illinois dentists advocate to administer flu and other vaccines. ADA News. 2013. https://www.ada.org/en/publications/ada-news/2013-archive/april/who-calls-the-shots. Accessed 10 June 2018.

Haughney MGJ, Devennie JC, Macpherson LMD, Mason DK. Integration of primary care dental and medical services: a three year study. Br Dent J. 1998;184(7):343–7.

Illinois State Medical Society (ISMS). 2013 Legislative issues. 2013. https://www.isms.org/Governmental_Affairs/Legislative_Action_Hub/2013_Legislative_Issues/. Accessed 10 June 2018.

Jones R, McConville J, Mason D, Macpherson L, Naven L, McEwen J. Attitudes towards, and utility of, an integrated medical-dental patient-held record in primary care. Br J Gen Pract. 1999;49(442):368–73.

Lewis DM, Krakow AM, Payne TF. An evaluation of the dental-medical history. Defense Technical Information Center. Accession Number ADA041260; 1977.

Lutka RW, Threadgill JM. Correlation of dental-record medical histories with outpatient medical records. Gen Dent. 1995;43(4):342–5.

Powell V, Din F. Rationale and need to articulate medical and dental data. In: Powell V, Din F, Acharya A, Torres-Urquidy MH, editors. Integration of medical and dental care and patient data. 1st ed. London, UK: Springer; 2012.

Ring ME. Dentistry: an illustrated history. New York: Harry N Abrams Inc; 1992.

Selzer MH, McDermott JH. Inaccuracies in patient medical histories. Compr Ther. 1999;25(5):258–64.

Sgobba C. A tooth infection suddenly killed this 26-year-old guy. Here's why you shouldn't ignore a throbbing toothache, either. Men's Health Magazine. 2017. https://www.menshealth.com/health/a19538456/deadly-tooth-infection/. Accessed 10 June 2018.

Starr P. Introduction, the social origins of professional sovereignty. In: Starr P, editor. The social transformation of American medicine: the rise of a sovereign profession and the making of a vast industry. 2nd ed. New York: Basic Books; 2017. p. 3–29.

Stilley KR, Berthelson CL. Automated personal health inventory for dentistry: a pilot study. J Am Dent Assoc. 2000;131(1):9–66.

Theis MK, Reid RJ, Chaudhari M, Newton KM, Spangler L, Grossman DC, Inge RE. Case study of linking dental and medical records. Am J Manag Care. 2010;16(2):e51–5.

Chapter 2
Achieving the 'True' Triple Aim in Healthcare

Aloksagar Panny, Kori Krueger, and Amit Acharya

2.1 Triple Aim

2.1.1 Definition and Overview

In the year 2007, the Institute of Healthcare Improvement (IHI) announced a system of interlinked goals to improve the health care system in the United States (U.S.): "improving the health of population, improving the experience of care and reducing the per capita cost of care" (Berwick et al. 2008). These goals were called the "Triple Aim". The three aims are shown in Fig. 2.1. The goals of triple aim are interdependent and changes to any goal could have an effect on the other two. For instance, improving the experience of care by introducing a new technology could increase the cost of care.

2.1.2 Components of "Triple Aim"

The triple aim initiative launched by IHI was designed to help health systems to achieve the three goals mentioned above. During the pilot phase, IHI worked with 15 organizations in U.S., England and Sweden that served as prototypes of 'Macro-integrators' (Brown 2008). Macro-integrators are entities that can bring together the

A. Panny · A. Acharya (✉)
Center for Oral and Systemic Health, Marshfield Clinic Research Institute, Marshfield, WI, USA
e-mail: panny.aloksagar@marshfieldresearch.org; acharya.amit@marshfieldresearch.org

K. Krueger
Institute for Quality Innovation and Patient Safety (IQIPS), Marshfield Clinic, Marshfield, WI, USA
e-mail: krueger.kori@marshfieldclinic.org

A. Acharya et al. (eds.), *Integration of Medical and Dental Care and Patient Data*, Health Informatics, https://doi.org/10.1007/978-3-319-98298-4_2

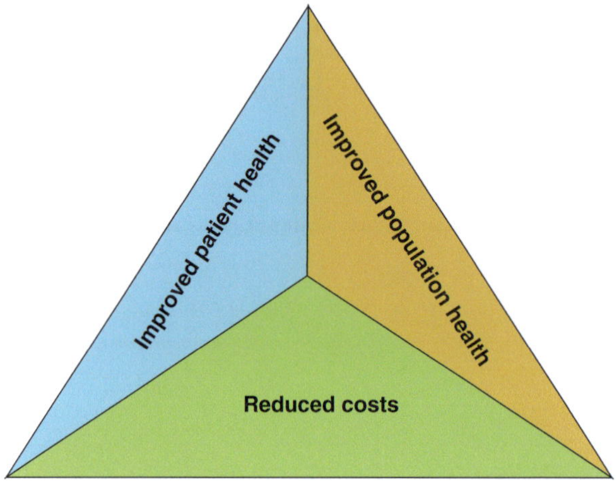

Fig. 2.1 Triple aim

Table 2.1 Initial triple aim sites (macro integrators)

Health plans	Capital health plan (FL) Care Oregon (OR) Blue Cross Blue Shield of Michigan (MI) Independent Health (NY)
Integrated Delivery Systems (w/ Health Plans)	Kaiser Permanente Mid-Atlantic region (MD) HealthPartners (MN) Presbyterian Healthcare (NM) Veterans Health System
Integrated Delivery Systems (w/o Health Plans)	Cincinnati Children's Hospital Medical Center (OH) Allegiance Health (MI) Erlanger Health System (TN) Fort Healthcare (WI)
Safety Net	Primary Care Coalition Montgomery County (MD) Colorado Access (CO) Nassau Health Care Corporation (NY) Contra Costa Health Services (CA)
International centers	Jonkoping county (Sweden) Bolton Primary Care Trust (England)

resources required to support a defined population (Brown 2008). These can be health plans, integrated delivery systems, safety net hospitals etc. (Table 2.1).

These systems build alliances and coalitions among various organizations across the continuum of care. The key functions of a macro integrator as described by Brown (2008) are as follows:

- Designing and implementing patient centered care models, new financial models and information technology for improving care and assessing performance.
- Developing, implementing and improving performance measures to accomplish triple aim goals.
- Integrating and improving the frontline systems like primary care providers, specialty services, hospitals and long term care services.
- Developing effective governance structures and establishing/enforcing accountability.

On the other hand care providers and teams on the front line which interact with individual patients and families to make sure the best and appropriate care is provided are called "Micro-integrators". A strong association between Macro and Micro integrators is essential to evaluate whether the available resources were efficiently utilized to meet the needs of defined populations.

2.1.3 *How to Achieve 'Triple Aim'?*

The national health expenditure of the U.S. is expected to rise from 17.8 to 19.9% of Gross Domestic Product (GDP) by 2025 (CMS 2018b). Aging population and the increase in lifestyle-related diseases like diabetes and obesity are driving health systems both in the U.S. and internationally to investigate new ways to obtain greater value for the resources that are devoted to health systems. As the triple aim involves system design that serves populations and requires simultaneously improving the three dimensions, this would entail in increasing the value of the healthcare resources.

A concept design was developed by IHI (IHI 2018) for health systems to achieve the triple aim. This included:

1. **Focusing on individuals and families**: Each individual has better knowledge about his/her state of health and his needs than professionals. This valuable data will help in redesigning the systems of care.
2. **Focusing on primary care**: Redesigning and expanding the primary care to make appropriate care services available all the time so as to prevent the need for emergency and acute care services and early identification of health problems by using risk assessments.
3. **Cost controlling**: Developing better cost control platforms by reducing overuse and providing financial incentives to providers for better health outcomes but not for more services.
4. **Prevention and health promotion**: Segmenting population in a community based on health risks to provide customized preventive services and advocating for health promotion and disease management.
5. **System integration**: Alignment of organizations and functions which are not usually under a single system to address the requirements for healthcare services among the defined population.

2.2 Physician Group Practice Demonstration (PGP) and Oral Health

2.2.1 *Background and Overview*

On 1 April 2005 the Centers for Medicare and Medicaid Services (CMS) initiated the Physician Group Practice (PGP) demonstration, the first legislatively mandated pay for performance initiative, which offers participating practices the opportunity to earn incentives for improving the quality and cost efficiency of health care (Pope et al. 2002). This was a pilot initiative to test whether a unique reimbursement mechanism of providing financial incentives to physician group practices could improve quality of health care delivery to Medicare-fee-for-service (FFS) beneficiaries and also prove to be cost-effective (Pope et al. 2002; Trisolini et al. 2006)

Initially ten PGPs were selected by CMS to participate in the PGP demonstration based on their organizational structure, geographic location and their proposed implementation strategy (Pope et al. 2002). Large PGPs were selected based on their administrative and clinical capabilities so that they could treat large number of Medicare beneficiaries and also would enable CMS to calculate the performance payments that are statistically reliable. Additionally the PGPs were required to be multispecialty groups and coordinate care across multiple providers and sites of care. Each of the PGPs had more than 200 physicians with a combined pool of more than 5000 physician's in all the PGP's (Kautter et al. 2007). The participant PGPs were:

- Dartmouth-Hitchcock clinic
- Billings clinic
- Geisinger clinic
- Middle sex health system
- Marshfield clinic
- Forsyth Medical group
- Park Nicollet health services
- St. Johns health system
- The Everett clinic
- University of Michigan. Faculty group practice

The beneficiary assignment for PGP demonstration was based on the PGPs ability to coordinate and manage the health care of the assigned beneficiary. The beneficiaries were identified retrospectively at the end of each year to be assigned to their respective PGPs in the following year. They did not have an option to accept or reject participation and their assignment to a PGP was based on the utilization of covered Medicare services (Pope et al. 2002). If a participating PGP had control over the beneficiary's utilization of services then it enables them to manage the health care of beneficiary. Because of this, the beneficiaries receiving at least one evaluation and management (E&M) service from the participating PGPs were eligible for assignment to them. Also if there are multiple beneficiaries qualifying under the above criteria, then one who is receiving largest share of E&M services from a PGP would be assigned to that particular PGP (Pope et al. 2002). Also beneficiaries were assigned to almost one participating PGP to avoid overpayments by CMS to multiple PGPs for serving overlapping Medicare population (Pope et al. 2002). The beneficiary assignment was re-determined at the end of each participating year based on the service utilization patterns. A total of 223,203 FFS beneficiaries were assigned to ten participating PGP's (Pope et al. 2002). The FFS beneficiaries with similar characteristics to assigned beneficiaries, residing in the PGPs market area and not assigned to the PGP will serve as a comparison population for the participating PGPs to provide a benchmark for assessing cost-control performance (Pope et al. 2002).

2.2.2 Payment Plan and Timeline for PGP's Demonstration

The PGP demonstration started on 1 April 2005 and it included a base year and five performance years. Initially the CMS designed the PGP demonstration for 3 years but later continued it for additional 2 years. The evaluation of demonstration is done every year to assess the strategies and interventions employed by PGPs in response to the demonstration's incentives. The final PGP performance report for each Performance Year (PY) would be available only after 9–12 months following the end of the year due to data availability and processing delays (Pope et al. 2002). An interim report on service utilization (like readmission rates etc.) in PY 1 versus base year would give participating PGPs a timely feedback on their performance (Pope et al. 2002). The timeline for baseline assessments and incentive payments to the PGPs is demonstrated in Table 2.2.

The PGP demonstration savings, also called Medicare savings are the dollar amounts that participating PGPs and the Medicare program share. The first step in calculating Medicare savings would be determining the per capita target expenditures for participating PGPs. These target expenditures are PGP-specific and are calculated based on the per capita base year expenditure of the PGPs (Kautter et al. 2007). The Medicare savings are calculated as the difference between PGPs per capita target expenditure and PGPs per capita actual expenditure in a given PY (Kautter et al. 2007). Both the target expenditure and actual expenditure of PGPs are

Table 2.2 Timeline for physician group practice demonstration

Demonstration year	Milestone
Base year (1st January 2004 to 31st December 2004)	• PGP Demonstration started.
Performance year one (1st April 2005 to 31st March 2006)	• Interim service utilization report submitted by participating PGPs.
Performance year two (1st April 2006 to 31st March 2007)	• Interim service utilization report submitted by participating PGPs. • 75% of the total incentive payments for Performance year one received by participating PGPs.
Performance year three (1st April 2007 to 31st March 2008)	• Interim service utilization report submitted by participating PGPs. • 75% of the total incentive payments for Performance year two received by participating PGPs.
Performance year four (1st April 2008 to 31st March 2009)	• Interim service utilization report submitted by participating PGPs. • 75% of the total incentive payments for Performance year two received by participating PGPs.
Performance year five (1st April 2009 to 31st March 2010)	• Interim service utilization report submitted by participating PGPs. • 75% of the total incentive payments for Performance year two received by participating PGPs. • Risk score cap was imposed to calculate the actual Expenditure of PGPs
Post demonstration year (After 31st March 2010)	• Rest of the 25% of the total incentive payments for all the performance years received by participating PGPs.

retrospective calculations as they are known only after the end of each PY (Kautter et al. 2007). Also case-mix adjustments were considered for changes in the types of patients treated by PGPs and comparison groups (Kautter et al. 2007).

$$\begin{aligned}\textbf{Medicare savings} &= \textbf{Target expenditures of PGPs}\left(\textbf{per capita}\right)\\ &\quad -\textbf{Actual expenditure of PGPs}\left(\textbf{per capita}\right)\end{aligned}$$

2.2.3 *Quality Metrics in PGP Demonstration*

The provision of financial incentives to participating PGPs is also based on quality improvement. A set of 32 measures were adopted for this demonstration drawn mainly from CMS Doctor's Office Quality (DOQ) Project which includes both process and outcome measures for five different conditions namely Diabetes Mellitus, Congestive heart failure, Coronary artery disease, Hypertension and assessment of preventive measures like breast cancer screening and colorectal cancer screening (Trisolini et al. 2005).

The implementation of measures occurred in a phased manner over the course of the PGP demonstration. Only the diabetes module was active in the PY1. Heart failure and coronary artery disease modules were included in PY2 and all the five modules were included in PY3, PY4 and PY5 (Trisolini et al. 2005). The quality performance of PGPs was calculated by analyzing the Medicare claims data and the beneficiary medical records. Predetermined threshold targets and improvement-over-time targets were laid down for PGPs by CMS to qualify for quality improvement incentives (Trisolini et al. 2005).

2.2.4 *Physician Group Practice Transition Demonstration*

The PGP transition demonstration was a continuation of PGP demonstration that ended in March 2010. The PGP transition demonstration started in January 2011 and concluded in December 2012 (CMS.gov 2018e). All ten participating PGPs of PGP demonstration were part of the PGP transition demonstration (CMS.gov 2018e). The major changes in the PGP transition demonstration compared to the original PGP demonstration were: (1) Changes in beneficiary assignment to PGP's, (2) Replacing the PGP-specific target expenditure benchmark with national target expenditure benchmark, (3) Changes in percentage of shared savings between PGP's and 4 CMS and (4) changes in CMS risk adjustment methods (CMS.gov 2018e). Also new quality metrics were added to the PGP transition demonstration. These included evaluation of Chronic Obstructive Pulmonary Disorder (COPD), care for frail elderly, monitoring transitions of care and also some of the meaningful use core clinical quality measures.

2.2.5 *Lack of Oral Health Integration Within the PGP Demonstration*

In the year 2000, well before the PGP demonstration initiative was launched by the CMS, a report titled "Oral Health in America: A Report of the Surgeon General" was released by the Surgeon general of the U.S Public Health Services to increase the oral health awareness among the medical community and the general population (U.S. Department of Health and Human Services Oral Health Coordinating Committee 2016). The report outlined the burden of oral diseases and disorders in the United States and also addressed the existing inequalities and disparities that prevent patients from obtaining optimal oral care. It indicated that around 46% adults in the U.S. have some type of periodontal disease (Eke et al. 2015).

It is estimated that around 48% of PGP beneficiaries were between 65 and 74 years of age and 36.7% of PGP beneficiaries were between 75 and 84 years of age (Trisolini et al. 2006). The load of poor oral health among PGP beneficiaries would impact the cost and quality of care. The non-inclusion of a comprehensive oral examination as a quality metric in both the PGP demonstration and the PGP transition demonstration was questionable. The care of frail elderly, which is one of the quality measures added in the PGP transition demonstration had no requirement for oral health screening although the data from the surgeon general's report suggest that there is an increasing number of adults in the age group of 65–74 years with some degree of periodontal disease. Studies also provide evidence of a growing oral health care crisis among the baby boomers affecting their oral health related quality of life (Yellowitz and Schneiderman 2014). The provision of oral care, especially to frail elderly, would improve the quality of care and also lower the cost of care by improving their overall health and also prevent unwanted emergency department visits for non-traumatic dental conditions. The report also emphasizes the relationship between the oral health and systemic health. It states that oral health is integral to general health and these two should not be interpreted as separate entities. The report had a broad review of the literature regarding the associations between oral diseases and systemic conditions including diabetes, heart diseases and adverse pregnancy outcomes.

2.2.5.1 Oral Health and Diabetes

The association between diabetes and periodontitis is so well accepted that it is called the sixth complication of diabetes (Löe 1993). Periodontitis is a chronic inflammatory disease affecting the supporting structures of the tooth. The surgeon general's report states that individuals with diabetes are at greater risk of periodontal diseases (USDHHS 2000). Type1 diabetes, also known as insulin dependent diabetes mellitus, is caused by the autoimmune destruction of β cells of the pancreas leading to insulin deficiency mainly in children and adolescents. Studies indicate that patients with poor periodontal health have increased values for HbA1c indicating poor glycemic control and also there is an increased susceptibility to periodontal diseases in individuals with type1 diabetes (Ajita et al. 2013). Type 2 diabetes, also known as non-insulin dependent diabetes mellitus is caused by insulin resistance as a consequence of complex pathophysiologic changes leading to disturbances in glucose metabolism. Inflammation plays a vital role in pathogenesis of both diabetes and periodontitis. Stumvoll et al. (2005) has indicated that increased concentrations of inflammatory cytokines (like TNFα and interlukin-6) inhibit insulin mediated glucose metabolism leading to poor glycemic control (Stumvoll et al. 2005). Studies also indicate that dysregulated cytokine secretion by the immune system during the periodontal bacterial infection leads to periodontal destruction (Seymour and Taylor 2004). Studies show that there is an increased concentration of cytokines in gingival crevicular fluid (GCF) leading to greater periodontal destruction in individuals with poor metabolic control (HbA1c > 9%). This indicates the association between these two diseases (Engebretson et al. 2004).

The oral health plays a greater role in glycemic control in patients with diabetes mellitus. As Fig. 2.2 illustrates, there is a bidirectional interrelationship between poor glycemic control and periodontal disease. The quality metrics laid down by CMS requires the PGP participants to report on the percentage of patients receiving HbA1c examination and percentage of patients with poor glycemic control (HbA1C > 9%). The report by the US surgeon general states that around 23% of adults between 65 and 74 years of age have moderate to severe periodontal disease (USDHHS 2010) and 48% of the PGP beneficiaries were in the age group of 65–74 years (Trisolini et al. 2006). The above data clearly states that majority of the PGP beneficiaries would have had some degree of periodontal disease. Therefore, the non-inclusion of oral examination as a quality metric in the management of diabetes mellitus (DM) patients is questionable. Periodontal health plays a vital role in blood glucose regulation of DM patients and focusing on the oral health of a DM patient would have greatly improved the quality and cost efficiency of care.

2.2.5.2 Oral Health and Heart Diseases

Coronary heart disease (CHD) is one of the main causes of mortality in the United States. The Centre for Disease Control and Prevention (CDC) reported around 28.4 million adults were diagnosed with heart diseases and 5.6% of them were diagnosed with CHD (USDHHS 2015). A large number of epidemiologic studies reported a strong association between periodontal disease and cardiovascular disease. A systemic review of the literature on the possible association of periodontal disease and other oral diseases, and CHD revealed that there is a 24–35% increase in the risk of CHD in people with periodontal disease (Humphrey et al. 2008). The mechanism of

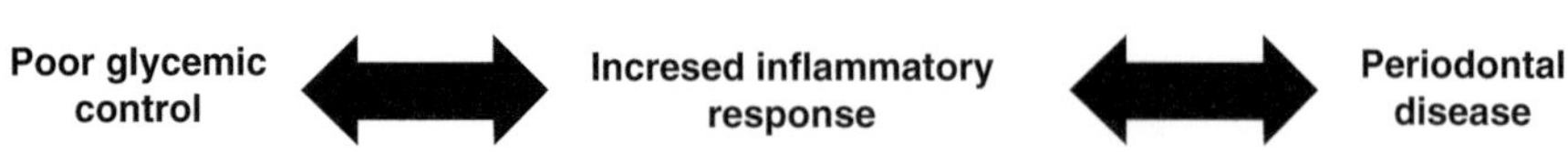

Fig. 2.2 Bidirectional relationship between poor glycemic control and periodontal disease

this association is varied. Studies have identified the presence periodontal pathogens like *Actinobacillus actinomycetemcomitans, B. forsythus and Porphyromonas gingivalis* in carotid atheroma's (Rath et al. 2014). Studies also have reported that periodontal bacteria like *Porphyromonas gingivalis* can invade the endothelium of both carotid and coronary arteries (Dorn et al. 1999). Lipopolysaccharide (LPS), an endotoxin and a potential stimulus to activate the release of inflammatory cytokines (like TNFα and Interleukin's) which directly or indirectly play a role in atherosclerotic heart disease, is present in subgingival plaque associated with periodontal disease (Castell et al. 1989; Yamauchi-Takihara et al. 1995). Studies also reported that periodontal pathogens are associated with acute phase proteins like C-reactive proteins (CRP) and fibrinogen which affect coagulation, platelet activation and aggregation leading to formation of atheroma (Wu et al. 2000). There is increasing evidence suggesting the role of periodontal pathogens in atheroma formation. The participants in the PGP demonstration were directed to improve the antiplatelet therapy, beta-blocker therapy and also drug therapy for lowering LDL cholesterol in PGP beneficiaries.

This was a preventative approach to prevent occurrence of acute conditions (like myocardial infarction (MI)) among the participating beneficiaries so as to avoid emergency department visits and hospitalizations eventually decreasing the cost of care and also improving the quality of life. Monitoring the oral health of the PGP beneficiaries and treating periodontal diseases would have been a preventative approach to addressing CHD as bad oral health greatly increases the risk of CHD.

2.2.5.3 Oral Health and Hypertension

Hypertension is one of the major risk factors for cardiovascular diseases. Around 75 million American adults are suffering from high blood pressure (Centers for Disease Control and Prevention (CDC) 2017). Vascular inflammatory processes are attributed as one of the causative factors for hypertension. The endothelial cells lining the blood vessels release various vasodilators and vasoconstrictors, playing a crucial role in the regulation of blood pressure (Leong et al. 2014). Increased expression of cellular adhesion molecules by endothelial cells and increased leukocyte infiltration and cytokine production during inflammation cause disturbances in the normal endothelial functioning and hence disturb the balance between vasoconstrictors and vasodilators in the blood (Leong et al. 2014) leading to an increase in blood pressure. Studies indicate periodontal disease pathogens like *Porphyromonas gingivalis* in the blood lead to expression of adhesion molecules by endothelial cells thus disrupting the normal endothelial function (Amar et al. 2003; Tsioufis et al. 2011). Results from the Oral Infections and Vascular Disease Epidemiology Study (INVEST) by Desvarieux et al. indicated a strong association between prevalent hypertension and periodontal pathogens like *A. actinomycetemcomitans*, *P. gingivalis*, *T. forsythia* and *T. denticola* among others (Desvarieux et al. 2010). Around 55% of the total Medicare population is hypertensive and there are around 40 million physician office visits per year with hypertension as a primary diagnosis

(CMS.gov 2017). A tremendous amount of medical and financial resource is used to manage this population of patients. In the context of increasing evidence suggesting the influence of periodontal pathogens on hypertension, improving the periodontal health of hypertensive patients and regularly monitoring their oral health will definitely play an important role in cost savings.

2.3 Accountable Care Organizations (ACO)

2.3.1 Background and Overview

The Patient Protection and Affordable Care Act (ACA), also called "Obama care", enacted on 23 March 2010 included a number of provisions to improve the quality of Medicare services and establishment of new payment models (Medicare Program 2011). Under these provisions, section 3022 of the ACA required the establishment of Medicare shared savings program (MSSP) to encourage the development of Accountable Care Organizations (ACO) (Medicare Program 2011). The ACO model was built on theories tested in the PGP demonstration and PGP transition demonstration, implemented by Medicare previously.

2.3.2 What Are ACOs?

ACOs are group of physicians, hospitals or other health care providers which volunteer to assume the responsibility for the care of a defined population of Medicare fee-for service beneficiaries (CMS.gov 2018a). These are entities that agree to be accountable for improving quality and cost outcomes. The term "Accountable Care Organization" was coined in 2006 by Elliot Fisher, MD, Director of Dartmouth Institute for Health Policy and Clinical Practice in Hanover, New Hampshire (Fisher 2018).

2.3.2.1 Organizational Requirements to Become an ACO

ACOs have been established by both CMS and private insurance companies to provide incentives to providers based on savings and outcomes. Group practices, networks of individual practices, federally qualified health centers, rural health clinics, provider health plan partnerships and large health systems are some of the groups of providers that can establish as an ACO (CMS 2018a). Some of the key requirements for an organization to become an ACO are (NCQA 2018):

- Ability to define the organizational structure and be able to manage resources and align provider incentives through arrangements.
- Ability to recruit and retain both primary care providers and specialists as per the requirement.
- Ability to provide patient centered primary care services.

- Ability to collect, integrate and use data from various sources for performance reporting.
- Ability to facilitate secure and timely exchange of information between the participating providers.
- Ability to measure and report on patient experience and cost and quality measures.

2.3.3 Payment Models in ACOs

The performance of ACOs is measured against an ACO-specific benchmark developed by CMS. This is an estimate of total Medicare fee-for-service (both part A and part B) expenditure of all the assigned ACO beneficiaries in the absence of an ACO, even if all the services were not provided (Douven et al. 2015).

Beneficiary characteristics and increases in national per capita expenditures for Medicare services are taken into account to adjust the specified benchmark (Douven et al. 2015).

Broadly the CMS proposed two models for calculating the shared savings and losses between the ACOs.

2.3.3.1 One-Sided Payment Model

In this model if the total expenditure of an ACO is below the benchmark then it will be eligible to share up to 50% of the savings with CMS (Douven et al. 2015). The ACO's in this model does not incur any penalty even if their total expenditure exceeds the benchmark and will still receive Medicare fee-for-service payments for all the services rendered (Douven et al. 2015). Figure 2.3 conceptually illustrates the concept of shared savings in terms of expenditure and efficiency. We can notice as the expenditure decreases the efficiency increases.

For one-sided (Track1) payment model:

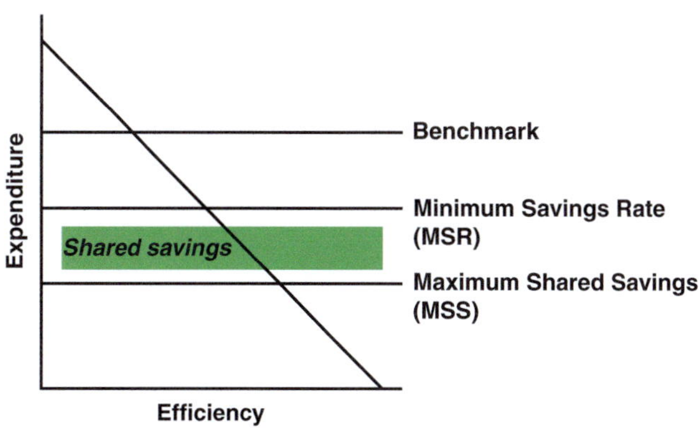

Fig. 2.3 One-sided payment model

- **Shared Savings** = (Assigned benchmark – Actual expenditure);
- **Minimum Saving Rate (MSR)**: The percentage of savings that ACO's must meet or exceed to qualify for the shared savings program. 'Exceed' in this context is less than or equal to the previously mentioned MSR rate. This rate is calculated by CMS as a function of total number of assigned beneficiaries and their associated expenses;
- **Maximum Shared Savings (MSS)**: The maximum percentage of saving that an ACO can receive during a given year.

2.3.3.2 Two-Sided Payment Model

In this model if the total expenditure of an ACO is well below the benchmark (savings) then it will be eligible to receive bonuses from CMS where as if the spending exceeds the benchmark (overruns) then they incur penalty and must repay the CMS (Douven et al. 2015). The maximum bonus or penalty is capped at 60% of the savings or overruns, respectively (Douven et al. 2015). Figure 2.4 conceptually illustrates the concept of minimum loss rate (MLR) and maximum owed losses-(MOL).

For two–sided (Track 2) payment model

- **Minimum Loss Rate (MLR)**: The percentage of losses the ACO must meet or exceed to be liable for the shared losses (Penalty);
- **Maximum Owed Losses (MOL)**: The Maximum percentage of losses owed by an ACO to CMS during a given year. This is the maximum amount an ACO owes as penalty to the CMS if it exceeds its spending above the MLR.

2.3.4 *Quality Metrics in ACO*

ACOs must completely and accurately report the quality data used to calculate and assess their quality performance. Also they must meet the required standards to qualify for shared savings payments. As of 2017 there are around 31 quality metrics across four domains namely patient experience, care coordination, preventive health

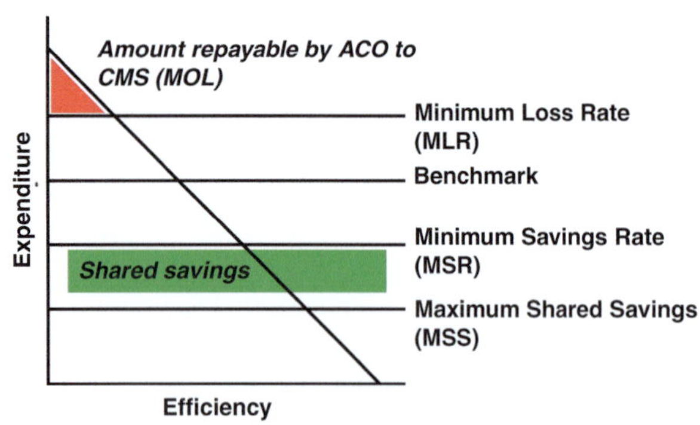

Fig. 2.4 Two-sided payment model

and at-risk population (ACO 2015). The data for all the measures is obtained from the *Consumer Assessment of Healthcare Providers and Systems* (CAHPS) survey, Medicare and Medicaid EHR incentive program data, claims data and ACO group practice reporting option (GPRO) web interface (ACO 2015).

2.3.5 ACO Programs

The contractual responsibility of ACOs is varied and includes both public and private payers. Each ACO has varied responsibilities depending on the nature of contracts. In a broad perspective an ACO may have contracts with public payers like Medicare and Medicaid and private payers like Kaiser Permanente, Aetna, and Delta Dental (Fig. 2.5). Medicare offers many ACO programs like the ones discussed in Sects. 2.3.5.1, 2.3.5.2 and 2.3.5.3.

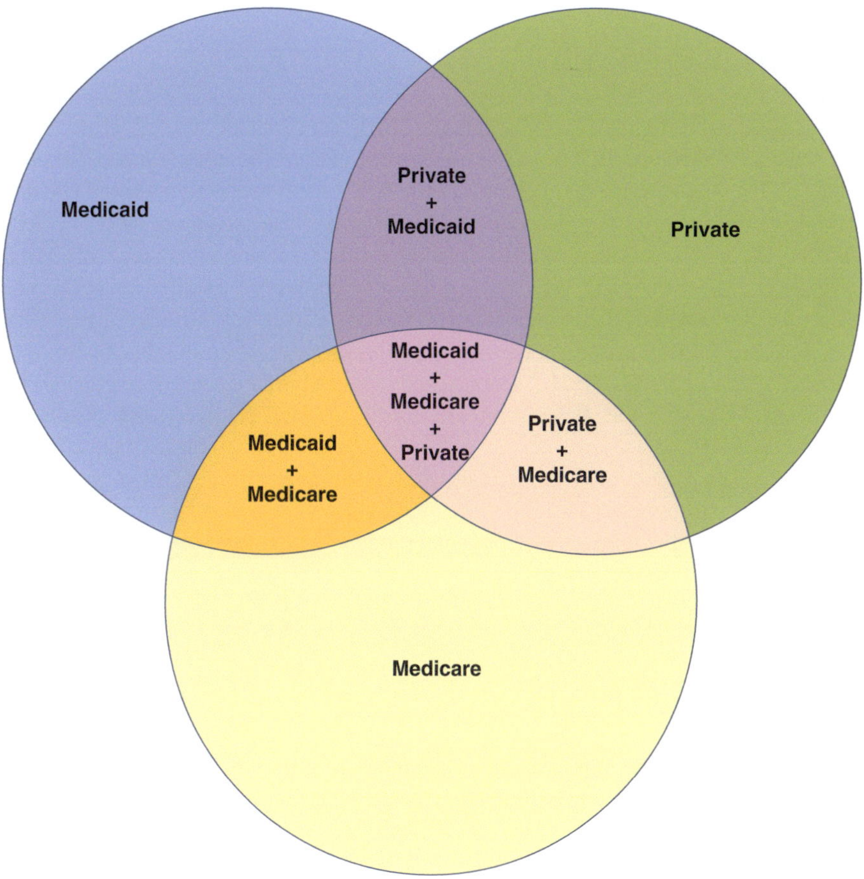

Fig. 2.5 Contractual structure of ACOs

2.3.5.1 Medicare Shared Savings Program (MSSP)

The MSSP is the earliest initiative by CMS established under the ACA. It is the basic mechanism where ACOs, which meet certain quality metrics, laid down by CMS and also increases their cost efficiency; receive incentives in form of shared savings. The ACOs in this program must serve a minimum of 5000 Medicare beneficiaries for 3 years (American College of Physicians 2011).

2.3.5.2 Advance Payment Model

These models are mainly designed to help rural providers and small group practices who volunteer to participate in MSSP by forming an ACO (CMS.gov 2018b). The CMS provides capital needed for these organizations to improve their infrastructure, staff and other facilities for better care coordination. These amounts will be deducted from the shared savings they receive from CMS (CMS.gov 2018c).

2.3.5.3 Pioneer ACO Model

This model was designed for organizations which have considerable experience and the required infrastructure for care–coordination across the continuum (CMS.gov 2018f). This would allow them to rapidly transition from receiving a shared savings payment to a capitation fee based model (population based payment model) (CMS 2018c). The participation is for 3 years and the organizations which receive shared savings in the first 2 years and also report and improve on quality measures will receive a set amount per each beneficiary assigned to them, per period of time (CMS 2018c). The ACOs in this program must serve a minimum of 15,000 Medicare beneficiaries for 3 years. The first 2 years would be based on the shared savings model but in the third year the ACOs which perform well will change to the capitation model (CMS 2018c).

Some of the other ACO models are ACO investment model, Next generation ACO model, Comprehensive end-stage renal disease care model and Advancing care coordination through episode payment models (cardiac and orthopedic bundled payment models) (CMS.gov 2018a).

2.4 Oral Health and ACO

Oral health is an important concern for health care policy makers, and increasing compilation of evidence shows links between oral and systemic health. It is therefore necessary for patients to have access to routine dental care and oral disease prevention as a strategy to improve overall health outcomes. The accessibility of dental care and the care delivery models are changing as a result of emergence of large dental practices and new health care reforms. Although ACOs formed under the MSSP of ACA were responsible for the overall health of the assigned beneficiaries, responsibility of oral health was not mandated under this provision (Vujicic and Nasseh 2013). A "National Survey of Accountable Care Organizations" (NSACO) created by University of California, Berkeley and administered by Dartmouth institute indicates that only 9% of the ACOs with commercial contracts and 25% of the ACOs with Medicaid contracts are accountable for the oral health of their beneficiaries (Colla et al. 2016). In the view of the report published by the surgeon general of United States indicating increasing burden of oral diseases, mainly the dental caries and periodontal diseases among children, adult and elderly population (U.S. Department of Health and Human Services Oral Health Coordinating Committee 2016), it is important to understand the challenges and identify the opportunities of incorporating oral and dental care into ACOs.

2.4.1 Barriers and Challenges to Incorporating Oral and Dental Care into ACOs

There are various organizational, financial and technical barriers to integrating oral health and dental services into ACOs. The key barriers identified are:

2.4.1.1 Medicare Population

One of the major reasons for non-inclusion of dental care services in ACOs is the fact that majority of the population served by ACOs are Medicare beneficiaries and Medicare does not offer dental benefits (Colla et al. 2016). Around 25% of the total Medicare population aged 65 or older have diabetes and around 27% of them have CHD (Brennan et al. 2012). Medicare has estimated that the spending on Medicare diabetes patients will increase many folds and has introduced programs like Medicare diabetes prevention program (MDPP) to decrease the amount of spending on diabetes (CMS.gov 2018d). A retrospective study conducted by Jeffcoat et al. provided evidence that there is an average reduction of 40.2% in the per capita total health care expenditure of a diabetic person and a 10.2% reduction in the per capita health care expenditure of a person with CHD who received both preventive and interventional oral care (Jeffcoat et al. 2014). Also, the results from the study indicated a 10.2% reduction in the total annual health care spending of a person with CHD who received timely oral care (Jeffcoat et al. 2014). This evidence suggests that not only will the delivery of oral health care to this cohort of the Medicare population improve their total quality of life but will also save per capita spending on these individuals.

2.4.1.2 Dental Care as a Primary Care Service

The results from the NSACO survey indicate that around 52% of the 168 ACOs that were not providing dental services did not consider dental care as a component of primary care (Colla et al. 2016). The lack of awareness among the payers and providers, on oral-systemic health relationship and the lack of proper mandates necessitating oral health as an important component of overall health lead to failure in recognizing dental care as a primary care service. Around 113.3 million diabetic patient visits to physician offices were reported in the year 2010 (Ashman et al. 2010) and 121.9 million patient visits with hypertension as primary diagnosis were reported in 2013–2014 (Ashman et al. 2017). The diabetes expenditure is expected to reach around $336 billion by the year 2034 (Huang et al. 2009). Apart from monitoring oral health of these patients during the dental office visit, monitoring chronic conditions like diabetes and hypertension should be considered. Several studies indicated that including blood glucose screening as a part of the dental visit can help in regular screening of diabetic patients leading to early interventions and thus preventing further complications and contributing to savings in health care expenditure.

2.4.1.3 Lack of Integrated Information Systems

Lack of an advanced integrated health information technology was the major reason for ACOs not integrating medical and dental care records. Around 55% of 168 providers from the NSACO survey reported a lack of technical infrastructure to integrate care (Colla et al. 2016). ACOs like Hennepin Health have reported data sharing between medical and dental providers as the major hurdle in care coordination (ADA 2015). Marshfield clinic, one of the largest private medical providers in the United States has developed a robust medical-dental integrated electronic health record (iEHR) (Acharya et al. 2011). A recent survey conducted by Marshfield Clinic provides evidence of a strong need for access to patient's dental information by medical providers to provide more comprehensive care (Acharya et al. 2011). The health system invested in the development of the iEHR for integrating medical and dental records of patients, an important step towards a holistic care approach.

2.4.1.4 Impact on Performance Measures and Cost Efficiency

The ACOs are required to report and improve their performance around 31 quality metrics across four domains (Leung et al. 2011) and these do not include any oral health related measures. As ACOs are not required to report on oral measures they find inclusion of dental care having negligible impact on both their performance measures and cost efficiency. Around 51% providers from the NSACO survey cited that negligible impact on performance measures and 42% providers from the NSACO survey cited negligible impact on cost efficiency as reasons for not including dental care as a part of their care coordination efforts (Colla et al. 2016). The Dental Quality Alliance, a multi stakeholder organization established by the American Dental Association (ADA) develops quality metrics for performance measurement as means to improve oral health care delivery (Ojha and Aravamudhan 2016). They also educate the providers and payers on performance measurement and also aid in the implementation of these measures. They include pediatric, maternal and adult oral health measures. They measure quality of care, access to care, timeliness of care delivery and cost of care delivery among various cohorts of populations (Ojha and Aravamudhan 2016). Incorporating these measures as a part of ACOs performance measurement would not only encourage them to provide oral care but will also increase the quality of care delivered. Some of the other reasons for not including oral health care measures are lack of insurance among the beneficiaries, difficulty recruiting dental providers and a perception of low need among beneficiaries (Colla et al. 2016).

2.4.2 Opportunities to Integrate Dental Care in an ACO

2.4.2.1 Improving the Payment Models and Implementing Pay for Performance

Most of the dental plans are stand-alone plans and lower reimbursements rates for dentists providing services to populations covered by Medicaid expansion under ACA is a big challenge. The adoption of new payment models would address this problem. As there is a shift from fee for service payment models to value-based models, there is an immense pressure on providers to provide quality of care and improve cost efficiency. The capitated payment models adopted by many of the ACOs providing dental care as a part of care coordination receive a fixed amount per member per month for all the beneficiaries assigned to them. The ACOs, in turn, reimburse the dental providers at a rate exceeding the usual Medicaid rates in order to increase the access to dental care for their beneficiaries. The dentist also receives a bonus for meeting certain quality metrics in addition to the regular fee-for-service reimbursement (ADA 2015). Figure 2.6 shows the shift in the Payment Models.

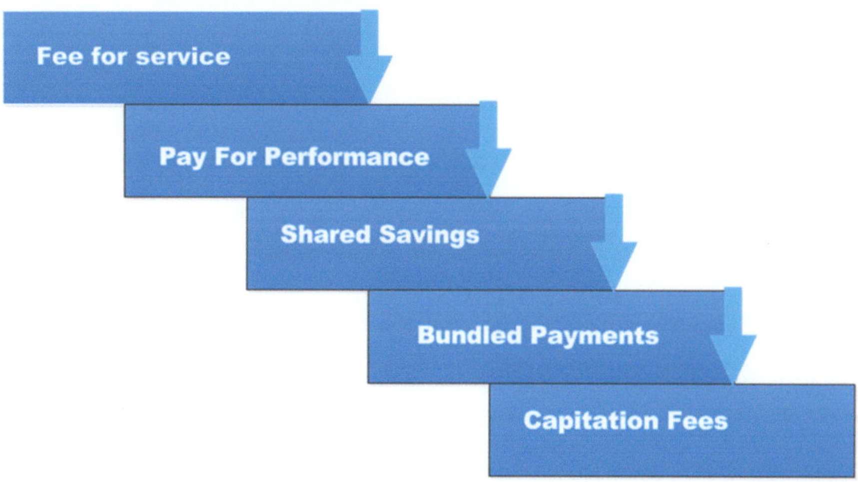

Fig. 2.6 Shift in the payment model

2.4.2.2 Identification of High Risk Population

To reduce the financial burden on ACOs due to increased dental service utilization, identification of a high-risk population among the assigned beneficiaries is recommended. Both Delta Dental of Iowa under its Delta Wellness Plan and Partners For Kids, an ACO created by Nationwide Children's Hospital have employed mechanisms to identify high-risk population to stratify patients as per their needs and establish care plans with emphasis on preventive and interventional care (ADA 2015). The providers in Dental Wellness Plan administered by Delta Dental of Iowa had to complete an online oral risk assessment for all the beneficiaries visiting the dental clinic (ADA 2015). Trillium Coordinated Care Organization, and ACO based in Oregon, has conducted caries management by risk assessment (CAMBRA) to identify children with a high risk of caries. This will also aid in cost savings by preventing emergency room (ER) visits for dental pain and other dental problems (ADA 2015).

2.4.2.3 Oral Health as a Quality Measure

The ACOs report on many performance measures including percentage of diabetic patients with poor glycemic control and percentage of patients with heart failure and respiratory disorders (COPD or asthma). Poor oral health in the individual with the above disorders would further worsen their condition. Including oral health as a quality measure will mandate the ACOs to include oral care as a part of their care coordination (ADA 2015). This not only will improve the overall health of the beneficiary but also will help lower costs. The Hennepin Health reports on the number of members with at least on dental visit in 1 year (ADA 2015). The Permanente Dental Associates also report on 40 measures ranging from process to outcome measures. Trillium Coordinated Care Organization reports on the number of patients receiving smoking cessation counselling (ADA 2015; Colla et al. 2016). Other opportunities include developing integrated information systems and awareness among the leadership about the Oral-Systemic connection.

2.5 Conclusion

The increasing evidence that oral health has an effect on a person's overall health is compelling. Although policy makers are recommending strategies to reform health care delivery to achieve Triple Aim, oral health is often overlooked. There is an immense opportunity to build projects which address the institutional, educational and legislative barriers of integrating oral and medical care. Both the PGP demonstration project and ACOs have focused on coordinating care and delivering whole-person care but not all of them have included oral health as a part of their care coordination. Poor oral health has physical, emotional and psychological effect on an individual. Studies indicate that addressing oral problems could result in significant cost savings. Professional training programs should be developed for medical care providers identify oral health diseases and provide preventive care (like fluoride treatment). The dental insurance coverage, especially coverage for adult dental care, should be significantly improved. Appropriate Health Information Technology (HIT) and informatics platforms to effectively enable sharing of information between medical and dental providers must be developed to establish a care continuum. The quality metrics to measure the oral health care delivery and its outcome and appropriate dashboards to visualize and monitor those quality improvement goals must be developed and efficiently implemented in all health systems. Also, the leadership of the health care organization must be educated on the effects of oral health on systemic health thereby creating an environment and culture of holistic care and care delivery. Accessibility to oral and dental services must be improved among the high-risk population. Incorporating oral health into health reform efforts is important to achieve triple aim of improving the patient experience of care, improving the health of populations, and reducing the per-capita cost of care. Only then the achieving the 'True' Triple Aim in Healthcare is possible.

References

Acharya A, Mahnke A, Chyou P-H, Rottscheit C, Starren JB. Medical providers' dental information needs: a baseline survey. Stud Health Technol Inform. 2011;169:387–91. http://www.ncbi.nlm.nih.gov/pubmed/21893778.

ACO. Quality-measures-standards. 2015. https://www.cms.gov/medicare/medicare-fee-for-service-payment/sharedsavingsprogram/quality_measures_standards.html.

ADA. Dental care in accountable care organizations: insights from 5 case studies. 2015. https://www.ada.org/~/media/ADA/Science and Research/HPI/Files/HPIBrief_0615_1.pdf?la=en.

Ajita M, Karan P, Vivek G, MA S, Anuj M. Periodontal disease and type 1 diabetes mellitus: associations with glycemic control and complications: an Indian perspective. Diabetes Metab Syndr. 2013;7(2):61–3. https://doi.org/10.1016/j.dsx.2013.03.001.

Amar S, Gokce N, Morgan S, Loukideli M, Van Dyke TE, Vita JA. Periodontal disease is associated with brachial artery endothelial dysfunction and systemic inflammation. Arterioscler Thromb Vasc Biol. 2003;23(7):1245–9. https://doi.org/10.1161/01.ATV.0000078603.90302.4A.

American College of Physicians. Detailed summary--Medciare Shared Savings/Accountable Care Organization (ACO) program. 2011. https://www.acponline.org/system/files/documents/running_practice/delivery_and_payment_models/aco/aco_detailed_sum.pdf

Ashman JJ, Talwalkar A, Taylor SA. Age differences in visits to office-based physicians by patients with diabetes: United States, 2010 key findings. 2010. https://www.cdc.gov/nchs/data/databriefs/db161.pdf

Ashman, J. J., Rui, P., Schappert, S. M., & Strashny, A.. Characteristics of visits to primary care physicians by adults diagnosed with hypertension. National Health Statistics Reports Number, 106. 2017. https://www.cdc.gov/nchs/data/nhsr/nhsr106.pdf

Berwick DM, Nolan TW, Whittington J. The triple aim: care, health, and cost. Health Affairs (Project Hope). 2008;27(3):759–69. https://doi.org/10.1377/hlthaff.27.3.759.

Brennan N, Bartee S, Wheatcroft G, Krometis J. Chronic conditions among medicare beneficiaries. 2012. https://www.cms.gov/research-statistics-data-and-systems/statistics-trends-and-reports/chronic-conditions/downloads/2012chartbook.pdf

Brown PC. Improving the performance curve in behavioral healthcare. 2008. https://www.ibhi.net/ref-lib-papers/Summary of the Triple Aim Symposium.pdf

Castell JV, Andus T, Kunz D, Heinrich PC. Interleukin-6. The major regulator of acute-phase protein synthesis in man and rat. Ann N Y Acad Sci. 1989;557:87–99; discussion 100–1. http://www.ncbi.nlm.nih.gov/pubmed/2472097.
Centers for Medicare & Medicaid Services (CMS), HHS. Medicare program, medicare shared savings program: accountable care organizations; final rule. Fed Regist. 2011;76(212):67801–990.
Centers for Disease Control and Prevention (CDC). FastStats - Hypertension. 2017. https://www.cdc.gov/nchs/fastats/hypertension.htm. Accessed 30 June 2018.
CMS. Accountable Care Organizations: what providers need to know. 2018a. https://www.cms.gov/Medicare/Medicare-Fee-for-Service-Payment/sharedsavingsprogram/Downloads/ACO_Providers_Factsheet_ICN907406.pdf
CMS. NHE-Fact-Sheet. 2018b. https://www.cms.gov/Research-Statistics-Data-and-Systems/Statistics-Trends-and-Reports/NationalHealthExpendData/NHE-Fact-Sheet.html. Accessed 30 June 2018.
CMS. Pioneer ACO model. Baltimore, MD: Center for Medicare & Medicaid Innovation; 2018c. https://innovation.cms.gov/initiatives/Pioneer-ACO-Model/PioneerACO-FactSheet.html.
CMS.gov. Chronic conditions overview. 2017. https://www.cms.gov/Research-Statistics-Data-and-Systems/Statistics-Trends-and-Reports/Chronic-Conditions/.
CMS.gov. Accountable Care Organizations (ACOs): general information. Center for Medicare & Medicaid Innovation. 2018a. https://innovation.cms.gov/initiatives/ACO/. Accessed 30 June 2018.
CMS.gov. Advance Payment ACO model. Baltimore, MD: Center for Medicare & Medicaid Innovation. 2018b. https://innovation.cms.gov/initiatives/Advance-Payment-ACO-Model/index.html. Accessed 1 July 2018.
CMS.gov. Advance Payment ACO Model. Baltimore, MD: Center for Medicare & Medicaid Innovation. 2018c. https://innovation.cms.gov/Files/fact-sheet/Advanced-Payment-ACO-Model-Fact-Sheet.pdf. Accessed 1 July 2018.
CMS.gov. Medicare Diabetes Prevention Program (MDPP) expanded model. Center for Medicare & Medicaid Innovation. 2018d. https://innovation.cms.gov/initiatives/medicare-diabetes-prevention-program/. Accessed 30 June 2018.
CMS.gov. Physician group practice transition demonstration. Center for Medicare & Medicaid Innovation. 2018e. https://innovation.cms.gov/initiatives/physician-group-practice-transition/. Accessed 30 June 2018.
CMS.gov. Pioneer ACO model. Center for Medicare & Medicaid Innovation. 2018f. https://innovation.cms.gov/initiatives/Pioneer-ACO-Model/index.html. Accessed 1 July 2018.
Colla CH, Stachowski C, Kundu S, Harris B, Kennedy G, Vujicic M. Dental care within accountable care organizations: challenges and opportunities. 2016. http://www.ada.org/~/media/ADA/Science and Research/HPI/Files/HPIBrief_0316_2.pdf
Desvarieux M, Demmer RT, Jacobs DR Jr, Rundek T, Boden-Albala B, Sacco RL, Papapanou PN. Periodontal bacteria and hypertension: the oral infections and vascular disease epidemiology study (INVEST). J Hypertens. 2010;28(7):1413–21. https://doi.org/10.1097/HJH.0b013e328338cd36.
Dorn BR, Dunn WA, Progulske-Fox A. Invasion of human coronary artery cells by periodontal pathogens. Infect Immun. 1999;67(11):5792–8. http://www.ncbi.nlm.nih.gov/pubmed/10531230.
Douven R, Mcguire TG, Mcwilliams JM. Avoiding unintended incentives in ACO payment models. Health Aff (Millwood). 2015;34(1):143–9. https://doi.org/10.1377/hlthaff.2014.0444.
Eke PI, Dye BA, Wei L, Slade GD, Thornton-Evans GO, Borgnakke WS, et al. Update on prevalence of periodontitis in adults in the United States: NHANES 2009 to 2012. J Periodontol. 2015;86(5):611–22. https://doi.org/10.1902/jop.2015.140520.
Engebretson SP, Hey-Hadavi J, Ehrhardt FJ, Hsu D, Celenti RS, Grbic JT, Lamster IB. Gingival crevicular fluid levels of interleukin-1β and glycemic control in patients with chronic periodontitis and type 2 diabetes. J Periodontol. 2004;75(9):1203–8. https://doi.org/10.1902/jop.2004.75.9.1203.
Fisher E. Elliott Fisher, MD, MPH::The Dartmouth Institute. 2018. http://tdi.dartmouth.edu/about/our-people/directory/elliott-s-fisher-md-mph. Accessed 30 June 2018.

Huang ES, Basu A, O'Grady M, Capretta JC. Projecting the future diabetes population size and related costs for the U.S. Diabetes Care. 2009;32(12):2225–9. https://doi.org/10.2337/dc09-0459.

Humphrey LL, Fu R, Buckley DI, Freeman M, Helfand M. Periodontal disease and coronary heart disease incidence: a systematic review and meta-analysis. J Gen Intern Med. 2008;23(12):2079–86. https://doi.org/10.1007/s11606-008-0787-6.

IHI. The IHI Triple Aim. 2018. http://www.ihi.org/Engage/Initiatives/TripleAim/Pages/default.aspx. Accessed 30 June 2018.

Jeffcoat MK, Jeffcoat RL, Gladowski PA, Bramson JB, Blum JJ. Impact of periodontal therapy on general health. Am J Prev Med. 2014;47(2):166–74. https://doi.org/10.1016/j.amepre.2014.04.001.

Kautter J, Pope GC, Trisolini M, Grund S. Medicare physician group practice demonstration design: quality and efficiency pay-for-performance. Health Care Financ Rev. 2007;29(1):15–29. http://www.ncbi.nlm.nih.gov/pubmed/18624077.

Leong X-F, Ng C-Y, Badiah B, Das S. Association between hypertension and periodontitis: possible mechanisms. Scientific World Journal. 2014;2014:1–11. https://doi.org/10.1155/2014/768237.

Leung M, Trisolini M, Trebino D, Pope G, Grund S, Roberson J, Landiza F. Physician group practice transition demonstration quality measurement and reporting specifications. 2011. https://innovation.cms.gov/Files/reports/PGP-Transition-Quality-Specs-Report.pdf

Löe H. Periodontal disease. The sixth complication of diabetes mellitus. Diabetes Care. 1993;16(1):329–34. http://www.ncbi.nlm.nih.gov/pubmed/8422804.

NCQA. ACO eligibility. 2018. http://www.ncqa.org/programs/accreditation/accountable-care-organization-aco/aco-eligibility. Accessed 30 June 2018.

Ojha D, Aravamudhan K. Leading the dental quality movement: a dental quality alliance perspective. J Calif Dent Assoc. 2016;44(4):239–44. http://www.ncbi.nlm.nih.gov/pubmed/27265980.

Pope GC, Michael Trisolini M, John Kautter M, Adamache W, Jerry Cromwell M. Physician Group Practice (PGP) demonstration design report. 2002. https://innovation.cms.gov/files/migrated-medicare-demonstration-x/pgp_full_demo_report.pdf

Rath S, Mukherjee M, Kaushik R, Sen S, Kumar M. Periodontal pathogens in atheromatous plaque. Indian J Pathol Microbiol. 2014;57(2):259. https://doi.org/10.4103/0377-4929.134704.

Seymour GJ, Taylor JJ. Shouts and whispers: an introduction to immunoregulation in periodontal disease. Periodontol 2000. 2004;35(1):9–13. https://doi.org/10.1111/j.0906-6713.2004.003555.x.

Stumvoll M, Goldstein BJ, van Haeften TW. Type 2 diabetes: principles of pathogenesis and therapy. Lancet. 2005;365(9467):1333–46. https://doi.org/10.1016/S0140-6736(05)61032-X.

Trisolini M, Kautter AJ, Gregory C, Pope B, Bapat MAE, Olmsted M, et al. Physician group practice demonstration quality measurement and reporting specifications Version 2. 2005. https://innovation.cms.gov/Files/reports/Quality-Specs-Report.pdf

Trisolini M, Pope G, Kautter J, Aggarwal J. Medicare physician group practices: innovations in quality and efficiency. 2006. https://www.commonwealthfund.org/sites/default/files/documents/___media_files_publications_fund_report_2006_dec_medicare_physician_group_practices__innovations_in_quality_and_efficiency_971_trisolini_medicare_physician_group_practices_i_pdf

Tsioufis C, Kasiakogias A, Thomopoulos C, Stefanadis C. Periodontitis and blood pressure: the concept of dental hypertension. Atherosclerosis. 2011;219(1):1–9. https://doi.org/10.1016/j.atherosclerosis.2011.04.030.

U.S. Department of Health and Human Services Oral Health Coordinating Committee. U.S. Department of Health and Human Services Oral Health Strategic Framework, 2014–2017. Public Health Rep. 2016;131(2):242–57. http://www.ncbi.nlm.nih.gov/pubmed/26957659.

USDHHS. Oral health in America: a report of the surgeon general. NIH Publication No. 00-4713. 2000. https://profiles.nlm.nih.gov/ps/retrieve/ResourceMetadata/NNBBJT/.

USDHHS. Oral health in America: a report of the surgeon general (Executive Summary). National Institute of Dental and Craniofacial Research. 2010. https://www.nidcr.nih.gov/research/data-statistics/surgeon-general. Accessed 30 June 2018.

USDHHS. Summary health statistics: National Health Interview Survey. 2015. https://ftp.cdc.gov/pub/Health_Statistics/NCHS/NHIS/SHS/2015_SHS_Table_A-1.pdf

Vujicic M, Nasseh K. Accountable Care Organizations present key opportunities for the dental profession. 2013. http://www.ada.org/~/media/ADA/Science and Research/HPI/Files/HPIBrief_0413_2.pdf?la=en.

Wu T, Trevisan M, Genco RJ, Falkner KL, Dorn JP, Sempos CT. Examination of the relation between periodontal health status and cardiovascular risk factors: serum total and high density lipoprotein cholesterol, C-reactive protein, and plasma fibrinogen. Am J Epidemiol. 2000;151(3):273–82. http://www.ncbi.nlm.nih.gov/pubmed/10670552.

Yamauchi-Takihara K, Ihara Y, Ogata A, Yoshizaki K, Azuma J, Kishimoto T. Hypoxic stress induces cardiac myocyte-derived interleukin-6. Circulation. 1995;91(5):1520–4. http://www.ncbi.nlm.nih.gov/pubmed/7867193.

Yellowitz JA, Schneiderman MT. Elder's oral health crisis. J Evid Based Dent Pract. 2014;14(Suppl):191–200. https://doi.org/10.1016/j.jebdp.2014.04.011.

Chapter 3
An Environmental Scan of the Various Oral-Systemic Contact Points

Amit Acharya, Shin-Mey Rose Yin Geist, Valerie Powell, and Miguel H. Torres-Urquidy

3.1 Introduction

The Institute of Medicine (IOM), National Academy of Sciences, released a report, "Dental Education at the Crossroads: Challenges and Change," in January 1995, calling for greater collaboration between medicine and dentistry. The report cited a need for closer integration between dentistry and medicine inclusive of all aspects of health care: research, education, and patient care. In 2000, Surgeon General David Satcher's report entitled "Oral Health in America" focused attention on a national problem which had gone largely unrecognized for decades: the oral health crisis (Satcher 2000).

Dr. Satcher emphasized that oral health does not only encompass teeth. He underlined the importance of recognizing the integration between oral and systemic health and the profound mutual impact one has on the other, stating that one cannot

A. Acharya (✉)
Center for Oral and Systemic Health, Marshfield Clinic Research Institute, Marshfield, WI, USA
e-mail: acharya.amit@marshfieldresearch.org

S.-M. R. Y. Geist
University of Detroit Mercy, Detroit, MI, USA
e-mail: geistsh@udmercy.edu

V. Powell
Robert Morris University, Moon Township, PA, USA
e-mail: powell@rmu.edu

M. H. Torres-Urquidy
Centers for Disease Control and Prevention, Atlanta, GA, USA
e-mail: miguel@forwardthinkingconcepts.org

A. Acharya et al. (eds.), *Integration of Medical and Dental Care and Patient Data*, Health Informatics, https://doi.org/10.1007/978-3-319-98298-4_3

have systemic health in the absence of oral health. To emphasize this point, he summarized the existing evidence that points to important links between oral disease, such as periodontal disease, and systemic diseases such as diabetes, heart disease, and stroke, and respiratory health and fetal health (miscarriage and stillbirth). The Surgeon General further exposed the access disparity to dental health care encountered by disparity-prone populations including low income individuals, those with no insurance, children, the elderly, handicapped, and institutionalized patients who experience what he dubbed the "silent epidemic" when referencing the high rate of oral disease prevalent among these populations.

The report revealed a struggling, stagnated, dental industry experiencing workforce shortages which exacerbated the problem by denying access to vulnerable populations without the ability to pay for services. His report revealed how, in addition to the systemic ramifications of poor oral health, far-reaching consequences were inflicted on those with limited or no access, including high social and economic cost to the individual, negative impact on quality of life and the burden this also placed on society. Importantly, the Surgeon General emphasized that this trend was reversible and preventable and pointed to the importance of bringing education and research to bear on the problem as actionable ways to advance oral-systemic health. Dr. Satcher called for further investigations into oral-systemic health connections, health disparity research, community based, public health, and behavioral health initiatives, health services research, and an expansion in diagnostic and treatment options which would emphasize proactive disease prevention. His report emphasized that for three decades, improvements in oral health had been a focus area of the U.S. Department of Health and Human Services's Healthy People initiative and that solving the problem would require a concerted effort between the health care industry, including professionals and health care entities, academia, the government, health insurers, and patients. Notably, 18 years later, oral health remains a priority focus in Healthy People 2020, with many objectives remaining to be achieved (Koh 2010).

A chasm currently persists between our perceptions, financing, and most importantly the delivery of oral health services and general medical services. Currently, proportionately fewer individuals annually access oral health services than medical services. The oral health service record for some of our most vulnerable citizens remains abysmal. The elderly, among whom chronic diseases are more prevalent, have the lowest rate of dental insurance coverage of any age group. Poor children on Medicaid/CHIP have public dental insurance, but low reimbursement rates and other problems have left most without annual oral health services.

This chapter serves as the introductory piece to the *Oral and Systemic Connection* section of the book which constitutes Chaps. 4–10. The following chapters will expand on the ideas presented in this chapter and discuss in depth the biological, epidemiological, informatics, technical, and clinical considerations for some of the important diseases that impact patients. The following sections provide an overview of the relationship between various oral and systemic health and disease, clinical practice considerations, and present a list of contact points between oral and systemic conditions.

3.2 Oral-Systemic Connections and Clinical Practice Considerations

The link between oral health and systemic health cannot be denied. The separation of dental and medical is no longer defensible or sustainable in modern healthcare. An efficient interdisciplinary communication model is required. However, an interdisciplinary agreement on the nature of such communication does not exist. When a periodontist receives a patient referred by a general dentist, it is clear what information should be sent to the referring dental provider. In many instances that same information is not meaningful or useful to a referring primary care physician or endocrinologist providing care for a patient with diabetes. A collaborative medical-dental approach to care would also lead to reciprocal best practice concepts for screening, such as the opportunities for dental providers to screen for eating disorders or oral cancer or for medical providers to screen for oral health as suggested by a number of sources. Providers in both silos sharing care of patients will benefit from accurate information on medications prescribed in the other silo (blood thinners, antibiotics, pain medications) and on tests ordered in one of the silos. The reader will be introduced to the case for integration, as well as some supporting evidence and clinical considerations, in the following sub sections.

3.2.1 Diabetes Mellitus

Diabetes mellitus (DM), along with its complications, is one of the most complex and difficult diseases for healthcare professionals to manage worldwide. Over the last decade, there has been a rapid rise in the incidence and prevalence of DM due to global changes in lifestyle. It was projected that by 2030, there will be an estimated 366 million patients with diabetes in the world. In the United States, currently at least 25.8 million children and adults—8.3% of the population—have diabetes. Among them, 18.8 million are diagnosed and 7.0 million are undiagnosed (American Diabetes Association 2011a).

Managing complications of diabetes such as heart disease and stroke, hypertension, retinopathy, chronic kidney disease, neuropathy, and lower-limb amputations demands a high expenditure of healthcare resources. The total cost of diabetes in the United States in 2007 was estimated at $218 billion. The cost of diagnosed diabetes care are estimated at $174 billion. The cost of undiagnosed diabetes, pre-diabetes, and gestational diabetes amount to an additional $44 billion (American Diabetes Association 2011b). Early diagnosis and treatment of diabetes will prevent or reduce complications and can save tremendous health care costs and improve quality of life. Dental records reporting periodontal disease hold promise for the diagnosis of diabetes. The association of diabetes and periodontal disease has been well established; diabetic individuals have a high prevalence of periodontitis. Many patients with severe periodontitis have been referred for diabetes evaluation and subsequently diagnosed with diabetes. Recently it was found that periodontitis could be an independent predictor for diabetes incidence. Physicians will find the benefit of patients' dental records of periodontitis and its progression helpful in diagnosing diabetes and monitoring the progression of the disease (Demmer et al. 2008; Choi et al. 2011).

3.2.2 *Xerostomia, Candidiasis, and Frequent Dental Infections*

Xerostomia, candidiasis, and frequent dental infections are common in patients with poorly controlled diabetes (Soysa et al. 2006; Borges et al. 2010; Khovidhunkit et al. 2009; Ueta et al. 1993). Records of these conditions can also be helpful in diagnosing diabetes as well as providing physicians with a picture of the patient's DM status.

There are indications that collaborative and coordinated dental care can reduce the expenditures in health care resources for diabetes. Due to immunity impairment, diabetes patients have a higher risk for infection and infection complications; timely elimination of the chronic odontogenic infections can prevent costly severe head and neck infection and even septicemia (Calvet and Yoshikawa 2001; Rajagopalan 2005; Huang et al. 2005; Rao et al. 2010). Evidence has shown, although with some controversy, that periodontal treatment improves glycemic control in diabetes (Taylor and Borgnakke 2008; Taylor 2003; Grossi 2001; Jones et al. 2007; Janket et al. 2005). Research on periodontal disease and increased risk for CVD in diabetes yields interesting results that periodontal bacteria are associated with coronary disease (Desvarieux et al. 2005; Janket et al. 2008). Although the direct cause and effect relationship is not yet fully established, such research has raised general awareness of the importance of oral health. Many dental offices monitor the A1c levels of diabetic patients, provide glucose checks, and a tobacco cessation program to collaborate and coordinate diabetic patients' healthcare. These provisions have shown a positive result (Geist et al. 2011).

3.2.3 *Chronic Kidney Disease*

Chronic kidney disease (CKD) is a major burden to the healthcare system. CKD is an irreversible and progressive disease for which diabetes and hypertension are major risk factors. There are 26 million people in the United States with this disease. CKD usually progresses to kidney failure (usually called end stage renal disease or ESRD). Once patients reach this stage, they need costly renal replacement therapy, either dialysis or a kidney transplant. Since 1972, the Medicare national insurance program for ESRD has paid 80% of the cost of renal replacement therapy including dialysis and transplantation for approximately 90% of patients in the United States (National Kidney Foundation 2002, 2009). It is reported by the National Institute of Diabetes and Digestive and Kidney Disease that the Medicare spending for patients with CKDs and age group 65 and older exceeded $50 billion in 2013 (NIDDK 2018). There were 158,739 US patients living with a functioning kidney transplant in 2007.

Every healthcare effort should be made to reduce mortality and morbidity due to kidney failure, improve the quality of life of patients, and reduce the attendant healthcare expenditures. Oral health care providers and nephrologists are encouraged to communicate often to provide good oral health and to reduce dental infection and its complications. Patients should have a coordinated oral health care program before and after kidney transplant to prevent dental infection and immunosuppressant-induced oral health problems (National Institute of Dental and Craniofacial Research 2011).

3.2.4 *HIV Infection and AIDS (HIV/AIDS)*

HIV/AIDS is another global epidemic. By the end of 2007, there were 33 million people in the world living with HIV infection (CDC 2011). In the United States, CDC estimates that more than one million people are living with HIV (Centers for Disease Control and Prevention 2010a). The cost of lifetime medical care for HIV infected individuals each year is estimated to be $20 billion (Centers for Disease Control and Prevention 2010b).

No other systemic diseases have as high an impact on oral health as HIV/AIDS. Early on in this epidemic, many studies demonstrated a wide variety of oral lesions in individuals with HIV/AIDS. These lesions, from infections to neoplasms, are common; studies have shown that about 40–50% of HIV positive persons have oral fungal, bacterial, or viral infections, often occurring early in the course of the disease (Petersen 2005). Manifestations of these infections have been used in diagnosing HIV infection and subsequent disease progression to AIDS (Greenspan and Greenspan 1987; van der Waal et al. 1991; Coogan et al. 2005). The presence of oral candidiasis, oral hairy leukoplakia, or Kaposi sarcoma strongly suggest HIV infection. After the inception of highly active anti-retroviral therapy (HAART), these oral lesions often change in frequency and severity to a certain degree; however, they are still valuable in monitoring the disease process and treatment response, especially in circumstances where viral load or CD4 counts are not easily or frequently accessible (Ramírez-Amador et al. 2007; Hodgson et al. 2006). With HAART, many oral lesions related to the HAART medications' adverse effects can affect patients' quality of life (Hodgson et al. 2006) and need to be treated collaboratively with physicians and other healthcare providers. In summary, dentists' knowledge of oral lesions and the advantages of the accessibility of oral manifestations in dental care can contribute valuable information in early disease diagnosis, progression, and/or treatment response, to the physicians who care for persons with HIV infection.

3.2.5 *Hemophilia*

It is estimated that 20,000 people in the United States have hemophilia. It is a rare disease, but its treatments are expensive and demand extensive coordination. Individuals with hemophilia are encouraged to enroll in the federal government sponsored hemophilia treatment centers (HTCs). More than 100 federally funded HTCs are located throughout the United States. Many HTCs are located at major university medical and research centers so all the treatment that a patient needs will be coordinated easily to increase effectiveness, and to reduce complications and costs. The hemophilia teams at these centers include nurse coordinators, hematologists (adult or pediatric), social workers, physical therapists, orthopedists, dentists, and nutritionists. A CDC study showed that people who used an HTC were 40% less likely to die of a hemophilia-related complication compared to those who did not receive care at a treatment center. It also demonstrated that people who used a treatment center were 40% less likely to be hospitalized for bleeding complications (Centers for Disease Control and Prevention 2017). Individuals with hemophilia are encouraged to maintain optimal oral health. Their oral health records are an important source of information for coordinated care, especially for surgical dental procedures such as wisdom teeth extractions. Recent recommendations specify that only a hematologist may prescribe factor concentrates to avoid complications, minimize costs, and optimize the treatment outcome.

3.2.6 Autoimmune Diseases

The NIH estimates that up to 23.5 million Americans have an autoimmune disease (AD). Depending on the classification system, there are 80–100 different autoimmune diseases. Many of them affect multiple organs and different parts of the body (systemic autoimmune diseases), giving affected individuals a variety of symptoms and signs (NIH National Institute of Allergy and Infectious Diseases 2005). This problem makes diagnosis difficult, particularly, when an individual affected by different autoimmune diseases exhibits an overlapping array of symptoms and signs. The most common systemic autoimmune disorders are systemic lupus erythematosus (SLE), rheumatoid arthritis, and Sjögren syndrome, and most of the time they occur in the same individual. Diagnosis and treatment can be challenging and require a multidisciplinary approach. These diseases often have oral manifestations in the early stage and many times the oral lesions provide important clues in establishing early diagnosis.

3.2.7 Sjögren Syndrome

Sjögren syndrome (SS) is one of the most common systemic autoimmune diseases. It can cause dysfunction of the exocrine glands and of other organs such as the kidneys, gastrointestinal system, blood vessels, lungs, liver, pancreas, and the central nervous system. The characteristic symptoms are dry mouth and dry eyes due to the reduction of flow from the salivary and lachrymal glands, but patients may also experience extreme fatigue and joint pain and have a 20 times higher risk of developing lymphoma compared to the general population (Zintzaras et al. 2005). Currently it is estimated that four million Americans are affected by this debilitating disease (Sjögren's Syndrome Foundation 2018). Of these, about 50% exhibit primary Sjögren syndrome. The other 50% of cases are secondary Sjögren syndrome, which involves the presence of other systemic autoimmune disorders such as rheumatoid arthritis, lupus, or scleroderma. Diagnosis of Sjögren syndrome can be challenging. The average time between first symptoms and diagnosis is 10 years, while patients are already suffering from physical, psychological, and social disabilities.

The early sign of dry mouth may not be perceived by the affected individuals because it takes 40–50% of salivary function loss to feel dry (Dawes 1987). However, the oral manifestations, mainly oral candidiasis and dental decay at the root surface and incisal edge, serve as signs of oral dryness. Some individuals may experience frequent oral traumatic ulcers due to lack of lubrication of food. These clinical signs along with easy access for a lower lip minor salivary gland biopsy may contribute valuable information in establishing a diagnosis in an early stage.

3.2.8 Systemic Lupus Erythematous (SLE)

SLE is another common systemic autoimmune disorder. SLE affects many organs and systems in the body, producing widely variable symptoms. Oral lesions occur in about 40% of the patients, and include involvement in Sjögren syndrome. SLE can appear as thinning and redness of the oral mucosa (erythema) with ulcers and white radiating lines at the border of the areas of redness. This observation is called lichenoid mucositis and assists in establishing the diagnosis.

3.2.9 Cancer

Coordination and collaborative care is crucial before, during, and after cancer therapy. It is especially important in chemotherapy and radiation therapy. Most chemotherapeutic agents used in cancer treatment interrupt cell metabolism, inhibit cell division, and cause biological cell death of rapidly proliferating cancer cells. They also kill normal cells that divide frequently, such as bone marrow cells, mucosal cells in the digestive tract (including the oral cavity), and hair follicle cells. These result in the most common side effects of chemotherapy: bone marrow suppression, immunosuppression, mucositis, and hair loss. Mucositis and increased risk for infection due to immunosuppression are major concerns. Although these side effects are mainly reversible, when they happen during therapy they can be too severe for the therapy to continue. They may delay or interrupt cancer therapy and decrease its effectiveness. For example, latent dental infection can become active due to immunosuppression, resulting in severe and sometimes lethal head and neck infections such as Ludwig angina. Before patients start chemotherapy, it is essential that they have a comprehensive oral examination. All infection sources must be removed to prevent inter-treatment dental infections.

For patients diagnosed with leukemia or lymphoma, pre-chemotherapy tooth extraction may be prohibitive due to the myelosuppression and immunosuppression of the disease itself. However, palliative measures can be taken to reduce or avoid chemotherapy complications.

Advanced medical technology has recently made hematologic stem cell transplant (HCT)—once the last resort treatment of blood cell malignancies such as leukemia and many solid tumors—a widely used and potentially curative procedure. This new procedure, in addition to traditional bone marrow transplant (BMT), has made oral health care a vital part of HCT management before, during, and after the course of therapy. Pre- and post-transplant immunosuppressant treatment may cause short-term or long-term oral complications. These complications include mucositis, infections, oral bleeding, graft-versus-host disease, salivary changes and dry mouth, taste alterations, secondary malignancies in the oral cavity, and jaw bone necrosis. Vigilant oral care can reduce mortality and morbidity, increase the success rate of engraftment and improve the quality of life of the recipients (Epstein et al. 2009).

3.2.10 Chronic Graft-Versus-Host Disease (cGVHD)

HCT, BMT, and kidney and other organ transplant recipients are expected to have degrees of graft-versus-host disease (GVHD) in the months to years following the transplant. GVHD is a condition in which alloreactive donor T-cells recognize host tissue antigens as foreign and mount an immune response against the host tissue similar to systemic autoimmune diseases. Acute GVHD is usually managed by the transplant team while the patient is still in the medical center. However, more than 50% of patients develop chronic GVHD, which usually appears within 6–12 months of transplantation. Oral manifestations may be the initial or only signs of this reaction. Dental records of these oral lesions, which can be ulcerative or erythematous, and can include reticular lichenoid mucositis and frequent mucocele formation, can help in the diagnosis of cGVHD in the community health care setting. Patients may quickly be referred back to the original medical center if necessary.

3.2.11 Bisphosphonate-Associated Osteonecrosis

Since 2003, a new disease entity, bisphosphonate-associated osteonecrosis (BON), has emerged in cancer patients who have received intravenous nitrogen-containing bisphosphonates (Geist et al. 2005). This form of bisphosphonate has been used in treating bone cancer such as multiple myeloma and solid tumors that are known to metastasize to bone such as prostate cancer, breast cancer, and lung cancer. It is used to reduce or prevent skeletal events. The disease mechanism is not fully understood, but current evidence indicates that BON almost exclusively involves the jawbone and is most prevalent in patients who have received intravenous nitrogen-containing bisphosphonates such as pamidronate and zoledronic acid for cancer therapy. In most cases, necrosis of the jawbones appeared after dental surgical procedures such as tooth extractions. Patients with a history of intravenous nitrogen-containing bisphosphonate therapy are advised to avoid invasive dental procedures, and oral healthcare providers are warned to take precautions in treating such patients. The oral healthcare community urges oncologists to refer patients for oral health care before initiating IV bisphosphonate use to avoid future surgical dental procedures that may increase the risk of bisphosphonate-associated jawbone necrosis (Migliorati et al. 2011).

3.2.12 Head and Neck Cancer

Oral healthcare providers have a long history of collaboration with surgeons, oncologists, otolaryngologists, and other specialists in managing head and neck cancer patients. This is probably due to the common treatment area of the oral cavity. It is probably more so in Taiwan, where there is a high prevalence of nasopharyngeal carcinoma (NPC). NPC is a common form of head and neck cancer among Southern Chinese and the treatment is almost exclusively high dose external irradiation with a minimal dosage of 65 Gy. In order to encourage compliance, increase the survival rate, and improve the quality of life of the survivors, complications of radiation therapy must be managed collaboratively among the radiation oncologist, ENT specialists, dentists, dental specialists, and other health professionals. In the early 1970s, tumor boards were established in major hospitals where NPC and other head and neck cancer patients were treated. It was in these tumor board conferences that the involved specialists contributed their expertise to help define the treatment plan for individual patients and resolve issues of complications. Because of the involvement of oral healthcare providers and ENT specialists, the most severe complication of radiation therapy, osteoradionecrosis, has been greatly reduced (Hahn 1983; Geist and Chen 1993; Chen et al. 2000). Today, oral health care of head and neck cancer patients before, during, and after radiation therapy has become the standard of care for head and neck cancer treatment worldwide (Vissink et al. 2003; National Cancer Institute 2011).

Due to the complexity of cancer patient management and the multidisciplinary care involved, a teamwork approach should be adopted in every health care system where any type of cancer patient is treated. Oral health care providers should be included in the team. Some hospitals do not have an oral health care component for their cancer management team. This omission can be detrimental to their patients' overall health during cancer therapy. Hospitals should be encouraged to maintain if not expand oral health care to incorporate emerging techniques and medicine to improve the outcome of cancer treatment (Parzuchowski et al. 2011).

Before patients start radiation or chemotherapy, it is essential that they have a comprehensive oral examination. All infection sources must be removed to prevent inter- and post-treatment dental infections. These infections may delay or interrupt cancer therapy and decrease its effectiveness. Before IV bisphosphonate use, patients should have appropriate dental treatment to avoid future surgical dental procedures, which may increase the risk of bisphosphonate-associated jawbone necrosis.

3.2.13 Gardner Syndrome

Gardner syndrome is an inherited disease complex with multiple abnormalities that may involve the skin, retina, skeleton, and teeth. One of the components of the syndrome is familial colorectal polyposis. These polyps have a high rate of malignant transformation into invasive adenocarcinoma. Studies have shown that by age 30, about 50% of patients with Gardner syndrome will develop colorectal carcinoma. It is crucial to diagnose this syndrome in early life so preventive removal of the polyps can be done early. Multiple osteomas of the mandible and multiple supernumerary teeth are common findings. Dental records of these lesions can contribute to early diagnosis and prevent malignancy in patients with this syndrome.

3.2.14 Bardet-Biedl Syndrome

Bardet-Biedl syndrome (BBS) is a pleiotropic, autosomal recessive, genetic disorder with vast genetic heterogeneity (Forsythe et al. 2003). First described by Georges Louis Bardet and Artur Biedl in the early 1920s, BBS is characterized as a condition with a large array of clinical characteristics (Forsythe et al. 2003). Truncal obesity, impaired vision, chronic kidney disease, genitourinary abnormalities, and cognitive impairment pose significant and common problems in patients with BBS. Common extra-oral manifestations are orbital hypertelorism, strabismus, philtrum discrepancies, hypotonic upper lip mouth breathing, retrognathia, incompetent lips, and bitemporal narrowing (Moore et al. 2005; Drugowick et al. 2007; Majumdar et al. 2012; Ferreira do Amaral et al. 2014; Hassona et al. 2017). The intra-oral manifestations reported to date include hypodontia, predominantly with absent maxillary and mandibular premolars, followed by lower lateral incisors, high-arched palate, microdontia, crowding and spacing problems, short dental roots in both anterior and posterior teeth with obliterated pulp chambers (Urben and Baugh 1999; Moore et al. 2005; Drugowick et al. 2007; Majumdar et al. 2012; Andersson et al. 2013; Ferreira do Amaral et al. 2014; Hassona et al. 2017). Being a rare disease, it is very important to have a comprehensive understanding of dental anomalies associated with BBS. This will inform proper dental treatment planning and providing supportive oral care for affected patients, which is most often complicated by co-existing renal, cardiac, metabolic, and developmental abnormalities.

3.3 Contact Points Between Medical and Dental Care and Research

This section presents a pertinent list of contact points [C-1 to C-36] in a tabular form (Table 3.1) between individual oral-systemic categories of diseases and conditions where medical-dental collaboration is valuable for patient care or research.

Table 3.1 Contact Points C-1–C-36 (Medical-Dental Care and Research)

Contact Point #	Contact Points
C-1	Diabetes, Metabolic Syndrome—Periodontal Diseases
C-2	[C] Cardiovascular Disease, [H] Heart Disease, [S] Stroke—Gingivitis and Periodontal Diseases
C-3	Oncology—[C] Cancer; [O] Oral Cancer Screening, Oral Premalignant Lesions, Oral Cancer Care; [T] Tobacco/Betel Use Screening and Cessation (Risk Factor for Oral Cancer)
C-4	[R] Respiratory diseases ([A] Asthma, [P] Pneumonia, [C] COPD)—Periodontal Diseases
C-5	Chronic Kidney Disease (CKD); End Stage Renal Disease (ESRD)—Periodontal Diseases; Oral Manifestations of Renal Disease, Dialysis
C-6	Organ Failure Patients and Transplant Candidates—Oral Health Care
C-7	Blood Disorders, Iatrogenic or Otherwise: von Willebrand disease, Neutropenia, Polycythemia, Aplastic Anemia, Sickle Cell Anemia, Hemophilia
C-8	Stomatognathic System and Body Posture
C-9	Hypertension
C-10	Dermatological Diseases
C-11	Archaeal Role in Disease
C-12	Bacterial Diseases
C-13	Fungal Diseases
C-14	Viral Diseases
C-15	Oral Health—Stillbirth, Low Birth Weight (LBW), Prenatal Care [Disputed]
C-16	Mental Health—Eating Disorder Screening
C-17	Oral Health and Mental Health
C-18	Dementia, Alzheimer's Disease
C-19	Immunology—Sjögren's Syndrome and Xerostomia—Dental Screening
C-20	Rheumatoid Arthritis (xerostomia)
C-21	Rheumatology—Ankylosing spondylitis and Periodontal Disease
C-22	Bisphosphonate Osteonecrosis ([B] BON) and Osteoradionecrosis ([R] ORN, Post-radiation osteonecrosis)
C-23	Periodontal Diseases and Bone Diseases (Osteoporosis, Osteopenia)
C-24	Obstructive Sleep Apnea—Anterior Mandibular Positioning (AMP) Devices
C-25	Manifestations of thyroid disease, HPT
C-26	Special Populations, Children
C-27	Special Populations, MR/DD (ND/ID)
C-28	Special Populations, Geriatric Care
C-29	Congenital Conditions, CL/CP, Hutchinson's Teeth, Macroglossia
C-30	HIV/AIDS—Dental Screening
C-31	Ectodermal Dysplasia and Severe Hypodontia
C-32	Reducing Disparities in Healthcare (Including Dental Care)
C-33	Periodontal Diseases—Systemic Inflammation [Research]
C-34	Biofilms: Cystic Fibrosis, Endocarditis, Cystitis, Dental Plaque, Indwelling Devices and Implants. [Research]
C-35	Anesthesia, Sedation
C-36	Oral and Craniofacial Anomalies, Bardet-Biedl Syndrome [BBS]

3.4 Conclusion

In closing, we would like to refer to what is a good example of how integration in the future will help transform care. On 8 April 2017 the Washington Post reported on a case that highlighted the need for this endeavor. The piece entitled, "The awful sores in her mouth were a symptom of something very serious" by Sandra G. Boodman described the case of a 52-year-old woman suffering from a combination of oral and systemic symptoms that had puzzled both dental and medical specialists. Over the course of almost a year, the patient experienced weight loss, thrush (*Candida fungus*), unresponsive to treatment with oral rinses, and had seen several healthcare providers. She later reported nosebleeds and developed stones in the salivary gland. Earlier she was offered a range of treatments including antidepressants and was treated with penicillin. After not reaching conclusive resolution to her condition, she continued visiting providers and different diagnoses were offered such as *Lichen planus*. By then, however, she started developing blisters on her chest. Finally, an oral medicine specialist suggested what ultimately would be the final diagnosis: *Pemphigus vulgaris*, a rare autoimmune condition. It is in these situations where the integration of dental and medical care can translate to direct benefits, for patients, payers, and society at large.

Disclaimer The views presented in this chapter are solely of the author/s and do not necessarily represent the views of the US Government, Department of Health and Human Services and/or the Centers for Disease Control and Prevention.

References

American Diabetes Association. Standards of medical care in diabetes – 2011. Diabetes Care. 2011a;34(Suppl 1):S11–61.

American Diabetes Association. Cost of diabetes, diabetes statistics. 2011b. http://www.diabetes.org/diabetes-basics/diabetes-statistics/. Accessed 10 June 2018.

Andersson EM, Axelsson S, Gjølstad LF, Storhaug K. Taurodontism: a minor diagnostic criterion in Laurence-Moon/Bardet-Biedl syndromes. Acta Odontol Scand. 2013;71(6):1671–4.

Borges BC, Fulco GM, Souza AJ, de Lima KC. Xerostomia and hyposalivation: a preliminary report of their prevalence and associated factors in Brazilian elderly diabetic patients. Oral Health Prev Dent. 2010;8(2):153–8.

Calvet HM, Yoshikawa TT. Infections in diabetes. Infect Dis Clin North Am. 2001;15(2):407–21, viii. Review.

CDC. HIV Global. Gateway to Health Communication. CDC. 2011. https://www.cdc.gov/healthcommunication/toolstemplates/entertainmented/tips/HivGlobal.html. Accessed 30 Aug 2018.

CDC. Hemophilia Treatment Centers (HTCs). Hemophilia. NCBDDD. CDC. 2017. https://www.cdc.gov/ncbddd/hemophilia/HTC.html. Accessed 30 Aug 2018.

Centers for Disease Control and Prevention. HIV in the United States, CDC fact sheet. 2010a. http://www.cdc.gov/hiv/resources/factsheets/us.htm. Accessed 18 June 2011.

Centers for Disease Control and Prevention. Projecting possible future courses of the HIV epidemic in the United States. 2010b. http://www.cdc.gov/hiv/resources/factsheets/us-epi-future-courses.htm. Accessed 18 June 2011.

Chen YP, Tsang NM, Tseng CK, Lin SY. Causes of interruption of radiotherapy in nasopharyngeal carcinoma patients in Taiwan. Jpn J Clin Oncol. 2000;30(5):230–4.

Choi YH, McKeown RE, Mayer-Davis EJ, et al. Association between periodontitis and impaired fasting glucose and diabetes. Diabetes Care. 2011;34(2):381–6.

Coogan MM, Greenspan J, Challacombe SJ. Oral lesions in infection with human immunodeficiency virus. Bull World Health Organ. 2005;83(9):700–6. Epub 2005 Sep 30.

Dawes C. Physiological factors affecting salivary flow rate, oral sugar clearance, and the sensation of dry mouth in man. J Dent Res. 1987;66 Spec No:648–53.

Demmer RT, Jacobs DR Jr, Desvarieux M. Periodontal disease and incident type 2 diabetes: results from the first national health and nutrition examination survey and its epidemiologic follow-up study. Diabetes Care. 2008;31(7):1373–9.

Desvarieux M, Demmer RT, Rundek T, et al. Periodontal microbiota and carotid intima-media thickness: the oral infections and vascular disease epidemiology study (INVEST). Circulation. 2005;111(5):576–82.

Drugowick RM, Da Rós Gonçalves L, Barrôso AS, Feres-Filho EJ, Maia LC. Treatment of gingival overgrowth in a child with Bardet-Biedl syndrome. J Periodontol. 2007;78(6):1159–63.

Epstein JB, Raber-Drulacher JE, Wilkins A, Chavarria MG, Myint H. Advances in hematologic stem cell transplant: an update for oral health care providers. Oral Surg Oral Med Oral Pathol Oral Radiol Endod. 2009;107(3):301–12.

Ferreira do Amaral CO, Logar Gde A, Parisi AG, Takahashi K, Straioto FG. General and stomatologic aspects of Bardet-Biedl syndrome. J Craniofac Surg. 2014;25(6):e575–8.

Forsythe E, Beales PL, Ross AJ, Waters MA. Bardet-Biedl Syndrome. In: Pagon RA, Adam MP, Ardinger HH, et al., editors. GeneReviews®. Seattle, WA: University of Washington; 2003.

Geist JR, Chen FH. Nasopharyngeal carcinoma. Computed tomographic imaging of four cases. Oral Surg Oral Med Oral Pathol. 1993;75(6):759–66.

Geist RY, Geist JR, Jaw AM. Osteonecrosis related to bisphosphonates: a new concern for dentistry. J Mich Dent Assoc. 2005;87(11):40–2.

Geist SR, Geist JR, Sordyl CM, LeBow J. Benefits of casual random blood glucose assessment of diabetic dental patients in an urban dental school clinic. J Dent Educ. 2011;75:212–3.

Greenspan D, Greenspan JS. Oral mucosal manifestations of AIDS? Dermatol Clin. 1987;5(4):733–7.

Grossi SG. Treatment of periodontal disease and control of diabetes: an assessment of the evidence and need for future research. Ann Periodontol. 2001;6(1):138–45. Review.

Hahn LJ. Osteoradionecrosis of the mandible: clinical observation and treatment in 45 cases. Taiwan Yi Xue Hui Za Zhi. 1983;82(3):451–60.

Hassona Y, Kasabreh N, Hammoudeh H, Scully C. Oral healthcare management in Bardet Biedl syndrome. Spec Care Dentist. 2017;37(1):47–50.

Hodgson TA, Greenspan D, Greenspan JS. Oral lesions of HIV disease and HAART in industrialized countries. Adv Dent Res. 2006;19:57–62.

Huang TT, Ttseng FY, Liu TC, et al. Deep neck infection in diabetic patients: comparison of clinical picture and outcomes with nondiabetic patients. Otolaryngol Head Neck Surg. 2005;132(6):943–7.

Janket SJ, Wightman A, Baird AE, et al. Does periodontal treatment improve glycemic control in diabetic patients? A meta-analysis of intervention studies. J Dent Res. 2005;84(12):1154–9.

Janket S-J, Jones JA, Meurman JH, Baird AE, Van Dyke TE. Oral infection, hyperglycemia, and endothelial dysfunction. Oral Surg Oral Med Oral Pathol Oral Radiol Endod. 2008;105(2): 173–9. https://doi.org/10.1016/j.tripleo.2007.06.027

Jones JA, Miller DR, Wehler CJ, et al. Does periodontal care improve glycemic control? The department of veterans affairs dental diabetes study. J Clin Periodontol. 2007;34(1):46–52. Epub 2006 Nov 24.

Khovidhunkit SO, Suwantuntula T, Thaweboon S, et al. Xerostomia, hyposalivation, and oral microbiota in type 2 diabetic patients: a preliminary study. J Med Assoc Thai. 2009;92(9):1220–8.

Koh H. A 2020 vision for Healthy People. N Engl J Med. 2010;362:1653–6.

Majumdar U, Arya G, Singh S, Pillai A, Nair PP. Oro-dental findings in Bardet-Biedl syndrome. BMJ Case Rep. 2012. pii: bcr1220115320; https://doi.org/10.1136/bcr.12.2011.5320.

Migliorati CA, Epstein JB, Abt E, Berenson JR. Osteonecrosis of the jaw and bisphosphonates in cancer: a narrative review. Nat Rev Endocrinol. 2011;7(1):34–42. Epub 2010.

Moore SJ, Green JS, Fan Y, Bhogal AK, Dicks E, Fernandez BA, Stefanelli M, Murphy C, Cramer BC, Dean JC, Beales PL, et al. Clinical and genetic epidemiology of Bardet-Biedl syndrome in Newfoundland: a 22-year prospective, population-based, cohort study. Am J Med Genet A. 2005;132A(4):352–60.

National Cancer Institute. PDQ® oral complications of chemotherapy and head/neck radiation. Bethesda: National Cancer Institute; 2011. http://cancer.gov/cancertopics/pdq/supportivecare/oralcomplications/HealthProfessional. Accessed 8 May 2011.

National Institute of Dental and Craniofacial Research. Dental management of the organ transplant patient. NIH Publication No 11-6270. 2011. http://www.nidcr.nih.gov/OralHealth/Topics/OrganTransplantationOralHealth/OrganTransplantProf.htm. Accessed 18 June 2011.

National Kidney Foundation. KDOQI clinical practice guidelines for chronic kidney disease: evaluation, classification, and stratification Part 3. Chronic kidney disease as a public health problem. Am J Kidney Dis. 2002;39(2 Suppl 1):S1–266.

National Kidney Foundation. Insurance choice for medicare ESRD patients. 2009. https://www.kidney.org/sites/default/files/docs/insurance_choice_medicare_esrd-msp_new.pdf. Accessed 10 June 2018.

NIDDK, National Institute of Diabetes and Digestive and Kidney Diseases. Kidney Disease Statistics for the United States. NIDDK. 2018. https://www.niddk.nih.gov/health-information/health-statistics/kidney-disease. Accessed 30 Aug 2018.

NIH National Institute of Allergy and Infectious Diseases. The autoimmune diseases coordination. Committee Rep Congr: Prog Autoimmune Dis Res. 2005. https://www.niaid.nih.gov/sites/default/files/adccfinal.pdf. Accessed 10 June 2018.

Parzuchowski JS, Jordon J, Burgess L, et al. Lead-time from diagnosis to start of radiation shortened by 44% for head and neck cancer when patients go through a multidisciplinary clinic. J Clin Oncol. ASCO Annual Meeting Proceedings (Post-Meeting Edition) 2011;29(15_suppl) (May 20):e16627. Accessed 18 June 2011.

Petersen P, Bourgeois D, Ogawa H, Estupinan-Day S, Ndiaye C. The global burden of oral diseases and risks to oral health. Policy and Practice. Bull World Health Organ. 2005. http://www.who.int/bulletin/volumes/83/9/661.pdf.

Rajagopalan S. Serious infections in elderly patients with diabetes mellitus. Clin Infect Dis. 2005;40(7):990–6. Epub 2005 Feb 24. Review.

Ramírez-Amador V, Ponce-de-León S, Anaya-Saavedra G, Crabtree Ramírez B, Sierra-Madero J. Oral lesions as clinical markers of highly active antiretroviral therapy failure: a nested case–control study in Mexico city. Clin Infect Dis. 2007;45(7):925–32. Epub 2007 Aug 23.

Rao DD, Desai A, Kulkarni RD. Comparison of maxillofacial space infection in diabetic and non-diabetic patients. Oral Surg Oral Med Oral Pathol Oral Radiol Endod. 2010;110(4):e7–12. Epub 2010 Jul 24.

Satcher D. Oral Health in America: a report of the Surgeon General (executive summary) US Department of Health and Human Services. National Institute of Dental and Craniofacial Research, National Institutes of Health. 2000. http://www.nidcr.nih.gov/datastatistics/surgeon-general/report/executivesummary.htm. Accessed 18 June 2018.

Sjögren's Syndrome Foundation. A letter from your CEO: Sjögren's Awareness Month. 2018. https://www.sjogrens.org/news/492-a-letter-from-your-ceo-sjoegren-s-awareness-month. Accessed 10 June 2018.

Soysa NS, Samaranayake LP, Ellepola AN. Diabetes mellitus as a contributory factor in oral candidosis. Diabet Med. 2006;23(5):455–9.

Taylor GW. The effects of periodontal treatment on diabetes. J Am Dent Assoc. 2003;134:41S–8.

Taylor GW, Borgnakke WS. Periodontal disease: associations with diabetes, glycemic control and complications. Oral Dis. 2008;14(3):191–203. Review.

Ueta E, Osaki T, Yoneda K, et al. Prevalence of diabetes mellitus in odontogenic infections and oral candidiasis: an analysis of neutrophil suppression. J Oral Pathol Med. 1993;22(4):168–74.

Urben SL, Baugh RF. Otolaryngologic features of Laurence-Moon-Bardet-Biedl syndrome. Otolaryngol Head Neck Surg. 1999;120(4):571–4.

van der Waal I, Schulten EA, Pindborg JJ. Oral manifestations of AIDS: an overview. Int Dent J. 1991;41(1):3–8.

Vissink A, Burlage FR, Spijkervet FK, et al. Prevention and treatment of the consequences of head and neck radiotherapy. Crit Rev Oral Biol Med. 2003;14(3):213–25.

Zintzaras E, Voulgarelis M, Moutsopoulos HM, et al. The risk of lymphoma development in autoimmune diseases: a meta-analysis. Arch Intern Med. 2005;165(20):2337–44.

Chapter 4
Interdisciplinary Care Model: Diabetes and Oral Health

Neel Shimpi, Jordan L. Ashton, Cynthia A. Sorenson, Louay O. Danial, John O'Brien, William Melms, and Amit Acharya

4.1 Definition and Prevalence

Diabetes is a disease in which blood glucose (sugar) levels are elevated (American Diabetes Association 2009). The most common etiology of this metabolic disorder is either insulin deficiency, insulin resistance, or both. Insulin, a hormone that controls blood glucose levels, works by facilitating the absorption of glucose into body cells (NIDDK 2018; Röder et al. 2016; Wilcox 2005). In this chronic condition, glucose builds up in the blood instead of being absorbed by the cells in the body which increases the risk of developing complications for various diseases (American Diabetes Association 2018b; Cade 2008; Casqueiro et al. 2012; Huang et al. 2017). The National Diabetes Statistics Report of 2017 estimates the prevalence of diabetes and prediabetes in the United States (U.S) as 30.3 million and 84.1 million, respectively (Centers for Disease Control and Prevention 2017). Among the 30.3

N. Shimpi · A. Acharya (✉)
Center for Oral and Systemic Health, Marshfield Clinic Research Institute,
Marshfield, WI, USA
e-mail: shimpi.neel@marshfieldresearch.org; acharya.amit@marshfieldresearch.org

J. L. Ashton · C. A. Sorenson
Marshfield Clinic-Stettin Medical Center, Stettin, WI, USA
e-mail: ashton.jordan@marshfieldclinic.org; sorenson.cynthia@marshfieldclinic.org

L. O. Danial
Marshfield Clinic-Park Falls Medical Center, Park Falls, WI, USA
e-mail: danial.louay@marshfieldclinic.org

J. O'Brien
Family Health Center Inc., Marshfield, WI, USA
e-mail: john@marshfieldclinic.org

W. Melms
Marshfield Clinic-Minocqua Medical Center, Minocqua, WI, USA
e-mail: melms.william@marshfieldclinic.org

A. Acharya et al. (eds.), *Integration of Medical and Dental Care and Patient Data*,
Health Informatics, https://doi.org/10.1007/978-3-319-98298-4_4

million, 23.1 million were diagnosed clinically and 7.2 million were unaware of their diabetic status (American Diabetes Association 2018c). According to the report, diabetes was also considered as the seventh leading cause of mortality in US. Based on recent epidemiologic trends, it is projected that one in three American adults will suffer from diabetes by 2050 (Boyle et al. 2010).

4.2 Systemic Manifestations of Diabetes

Classic symptoms associated with diabetes include polyuria, polydipsia and polyphagia. Other systemic manifestations comprises of manifestations such as extreme fatigue, weight loss, blurry vision, delayed healing and tingling, pain or numbness in extremities (Steffes et al. 2003; World Health Organization 2014). Figure 4.1 illustrates the systemic manifestations of diabetes.

Uncontrolled diabetes could exacerbate the underlying inflammatory processes increasing the risk of developing acute or chronic complications (Steffes et al. 2003; Wu et al. 2014). The acute metabolic complications resulting in hyperglycemic emergencies include Diabetic Ketoacidosis (DKA) majority of times seen in patients with Type 1 diabetes, while Hyperosmolar hyperglycemic state (formerly known as Hyperosmolar hyperglycemic non-ketotic state (HONK)) is most of the times seen in patients with Type 2 diabetes and lactic acidosis (American Diabetes Association 2018a, b, c, d, e, f, g; Kitabchi et al. 2009). DKA is characterized by a triad of uncontrolled hyperglycemia, metabolic acidosis and increased total body ketone concentration while HHS shows characteristics signs like severe hyperglycemia, hyper osmolality and dehydration in the absence of significant ketoacidosis (American Diabetes Association 2018a, b, c, d, e, f, g). Lactic acidosis is often predisposed by conditions such as myocardial infarction with hypoxia or septic shock (Andersen et al. 2013). Acute complications also include hypoglycemia that follows when an imbalance occurs between insulin/hypoglycemic agent's intake and body's physiological needs (Shafiee et al. 2012). Chronic complications are divided into micro-vascular and macro-vascular components. Micro-vascular complications include nephropathy, neuropathy and retinopathy while macro-vascular complications include disorders of heart and blood vessels such as myocardial infarction and stroke (Mauri-Obradors et al. 2018).

4.3 Oral Manifestations

The exaggerated host response to the local microbial factors associated with uncontrolled diabetes can result in various inflammatory and soft tissue pathologies in oral cavities (Mauri-Obradors et al. 2018). Studies have shown that diabetes affects salivary glands leading to salivary dysfunction by reducing the secretory capacity of salivary glands (Lilliu et al. 2015; Mata et al. 2004). A case control study conducted in 70 diabetic patients, divided in to controlled and uncontrolled patients, showed

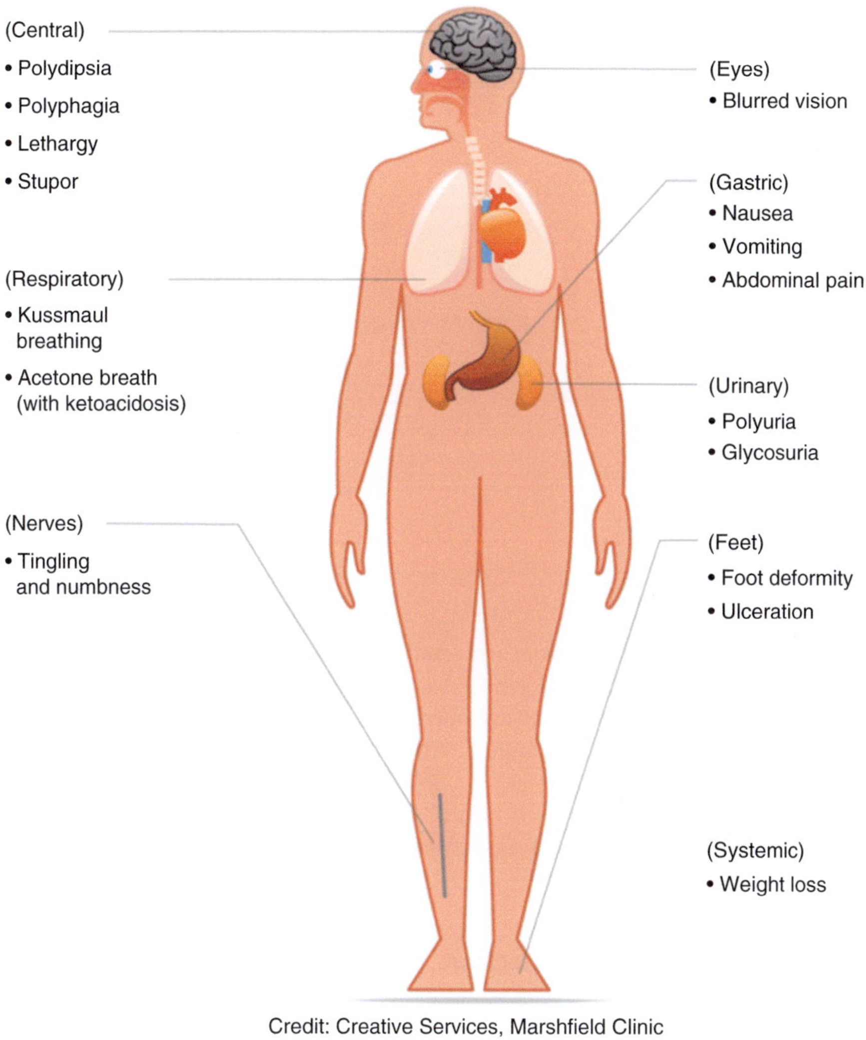

Fig. 4.1 Systemic manifestation of diabetes

parotid enlargement, hyposalivation, taste alterations and burning mouth syndrome were more common in uncontrolled patients as compared to controlled patients. It was also observed these patients frequently complain of candidiasis, herpes and proliferative lesions (Quirino et al. 1995). The concomitant manifestation of diabetes also includes fungal and bacterial infections, tooth loss and dental caries (Leite et al. 2013). Figure 4.2 shows the oral manifestations of diabetes.

Periodontitis has been identified as one of the most common oral manifestations of diabetes. Periodontitis is defined as the inflammation of the periodontium caused by a complex reaction initiated when subgingival plaque bacteria are in close contact with the epithelium of the gingival sulcus (Loesche 1996). Periodontitis is

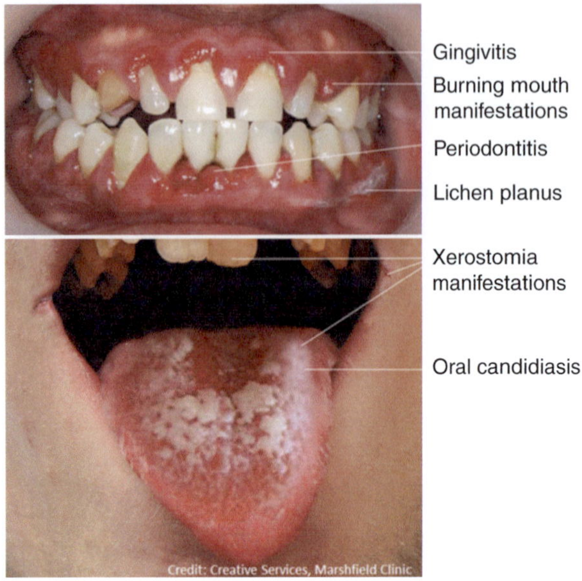

Fig. 4.2 Oral manifestations of diabetes

characterized by swollen gingivae, increased pocket depth, loss of alveolar bone and attachment loss with the apical movement of the junctional epithelium caused by the injury arising from toxins and enzymes produced by the bacteria and from host-mediated defense responses (Loesche 1996).

Recent estimates project about 64.7 million American adults suffer from mild, moderate or severe periodontitis (Eke et al. 2015). It was also reported that the prevalence rate increased to 64% for adults more than 65 years of age (Eke et al. 2015).

4.4 Oral-Systemic Connection

The relation between periodontal disease and diabetes has been recognized in the literature for many years (Bascones-Martínez et al. 2015; Borgnakke et al. 2013; Casanova et al. 2014; Mealey 2006; Preshaw et al. 2012). There is emerging evidence showing bi-directional relationship between diabetes and periodontal disease (Casanova et al. 2014; Eke et al. 2015; Mealey 2006). A review conducted on inter-relationships between diabetes and periodontal disease showed that glycemic control in Type 2 diabetic patients may be exacerbated by PD (Bascones-Martinez and Matesanz-Perez 2011; Chang and Lim 2012). The review explains two mechanisms of developing complications of diabetes. According to one mechanism, complications are caused by formation of sorbitol by action of aldose reductase on glucose while the other mechanism proposes production of advanced glycosylation end products (AGEs). AGEs are produced when glucose binds to proteins, lipids and nucleic acid. This binding of glucose to hemoglobin, collagen or albumin is deposited in organs resulting in alteration of their function. Although periodontal disease has a multifactorial etiology, it is widely accepted that it results from action of bacterial biofilm in the periodontium resulting in resistance to host defense mechanism.

Several mechanisms of interactions have been investigated for the correlation between diabetes and periodontal disease. The central feature of pathogenesis of PD and diabetes is elevated levels of inflammatory mediators. In case of poorly controlled diabetes; high levels of irreversibly AGEs are accumulated in the tissues including periodontium (Preshaw et al. 2012). These AGEs induce changes in extracellular matrix components and the microvascular integrity resulting in abnormal endothelial cell function, capillary growth and vessel proliferation. This change results in activation of pathways that increase inflammation, oxidative stress and apoptosis (Brownlee 2005). In response to the presence of inflammation, cells of periodontal and diabetic patients release cytoactive chemicals that result in destruction of connective tissue (Bascones-Martinez and Matesanz-Perez 2011).

The level of glycemic control is of key importance in determining increased risk. Studies have shown that chronic PD exacerbate insulin resistance and worsen glycemic control, while periodontal treatment that decreases inflammation may help diminish insulin resistance (Bascones-Martinez and Matesanz-Perez 2011; Borgnakke et al. 2013; Brownlee 2005). Patients with inflammatory PD often have elevated serum levels of proinflammatory cytokines. In patients with diabetes, hyper inflammatory immune cells can exacerbate the elevated production of proinflammatory cytokines. One of the study found out that periodontal treatment significantly reduced the Tumor Necrosis Factor alpha levels and also the mean HbA1c values from 8% to 7.1% (Allen et al. 2011). The study suggested that reduction in periodontal inflammation may help decrease the inflammatory mediators in the serum that are associated with insulin resistance thereby improving glycemic control (Brownlee 2005).

Many cross sectional and longitudinal epidemiologic studies have consistently found greater prevalence and incidence of PD in patients with Type 1 and Type 2 diabetes. One of the reports of the US National Health and Nutrition Examination Survey (NHANES) III showed that there was a higher prevalence of severe periodontitis with adult patient having HbA1C greater that 9% (Poretsky and Liao 2013). A longitudinal study carried out by the residents of the Gila River Indian Community identified that there was an association of poor glycemic control and periodontitis. The study also assessed the effect of periodontitis on developing nephropathy and they came up with the results that the incidence of developing nephropathy was more in patients with diabetes was greater than the non-diabetic patients (Shultis et al. 2007). One of the case control studies evaluated the level of oral disease in children and adolescent with diabetes in terms of PD and dental caries (Lalla and Papapanou 2011). The study suggested that diabetic children can start PD early in life and gradually increase in severity. With respect to dental caries, the study did not find any difference between the control and cases.

A meta-analysis based on 18 comparative cross sectional studies, 3 prospective cohort studies and 2 baseline clinical trials was conducted to assess the association between diabetes and PD (Khader et al. 2006). A literature search was performed from 1970 to 2003 that compared oral hygiene, gingival and periodontal status between diabetics and nondiabetics. After comparing the extent and severity of PD between diabetics and nondiabetics, the study demonstrated that diabetics had significantly worse oral hygiene status than nondiabetics (Khader et al. 2006).

Another meta-analysis carried out suggested that periodontal treatment leads to improvement of glycemic control in type 2 diabetic patients for at least 3 months (Engebretson and Kocher 2013). In this study, a literature search was done from 1960 to 2009 that included criteria such as original investigation done on human population with 3 or more than 3 months, intervention studies containing diabetic patients with periodontitis receiving periodontal treatment and diabetic patients with periodontitis receiving no treatment and outcomes related to metabolic control. The study showed that the effect of periodontal treatment reduced A1C levels in range of −1.9 to −0.14, while the untreated group showed a range of −0.8 to 0.31%.

Similarly, a systematic review was carried out to establish an effect of periodontal therapy on diabetes outcome (ICD10Data.com 2018). In this study the mean change of HbA1c from baseline was compared across treatment groups. The meta-analysis indicated that the mean treatment effect was −0.36% HbA1c as compared to no treatment. Due to small sample size and varied periodontal therapy, there was a limited confidence that periodontal therapy lowers the HbA1c index.

4.5 Diagnostic Codes

The range of diabetes diagnostic ICD9 Codes is from 250.00 to 250.93 comprising about 40 ICD 9 Codes. These include diabetes mellitus Type 1 or Type 2 with or without mention of complications. The complications include ketoacidosis, hyperosmolarity, coma, renal manifestations, ophthalmic manifestations, neurological complications, peripheral and circulatory disorders, other specified manifestations that includes diabetic hypoglycemia NOS, hypoglycemic shock NOS and unspecified complication. It is seen that oral complications of Diabetes are not mentioned in ICD 9 CM Codes.

The 2015 version of ICD 10 CM Codes have incorporated newer signs such as skin complications and oral complications.

Table 4.1 shows various ICD 10 codes for diabetes and oral complications.

SNOMED CT® has concepts ID that include education score-diabetes (309593006), refuse diabetes monitoring (185754009), and diabetes well-being questionnaire (273413007) that can be used in dental clinics (Tuso 2014).

4.6 Risk Assessment

Early intervention and lifestyle modifications effectively delay or prevent type 2 diabetes in individuals (American Diabetes Association 2018b). Leveraging informatics in developing tools can serve as screening tools (Acharya et al. 2018; Hegde et al. 2018). American Diabetes Association have started an online diabetes risk assessment tool that takes into consideration different factors such as age, gender,

Table 4.1 ICD 10 Codes for diabetes and oral complications

ICD 10 Code		Description
E10.63		**Type 1 diabetes mellitus with oral complications**
	E10.630	Type 1 diabetes mellitus with periodontal disease
	E10.638	Type 1 diabetes mellitus with other oral complications
E11.63		**Type 2 diabetes mellitus with oral complications**
	E11.630	Type 2 diabetes mellitus with periodontal disease
	E11.638	Type 2 diabetes mellitus with other oral complications
E13.63		**Other specified diabetes mellitus with oral complications**
	E13.630	Other specified diabetes mellitus with periodontal disease
	E13.638	Other diabetes mellitus with other oral complications

family history, high blood pressure, physically active and weight status (American Diabetes Association 2018b). The tool comprises of seven questions with two options to select a value of either '0' or '1'. If the sum of all the seven questions exceeds 5, the person is considered to be at a high risk (Douglass 2006). Based on the numbers, the interactive tool estimates the risk of diabetes.

Similarly, the American Academy of Periodontology has an online gum disease risk assessment tool that determines a risk of a patient based on few questions (American Academy of Periodontology 2008). There are 12 questions with two or three options. Once the person completes the question, the algorithm computes the values and provides with the risk of developing PD (Perio-Tools.com 2018). Lang and Tonetti developed an individual risk assessment tool for patients in supportive periodontal therapy (Lang et al. 2015). The risk assessment tool estimates the risk of progression of the periodontal disease when is patient is undergoing supportive therapy. The risk is determined by assessing the level of infection, attachment loss, periodontal pockets and evaluation of environmental, behavioral and systemic conditions. Based on scientific evidence available, vectors are formed.

4.7 Systems Biology: Genomics, Proteomics, Microbiomics, Phenotypes

A genome-wide search study used semi-automated fluorescence-based technology and linkage analysis to identify human genomes that predispose to type diabetes mellitus (Zeggini et al. 2007). The study witnessed major histocompatibility complex on chromosome 6p21 and chromosome llp15 in case of Type 1 and Type diabetes respectively. Another study noticed diabetes susceptibility loci in and around the genes CDKAL1, CDKN2A/CDKN2B, and IGF2BP2 by analyzing 3757 cases and 5346 controls (Scott et al. 2007).

Other genome-wide study carried out in 1161 Finnish type 2 diabetics cases and 1174 Finnish normal glucose-tolerant controls with more than 315,000 single-nucleotide polymorphisms (SNPs) identified type 2 diabetes associated variants in the intergenic region of chromosome 11p12 (Engebretson and Kocher 2013).

It is noteworthy that studies have also investigated the association between diabetes and periodontitis at the cellular level. Studies have shown that poor glycemic control is associated with elevated gingival crevicular fluid (GCF) Interleukin-1 beta. GCF samples, plaque index, bleeding on probing, probing depth and attachment level were collected from 45 patients suffering type 2 diabetes mellitus and untreated chronic periodontitis (Mohan et al. 2014). Along with this glycated hemoglobin levels were measured from anti coagulated whole blood. The study results showed that patients with HbA1c greater than 8% had significantly higher mean GCF IL-1 beta levels.

4.8 Treatment

According to the American Diabetes Association, treatment and care for managing diabetes includes oral health and hygiene, healthy lifestyle and good communication with the diabetic care team for responding to the changing needs. This includes brushing, flossing and regular follow up with the dentists (American Diabetes Association 2018a). Evidence indicates that C-reactive protein levels in GCF and blood serum level decreases with scaling and root planing (Mohan et al. 2014). The study participants in (Mohan et al. 2014) were divided into ‘experimental group’ comprising of 24 participants with type 2 diabetes, random blood sugar level of more than 200 and chronic periodontitis and ‘other group’ including 24 participants without type 2 diabetes mellitus, random blood sugar level less than 200 and chronic periodontitis. It was seen that the mean improvement in periodontal health parameters, CRP levels in serum and GCF was greater in ‘experimental group’ than the ‘other group’.

Interdisciplinary awareness needs to be increased amongst the providers to set a stage for integration such as monitoring blood glucose levels before carrying out any dental procedure. Depending on the blood glucose level, the patient should be managed accordingly. For example in cases of hypoglycemia, 15 g of glucose should be given orally while blood glucose level more than 200 should be considered for referral to medical provider. If the blood sugar level is more than 400, it is not advisable to continue with dental treatment and it such cases, the dental provider should refer the patient to medical provider right away.

4.9 Prognosis

Studies have shown that Type 1 and Type 2 diabetes are associated with elevated levels of systemic markers of inflammation (Dorcely et al. 2017). Increased level of inflammation in diabetes contributes to the micro-vascular and macro-vascular diabetic complications. Studies have demonstrated that diabetes alters the inflammatory response to oral pathogens. Oral bacteria such as Aggregatibacter actinomycetemcomitans, Porphyromonas gingivalis and Tannerella forsythia increase the risk of periodontitis. It is also been shown that genetic polymorphisms such as single nucleotide peptide modulates the host response against these pathogens while diabetes contributes to increasing the risk of developing periodontitis (American Diabetes Association (ADA) 2016).

Prognosis of patients with diabetes depends on how well an individual alters his or her risk of complications. Studies have shown that life expectancy has improved with insulin discovery for type 1 diabetic patient and with better prevention and treatment of complications (American Diabetes Association (ADA) 2016). Prognosis of diabetes mainly depends on glycemic control. As PD represents a modifiable risk factor that may reduce onset and progression of diabetes, periodontal therapy also plays a significant role in managing glycemic control and thus improving the prognosis.

4.10 Interdisciplinary Care Team

The interdisciplinary care team includes Medical providers, Dental providers including dentists, dental hygienists, Diabetes educators, Nurse practitioners, Pharmacist, Social Worker and Nutritionist.

4.11 Guidelines

Despite the evidence that PD is a complication of type 2 diabetes mellitus, siloed medical-dental healthcare and management of patients with diabetes persists. There are gaps in diabetes clinical care which need to be addressed. Knowledge gap, attitude and behavior amongst healthcare providers cause a substantial gap in diabetic treatment (Glurich et al. 2017; Shimpi et al. 2016a, b). Especially neglect of oral health among diabetic patients has been a hallmark for long time; this gap needs to be narrowed down.

Guidelines published by the American Diabetes Association recommend an annual oral examination to be done by the primary care provider or the physician (American Diabetes Association 2018a). For drawing attention between healthcare providers for the bi-directional relationship, it becomes necessary to develop educational modules in form of computer based training and continuing medical educations. For timely recognition of diabetic patients amongst the population requires real time identification. Screening for diabetes in dental and medical settings will help in increasing the standards of care.

4.12 Technology Implications

4.12.1 Electronic Health Records

Apart from maintaining the electronic version of patient's medical clinical data, the EHRs support care-related activity directly or indirectly including evidence-based decision support, quality management and outcomes reporting (HealthIT.gov 2017).

Having diabetes and periodontal registry will help the care team to track number of interventions and clinical parameters important in management of diabetes and periodontal disease. This will improve the disease management process and increase the quality of care.

Implementing data quality measures for healthcare delivery will enable healthcare providers to instantly quantify treatment outcomes, patient's perceptions, population health and efficient use of health care resources. A real time clinical guideline can be introduced in the EHR will aid the care team in efficient patient management (Centers for Disease Control and Prevention National Center for Health Statistics National Vital Statistics System 2018; Hegde et al. 2017).

With the advent in computer technology, a more personalized and tailored information is now made available for the end users through health assessments in form of Computer Assisted Survey Interviewing software, automated telephone diseases management among others. Collecting information on diabetes and periodontal disease in electronic health record can help in discovering medical conditions associated with the periodontal health (Hegde et al. 2017).

4.13 Ontology

Personalizing guidance service for management of diabetes was developed as a part of project by one of the study team at UK. The application on smart phones enabled diabetic patients to record blood glucose readings, carbohydrates consumed, insulin dosage, physical activity and other activities. Based on these observations ontology was developed (Cantais et al. 2005).

A knowledge based temporal abstraction (KBTA) was developed that provided communication among three agents, specialist agent, patient agent and WWW agent. DM ontology was developed that aimed in guiding decision and criteria regarding the diagnosis, management and treatment in Diabetes mellitus (Yu et al. 2011).

4.14 Care Plan

There needs awareness of the bidirectional connection of diabetes and periodontitis between healthcare providers. The dental and medical providers play an active and an important role in communicating clinical management of oral and systemic health. A proper referral mechanism will play a significant role in the delivering this interdisciplinary care.

Dental providers should check for fungal infections such as oral candidiasis. Oral candidiasis commonly called as thrush is characterized by presence of a creamy white patch and bleeding oral mucosa, mostly affects soft palate followed by cheek, tongue and gingivae. Dental providers should screen for diabetes and pre diabetes in their dental offices. Blood glucose level should be checked before proceeding with a dental treatment. Guidelines should be followed accordingly for the blood glucose levels.

Similarly, patients with diabetes should be informed about increased risk of periodontitis. Also, medical providers should evaluate patient's oral cavity for the oral status. Oral health education should be provided to all the patients. Patients with diabetes should be referred to dental providers for further evaluation of oral status. Identifying women with gestational diabetes mellitus requires glucose testing. Woman should be screened for risk of diabetes at initial prenatal visit (USPTF 2014).

Diabetic oral complications need to be identified and included in the ultimate care of diabetes in order to fight this chronic metabolic disease effectively. Salivary dysfunction has been reported in patients with diabetes (Al-Maskari et al. 2011). Findings of a systematic review demonstrated increased prevalence of xerostomia and hyposalivation amongst T2DM patients as compared to patients without T2DM (López-Pintor et al. 2016). Xerostomia resulting from reduced salivary rate, was more frequently reported by patients with diabetes (Lima et al. 2017; López-Pintor et al. 2016; Mortazavi et al. 2014).

4.15 Recommendations on Dental Diagnosis of Diabetes

- The American Diabetes Association has given the following guidelines for clinical care for people with diabetes. This global guideline for Type 2 Diabetes provides with recommendations for managing diabetes in older people. The guideline recommends including prevention of oral diseases and promotion of oral health as an essential component of diabetes management. Dental disease is mentioned as a risk of malnutrition in older people with diabetes. Establish PD as a routine complication of diabetes and increase awareness amongst health professionals and policy makers. Initiate and support research leading to evidence based treatment to improve health and oral health of people with diabetes. Increasing the focus of dental education amongst medical students will help in increasing quality of care (American Diabetes Association 2018d).
- Wisconsin State Guidelines for Diabetes and Oral Health. These guidelines serve as a tool to support and influence health care provider decision making to promote consistent, comprehensive and preventive diabetes care that includes oral health (DHS 2018).
- Educational materials based on association of diabetes and PD should be provided to patients.

References

Acharya A, Cheng B, Koralkar R, Olson B, Lamster I, Kunzel C, Lalla E. Secondary analysis of EHR data to enhance care of dental patients with diabetes. JDR Clin Transl Res. 2018;3(2):188–94. https://doi.org/10.1177/2380084418759496.

Allen E, Matthews J, O'Halloran D, Griffiths H, Chapple IL. Oxidative and inflammatory status in Type 2 diabetes patients with periodontitis. J Clin Periodontol. 2011;38(10):894–901. https://doi.org/10.1111/j.1600-051X.2011.01764.x.

Al-Maskari A, Al-Maskari M, Al-Sudairy S. Oral manifestations and complications of diabetes mellitus: a review. Sultan Qaboos Univ Med J. 2011;11(2):179–86. Retrieved from http://www.ncbi.nlm.nih.gov/pubmed/21969888

American Academy of Periodontology. American Academy of Periodontology statement on risk assessment. J Periodontol. 2008;79(2):202. https://doi.org/10.1902/jop.2008.082001.

American Diabetes Association. Diagnosis and classification of diabetes mellitus. Diabetes Care. 2009;33(Suppl 1):S62–7. https://doi.org/10.2337/dc09-S062.

American Diabetes Association. American Diabetes Association Releases 2018 standards of medical care in diabetes, with notable new recommendations for people with cardiovascular disease and diabetes. American Diabetes Association®; 2018a. http://www.diabetes.org/newsroom/press-releases/2017/american-diabetes-association-2018-release-standards-of-medical-care-in-diabetes.html. Accessed 1 July 2018.

American Diabetes Association. Diabetes complications. 2018b. http://www.diabetes.org/living-with-diabetes/complications/. Accessed 1 July 2018.

American Diabetes Association. Hyperosmolar hyperglycemic nonketotic syndrome (HHNS). American Diabetes Association®; 2018c. http://www.diabetes.org/living-with-diabetes/complications/hyperosmolar-hyperglycemic.html. Accessed 1 July 2018.

American Diabetes Association. Statistics about diabetes: American Diabetes Association®; 2018d. http://www.diabetes.org/diabetes-basics/statistics/. Accessed 1 July 2018.

American Diabetes Association. 2. Classification and diagnosis of diabetes: standards of medical care in Diabetes-2018. Diabetes Care. 2018e;41(Suppl 1):S13–27. https://doi.org/10.2337/dc18-S002.

American Diabetes Association. Type 2 diabetes. 2018f. http://www.diabetes.org/diabetes-basics/type-2/. Accessed 1 July 2018.

American Diabetes Association. Type 2 diabetes risk test. American Diabetes Association®; 2018g. http://www.diabetes.org/are-you-at-risk/diabetes-risk-test/. Accessed 1 July 2018.

American Diabetes Association (ADA). American Diabetes Association standards of medical care in diabetes - 2016. Diabetes Care. 2016;39(Suppl):S1–S112. https://doi.org/10.2337/dc16-S003.

Andersen LW, Mackenhauer J, Roberts J, Berg K, Cocchi M, Donnino M. Etiology and therapeutic approach to elevated lactate levels. Mayo Clin Proc. 2013;88(10):1127–40. https://doi.org/10.1016/j.mayocp.2013.06.012.

Bascones-Martinez A, Matesanz-Perez P. Periodontal disease and diabetes-review of the literature. Med Oral Patol Oral Cir. 2011;16(6):e722–9.

Bascones-Martínez A, Muñoz-Corcuera M, Bascones-Ilundain J. Diabetes y periodontitis: una relación bidireccional. Med Clin. 2015;145(1):31–5. https://doi.org/10.1016/j.medcli.2014.07.019.

Borgnakke W, Ylostalo P, Taylor G, Genco R. Effect of periodontal disease on diabetes: systematic review of epidemiologic observational evidence. J Periodontol. 2013;84(4 Suppl):S135–52. https://doi.org/10.1902/jop.2013.1340013.

Boyle J, Thompson T, Gregg E, Barker L, Williamson D. Projection of the year 2050 burden of diabetes in the US adult population: dynamic modeling of incidence, mortality, and prediabetes prevalence. Population Health Metrics. 2010;8(1):29. https://doi.org/10.1186/1478-7954-8-29.

Brownlee M. The pathobiology of diabetic complications: a unifying mechanism. Diabetes. 2005;54(6):1615–25. https://doi.org/10.2337/DIABETES.54.6.1615.

Cade W. Diabetes-related microvascular and macrovascular diseases in the physical therapy setting. Phys Ther. 2008;88(11):1322–35. https://doi.org/10.2522/ptj.20080008.

Cantais J, Cantais J, Dominguez D, Gigante V, Laera L, Tamma V. An example of food ontology for diabetes control. Proceedings of the International Semantic Web Conference 2005 Workshop on Ontology Patterns for the Semantic Web. 2005. http://citeseerx.ist.psu.edu/viewdoc/summary?doi=10.1.1.137.8373

Casanova L, Hughes F, Preshaw P. Diabetes and periodontal disease: a two-way relationship. BDJ. 2014;217(8):433–7. https://doi.org/10.1038/sj.bdj.2014.907.

Casqueiro J, Casqueiro J, Alves C. Infections in patients with diabetes mellitus: a review of pathogenesis. Indian J Endocrinol Metab. 2012;16(Suppl 1):S27–36. https://doi.org/10.4103/2230-8210.94253.

Centers for Disease Control and Prevention. National Diabetes Statistics Report, 2017 estimates of diabetes and its burden in the United States background. 2017.

Centers for Disease Control and Prevention National Center for Health Statistics National Vital Statistics System. ClinicalQualityMeasures. 2018. https://www.cms.gov/Regulations-and-Guidance/Legislation/EHRIncentivePrograms/ClinicalQualityMeasures.html

Chang P, Lim L. Interrelationships of periodontitis and diabetes: a review of the current literature. J Dent Sci. 2012;7(3):272–82. https://doi.org/10.1016/J.JDS.2012.02.002.

DHS. Diabetes: Part of the Wisconsin chronic disease prevention program. Wisconsin: Wisconsin Department of Health Services; 2018.

Dorcely B, Katz K, Jagannathan R, Chiang S, Oluwadare B, Goldberg I, Bergman M. Novel biomarkers for prediabetes, diabetes, and associated complications. Diabetes Metab Syndr Obes. 2017;10:345–61. https://doi.org/10.2147/DMSO.S100074.

Douglass C. Risk assessment and management of periodontal disease. J Am Dent Assoc. 2006;137(Suppl):27S–32S. Retrieved from http://www.ncbi.nlm.nih.gov/pubmed/17035673

Eke P, Dye B, Wei L, Slade G, Thornton-Evans G, Borgnakke W, et al. Update on prevalence of periodontitis in adults in the United States: NHANES 2009 to 2012. J Periodontol. 2015;86(5):611–22. https://doi.org/10.1902/jop.2015.140520.

Engebretson S, Kocher T. Evidence that periodontal treatment improves diabetes outcomes: a systematic review and meta-analysis. J Clin Periodontol. 2013;40:S153–63. https://doi.org/10.1111/jcpe.12084.

Glurich I, Schwei K, Lindeberg S, Shimpi N, Acharya A. Interdisciplinary diabetes management: qualitative assessment of Medical/Dental Practitioners' Perspectives. San Francisco: International Association for Dental Research; 2017.

HealthIT.gov. Improved diagnostics & patient outcomes. HealthIT.gov; 2017. https://www.healthit.gov/topic/health-it-basics/improved-diagnostics-patient-outcomes. Accessed 1 July 2018.

Hegde H, Steinmetz A, Theisen J, Koralkar R, Finnamore J, Halstead S, et al. Dental quality analytics: dental measures and provider performance dashboard. J Dent Res. 2017;96:566.

Hegde H, Koralkar R, Shimpi N, Glurich I, Panny A, Acharya A. Diabetes mellitus prediction using machine learning in a dental setting. AADR/CADR Annual Meeting. Fort Lauderdale. 2018. https://doi.org/10.3233/THC-171127

Huang D, Refaat M, Mohammedi K, Jayyousi A, Al Suwaidi J, Abi Khalil C. Macrovascular complications in patients with diabetes and prediabetes. Biomed Res Int. 2017;2017:7839101. https://doi.org/10.1155/2017/7839101.

ICD10Data.com. The Web's free 2018 ICD-10-CM/PCS Medical Coding Reference. 2018. https://www.icd10data.com/. Accessed 1 July 2018.

Khader Y, Dauod A, El-Qaderi S, Alkafajei A, Batayha WQ. Periodontal status of diabetics compared with nondiabetics: a meta-analysis. J Diabetes Complications. 2006;20(1):59–68. https://doi.org/10.1016/j.jdiacomp.2005.05.006.

Kitabchi A, Umpierrez G, Miles J, Fisher J, Kreisberg R, Malone J, Wall B. Hyperglycemic crises in adult patients with diabetes. Diabetes Care. 2009;32(7):1335–43. https://doi.org/10.2337/dc09-9032.

Lalla E, Papapanou P. Diabetes mellitus and periodontitis: a tale of two common interrelated diseases. Nat Rev Endocrinol. 2011;7(12):738–48. https://doi.org/10.1038/nrendo.2011.106.

Lang N, Suvan J, Tonetti M. Risk factor assessment tools for the prevention of periodontitis progression a systematic review. J Clin Periodontol. 2015;42:S59–70. https://doi.org/10.1111/jcpe.12350.

Leite R, Marlow N, Fernandes J, Hermayer K. Oral health and Type 2 diabetes. Am J Med Sci. 2013;345(4):271–3. https://doi.org/10.1097/MAJ.0b013e31828bdedf.

Lilliu M, Solinas P, Cossu M, Puxeddu R, Loy F, Isola R, et al. Diabetes causes morphological changes in human submandibular gland: a morphometric study. J Oral Pathol Med. 2015;44(4):291–5. https://doi.org/10.1111/jop.12238.

Lima D, Carneiro S, Barbosa F, Saintrain M, Moizan J, Doucet J. Salivary flow and xerostomia in older patients with type 2 diabetes mellitus. PLoS One. 2017;12(8):e0180891. https://doi.org/10.1371/journal.pone.0180891.

Loesche W. Microbiology of dental decay and periodontal disease. Medical microbiology. Galveston, TX: University of Texas Medical Branch at Galveston; 1996. http://www.ncbi.nlm.nih.gov/pubmed/21413316

López-Pintor R, Casañas E, González-Serrano J, Serrano J, Ramírez L, de Arriba L, Hernández G. Xerostomia, hyposalivation, and salivary flow in diabetes patients. J Diabetes Res. 2016;2016:4372852. https://doi.org/10.1155/2016/4372852.

Mata A, Marques D, Rocha S, Francisco H, Santos C, Mesquita MF, Singh J. Effects of diabetes mellitus on salivary secretion and its composition in the human. Mol Cell Biochem. 2004;261(1):137–42. https://doi.org/10.1023/B:MCBI.0000028748.40917.6f.

Mauri-Obradors E, Merlos A, Estrugo-Devesa A, Jané-Salas E, López-López J, Viñas M. Benefits of non-surgical periodontal treatment in patients with type 2 diabetes mellitus and chronic periodontitis: a randomized controlled trial. J Clin Periodontol. 2018;45(3):345–53. https://doi.org/10.1111/jcpe.12858.

Mealey B. Periodontal disease and diabetes. A two-way street. J Am Dent Assoc. 2006;137(Suppl):26S–31S. https://doi.org/10.14219/JADA.ARCHIVE.2006.0404.

Mohan M, Jhingran R, Bains V, Gupta V, Madan R, Rizvi I, Mani K. Impact of scaling and root planing on C-reactive protein levels in gingival crevicular fluid and serum in chronic periodontitis patients with or without diabetes mellitus. J Periodontal Implant Sci. 2014;44(4):158–68. https://doi.org/10.5051/jpis.2014.44.4.158.

Mortazavi H, Baharvand M, Movahhedian A, Mohammadi M, Khodadoustan A. Xerostomia due to systemic disease: a review of 20 conditions and mechanisms. Ann Med Health Sci Res. 2014;4(4):503–10. https://doi.org/10.4103/2141-9248.139284.

NIDDK. Insulin resistance & prediabetes. NIDDK; 2018. https://www.niddk.nih.gov/health-information/diabetes/overview/what-is-diabetes/prediabetes-insulin-resistance. Accessed 1 July 2018.

Perio-Tools.com. Risk assessment. Department of Periodontology, University of Bern Switzerland; 2018. http://www.perio-tools.com/pra/en/index.asp. Accessed 1 July 2018.

Poretsky L, Liao EP. Acute and chronic complications of diabetes. Amsterdam: Elsevier; 2013.

Preshaw P, Alba A, Herrera D, Jepsen S, Konstantinidis A, Makrilakis K, Taylor R. Periodontitis and diabetes: a two-way relationship. Diabetologia. 2012;55(1):21–31. https://doi.org/10.1007/s00125-011-2342-y.

Quirino M, Birman E, Paula C. Oral manifestations of diabetes mellitus in controlled and uncontrolled patients. Braz Dent J. 1995;6(2):131–6. http://www.ncbi.nlm.nih.gov/pubmed/8688658

Röder P, Wu B, Liu Y, Han W. Pancreatic regulation of glucose homeostasis. Exp Mol Med. 2016;48(3):e219. https://doi.org/10.1038/emm.2016.6.

Scott L, Mohlke K, Bonnycastle L, Willer C, Li Y, Duren W, et al. A Genome-Wide Association Study of Type 2 Diabetes in Finns detects multiple susceptibility variants. Science. 2007;316(5829):1341–5. https://doi.org/10.1126/science.1142382.

Shafiee G, Mohajeri-Tehrani M, Pajouhi M, Larijani B. The importance of hypoglycemia in diabetic patients. J Diabetes Metab Disord. 2012;11(1):17. https://doi.org/10.1186/2251-6581-11-17.

Shimpi N, Schroeder D, Kilsdonk J, Chyou P, Glurich I, Penniman E, Acharya A. Medical providers' oral health knowledgeability, attitudes, and practice behaviors: an opportunity for interprofessional collaboration. J Evid Based Dent Pract. 2016a;16(1):19–29. https://doi.org/10.1016/j.jebdp.2016.01.002.

Shimpi N, Schroeder D, Kilsdonk J, Ph C, Glurich I, Acharya A. Assessment of dental providers' knowledge, behavior and attitude towards incorporating chairside screening for medical conditions: a pilot study. J Dent Oral Care Med. 2016b;2(1):102. https://doi.org/10.15744/2454-3276.2.102.

Shultis WA, Weil EJ, Looker HC, Curtis JM, Shlossman M, Genco RJ, et al. Effect of periodontitis on overt nephropathy and end-stage renal disease in type 2 diabetes. Diabetes Care. 2007;30(2):306–11. https://doi.org/10.2337/dc06-1184.

Steffes M, Sibley S, Jackson M, Thomas W. Beta-cell function and the development of diabetes-related complications in the diabetes control and complications trial. Diabetes Care. 2003;26(3):832–6. http://www.ncbi.nlm.nih.gov/pubmed/12610045

Tuso P. Prediabetes and lifestyle modification: time to prevent a preventable disease. Perm J. 2014;18(3):88–93. https://doi.org/10.7812/TPP/14-002.

USPTF. Understanding task force recommendations screening for gestational diabetes what is gestational, (January), 1–4; 2014.

Wilcox G. Insulin and insulin resistance. Clin Biochem Rev. 2005;26(2):19–39. http://www.ncbi.nlm.nih.gov/pubmed/16278749

World Health Organization. WHO. About diabetes. Geneva: WHO; 2014. http://www.who.int/diabetes/action_online/basics/en/index1.html

Wu Y, Ding Y, Tanaka Y, Zhang W. Risk factors contributing to type 2 diabetes and recent advances in the treatment and prevention. Int J Med Sci. 2014;11(11):1185–200. https://doi.org/10.7150/ijms.10001.

Yu H, Liaw S, Taggart J, Khorzoughi AR. Using ontologies to identify patients with diabetes in electronic health records. CEUR Workshop Proceedings; 2011.

Zeggini E, Weedon M, Lindgren C, Frayling T, Elliott K, Lango H, et al. Replication of genome-wide association signals in UK samples reveals risk loci for type 2 diabetes. Science (New York, NY). 2007;316(5829):1336–41. https://doi.org/10.1126/science.1142364.

Chapter 5
Interdisciplinary Care Model: Papillon-Lefèvre Syndrome and Oral Health

Robert H. Posteraro

5.1 Definition and Prevalence

Papillon-Lefèvre syndrome (PLS) is a rare, autosomal recessive disease, characterized by symmetrical palmoplantar hyperkeratosis and severe, osteodestructive periodontitis. The disease was first described by Papillon and Lefèvre in 1924 (Papillon and Lefèvre 1924). The reported incidence is approximately 1–4 per million and the carrier rate is 2–4 per 1000 (Pratchyapruit and Kullavanijaya 2002). There is no sex or race preference. Approximately 30–50% of patients are the offspring of consanguineous relationships (Meyle and Gonzales 2001; Nagy et al. 2014).

5.2 Systemic Manifestations

Associated findings that have been described in some PLS patients include, psoriasiform lesions on the elbows, knuckles and knees, hyperhidrosis, fine body hair, dirty colored skin in the affected areas, mild mental retardation, calcification of the falx, dura, and tentorium. The disorder can predispose patients to pyoderma in the hyperkeratotic lesions, pyogenic abscesses of internal organs including the liver (most commonly reported), kidney (Morgan et al. 2011), and brain (Kanthimathinathan et al. 2013). Squamous cell carcinoma (rare) (Al-Benna et al. 2009) and melanoma (rare) (Cook 2009) have been reported within the hyperkeratotic lesions. Ocular surface squamous neoplasia (rare) was also reported in a patient with PLS (Murthy et al. 2004). In addition, oculocutaneous albinism type 1 (rare) has been reported in individuals with PLS in two, unrelated, families (Hewitt et al. 2004).

R. H. Posteraro
Department of Healthcare Management and Leadership, Texas Tech University Health Sciences Center School of Health Professions, Lubbock, TX, USA
e-mail: robert.posteraro@ttuhsc.edu

A. Acharya et al. (eds.), *Integration of Medical and Dental Care and Patient Data*, Health Informatics, https://doi.org/10.1007/978-3-319-98298-4_5

5.3 Oral Manifestations

Hyperkeratosis develops between ages 0 and 4 years, with periodontitis developing between 3 and 4 years of age (Morgan et al. 2011), at the time of eruption of the primary dentition. Late onset PLS has also been reported. At the time of eruption of the primary dentition, gingivitis and periodontitis develop, resulting in destruction of alveolar bone with loosening and ultimate exfoliation of the primary dentition. In most cases, periodontitis undergoes resolution, but recurs with eruption of the permanent dentition which undergoes the same alveolar bone loss and exfoliation as the primary dentition (Khan et al. 2014). Oral manifestations include gingival enlargement, gingival ulceration, and the formation of deep periodontal pockets (Posteraro 1992). Patients lose most, if not all, of their teeth by the time of their teenage years. The skin lesions and periodontitis with loss of teeth at such an early age have serious negative social and psychological consequences.

5.4 Oral Systemic Connections

Cathepsin C is important in the zymogen activation of serine proteases and is felt to be important in epithelial differentiation and desquamation. Disruption with this activity is presumed to be causative in the production of keratoderma and also in the dental manifestations of PLS, since cathepsin C is also found in the junctional epithelium that develops around the teeth during tooth eruption. The breakdown of the junctional epithelium could result in disruption of tooth eruption and could contribute to breakdown of the periodontal barriers to infection, leading to gingivitis and periodontitis that are characteristic of PLS. The fact that junctional epithelium is present only during tooth eruption would explain the periodontitis free interval following exfoliation of the primary dentition and its recurrence during the eruption of the permanent teeth. In addition, cathepsin C is found in osteoclasts and lack of cathepsin C could be an etiologic factor in the alveolar bone destruction seen in PLS. Cathepsin C is also found in polymorphonuclear leukocytes, and natural killer (NK) cells. Lack of cathepsin C activity could then explain the predilection of PLS patients to develop infections and pyogenic abscesses (Lundgren et al. 2005), and possibly their susceptibility to various tumors due to immunodeficiency (Cook 2009).

5.5 Diagnostic Codes

Table 5.1 lists all the ICD 9 CM and ICD 10 CM codes for PLS.

Table 5.1 ICD 9 CM and ICD 10 CM codes for PLS

Diagnostic codes	Codes	Description
ICD 9 CM	757.2	Dermatoglyphic anomalies
ICD 9 CM	757.39	Other specified anomalies of skin
ICD 10 CM	Q82.8	Papillon-Lefèvre Syndrome (PLS)

5.6 Risk Assessment

Methods are still being evaluated for developing risk assessment tools for PLS.

5.7 Systems Biology: Genomics, Proteomics, Microbiomics, Phenotypes

The genetic etiology of the disorder has been identified as a mutation in the cathepsin C gene (CTSC), located on chromosome 11q14q21 (Hart et al. 1998, 1999, 2000). There are a number of similar conditions that have been described, differing from PLS in some respects, which suggests that there are several variant mutations within the same gene, or in other genes that are influential in the regulation of the cathepsin C gene or in the formation or activation of cathepsin C. Identical mutations can give rise to a variety of different phenotypes, which may be due to other genetic and/or environmental factors (Nagy et al. 2014). Most of the mutations that have been identified are missense (53%), nonsense (23%), and frameshift (17%) mutations, although inframe deletions, one splicing variant, and one 5′ untranslated region mutation have also been reported (Nagy et al. 2014). The cathepsin C molecule is a tetramer, and tetramerization is important in the enzymatic functioning of the molecule. The mutations that result in PLS block formation of the enzyme.

5.8 Proteomics

Cathepsin C protein (dipeptidylpeptidase I) is a lysosomal exocysteine proteinase of the peptidase C1 family. It is an oligomeric enzyme, having a tetramer form, composed of four identical subunits. Cathepsin C functions by removing dipeptides from the amino terminus of proteins and is involved in the zymogen activation of neutrophil serine proteases (Nagy et al. 2014) which are important in modulating immune responses which may be contributory to the periodontitis of PLS (Cook 2009). This activity may be important in epithelial differentiation and desquamation, which could explain the hyperkeratosis of PLS.

5.9 Cytology

Immunologic changes are the likely cause of susceptibility to infection, resulting in the association of periodontitis, pyodermic infections, abscesses, and of peri-implantitis in PLS patients in whom dental implants have been inserted (Nickles et al. 2013).

5.10 Microbiology

A number of pathogens have been associated with the periodontitis of PLS. These include Aggregatibacter actinomycetemcomitans (commonly reported), other gram negative anaerobic bacteria, and Epstein-Barr type 1 virus (Pacheco et al. 2002).

5.11 Treatment

Various treatments, focused on the skin lesions and loss of dentition, have been described with varying rates of success. No treatment regimen has been shown, conclusively, to be greatly effective, however. The treatments are, essentially, symptomatic and functional. Treatment of the skin lesions includes topical emollients and systemic retinoids, such as acitretin (Lee et al. 2005).

5.12 Interdisciplinary Care Team

Because of its dermatologic and periodontal manifestations, treatment of patients who have PLS requires a multidisciplinary approach, involving a dermatologist, dentist, and oral surgeon. A psychologist or psychiatrist and genetic counselor are also important members of the team.

5.13 Guidelines

Close follow-up and regular attention to dental hygiene is important. Patients who have had dental implants are susceptible to develop periimplantitis unless regular followup and a program of dental hygiene is maintained (Nickles et al. 2013).

It is important to recognize the disease early and institute treatment, as well as initialize psychological counseling for the patient and genetic counseling for the patient and family members.

5.14 Existing Gaps and Suggestions

The patient may present, initially, to the pediatrician, the general dentist, or the pedodontist. Early specialist referral will include the dermatologist, periodontist, and oral surgeon. Each of these healthcare providers should be aware of the nature of the condition, and be able to diagnose it, or come to a differential diagnosis based on clinical symptoms and family history. Appropriate referral to specialists (dermatologist, oral surgeon, geneticist, and psychologist or psychiatrist) is indicated.

5.15 Technology Implications

Translational application using technology can improve the clinical care of patients suffering from PLS. These may include incorporating clinical decision support tools to facilitate diagnosis, and developing an automated disease prevention strategy and treatment of patients with PLS. Studies have shown researchers using an array of tools to characterize gene function for various diseases which can be applied to PLS. For example identifying the genetic basis of PLS, tools can be developed in addition to existing DNA based testing, and cytogenetic testing (Hart and Hart 2009).

5.16 Ontology

Human Phenotype Ontology is a database that collects information on symptoms described in the medical field (NIH 2018). According to HPO, 80–99% of patients suffering from PLS have the following symptoms. Table 5.2 describes the medical terms and associated HPO IDs.

5.17 Care Plan

Papillon-Lefèvre syndrome is multifactorial and may present to either medical or dental providers. The ability of both physicians and dentists to recognize the condition or, at least, develop a differential diagnosis is important. The knowledge that this condition has both medical and dental aspects is necessary to insure complete patient care (Muppa et al. 2011). Appropriate referrals and teamwork among medical and dental providers is important, not only for proper treatment but for genetic counseling and psychological counseling as well.

Patient education should insure an understanding of the condition, the options and limitations of various treatment plans, and the genetic basis and inheritance factors of the disease. Supportive and caring treatment of the patient and the patient's family are important for the dental and medical prognosis for the patient as well as for the patient's psychological and social development.

Table 5.2 Medical terms and associated HPO IDs

Medical terms	HPO ID
Palmoplantar hyperkeratosis	0000972
Palmoplantar keratoderma	0000982
Abnormality of fingernails	0001231
Atrophy of alveolar ridges	0006308
Gingivitis	0000230
Premature loss of deciduous teeth	0006323
Reduced number of teeth	0009804
Severe periodontitis	0000166

5.18 Recommendations on Dental Diagnosis of Papillon-Lefèvre Syndrome

Conventional periodontal treatments have usually been ineffective (de Vree et al. 2000). Treatment of the dental manifestations of the disease include total tooth extraction with prosthetic replacement with implant secured dentures; a combination of mechanical and antibiotic periodontal treatment with regular microbiological monitoring to insure efficacy of the antibiotic regimen, and intensive maintenance therapy, combined with regular attention to dental hygiene (Nickles et al. 2013). Systemic retinoids have also been found to be effective in treating the periodontitis.

5.19 Differential Diagnosis

Haim-Munk syndrome (HMS), is a CTSC mutation characterized by palmoplantar hyperkeratosis, periodontal inflammation, but also arachnodactyly, acralosteolysis, pes planus, and onychogryphosis (Rai et al. 2010).

Hypotrichosis-(acro)osteolysis-periodontitis-palmoplantar keratoderma (HOPP) syndrome is a syndrome that is similar in many respects to Haim-Munk syndrome but is not associated with a CTSC mutation and, therefore, is not a variant of HMS or PLS. The reported cases were also characterized by onychogryphosis, lingua plicata (furrowed tongue), and ventricular arrhythmias. HOPP syndrome lacks the pes planus deformity that is found in HMS. Two cases were reported by van Steensel et al. (2002) and a third case reported by Brun and van Steensel (2004). The mode of inheritance is uncertain.

Variant Carvajal syndrome is a condition characterized by prepubertal periodontitis, premature root resorption of the primary teeth, and palmoplantar keratosis, but also angular cheilitis, striae keratoderma, wiry hair, sparse eyebrows and eyelashes, small, white finger nails, thickened toe nails, reduced sweating, and cardiomyopathy (Barber et al. 2012). The index patient in the cited study died, suddenly, of unsuspected cardiomyopathy. The association of unsuspected cardiomyopathy in this patient makes this a serious dental-systemic condition. If the dentist suspects this diagnosis, say, on the basis of prepubertal periodontitis, palmoplantar keratosis, and the associated findings, attention should be paid and the patient referred to a cardiologist for evaluation for possible cardiomyopathy.

A variant of Carvajal/Naxos syndrome associated with hypo/oligodontia was described by Chalabreysse et al. in 2011. In this variant of Carvajal/Naxos syndrome, the affected patients had palmoplantar keratoderma, wooly hair, and biventricular dilated cardiomyopathy characteristic of Carvajal/Naxos syndrome, but also had many missing teeth (hypo/oligodontia). While this latter finding is different from the early dental loss of PLS, the loss of teeth could be mistaken for early exfoliation and a search for the other manifestations of this disease should be made in order to distinguish it from PLS. This is important because this variant of Carvajal/

Naxos syndrome is associated with cardiomyopathy and a cardiology referral to evaluate that possibility would be essential.

An unnamed syndrome of congental atrichia, palmoplantar hyperkeratosis, mental retardation, and early loss of teeth was described by Steijlen et al. (1994). The associated findings of atrichia and mental retardation distinguish this condition from PLS.

A rare case of arsenicosis was reported in which the patient presented with palmoplantar keratosis and early exfoliation of both primary and permanent teeth (Das et al. 2012). A provisional diagnosis of PLS was made, but arsenicosis was also included in the differential due to the fact that the patient's parents and neighbors also demonstrated palmoplantar keratosis without the other manifestations of PLS. The diagnosis of arsenicosis was confirmed by analysis of samples of the patient's hair and nails. A genetic test for the mutation of the cathepsin C gene couldn't be done in this patient, however, so the final differential diagnosis included: a Papillon-Lefèvre type presentation of chronic arsenicosis, or the theoretical possibility that chronic arsenicosis might have caused a mutation of the cathepsin C gene.

Olmsted syndrome is a rare palmoplantar keratodermal disease. A single case has been described in which the patient also presented with severe periodontal disease and loss of teeth (Alotaibi et al. 2015). The adult patient had been diagnosed as having Olmsted syndrome with palmoplantar keratosis and periorificial hyperkeratosis. He presented to the dental clinic in order to have his missing teeth replaced. The patient could not recall when he had begun to lose his permanent teeth. Panorex examination showed three remaining teeth and greater than 50% bone loss. The patient had a long history of poor oral hygiene, and the authors raise the question as to whether his loss of teeth was an unusual manifestation of Olmsted syndrome, or whether it was due to poor oral hygiene. They posit as a possible genetic etiology a mutation in the TRPV3 receptor resulting in inflammatory cytokine release with an increase in IL1β producing bone loss. However, the actual cause of loss of teeth in this patient could not be determined.

References

Al-Benna S, Hasler R, Stricker I, et al. Papillon-Lefèvre syndrome and squamous cell carcinoma: a case report. Cases J. 2009;2:7067.

Alotaibi A, Alotaibi M, Alsaeed S, et al. Olmsted syndrome with oral involvement, including premature teeth loss. Odontology. 2015;103(2):241–5.

Barber S, Day P, Judge M, et al. Variant Carvajal syndrome with additional dental anomalies. Int J Paediatr Dent. 2012;22(5):390–6.

Brun A, van Steensel M. A third case of HOPP syndrome – confirmation of the phenotype. Br J Dermatol. 2004;150(5):1032–3.

Chalabreysse L, Senni F, Bruyère P, et al. A new hypo/oligodontia syndrome: Carvajal/Naxos syndrome secondary to desmoplakin-dominant mutations. J Dent Res. 2011;90(1):58–64.

Cook G. Papillon-Lefèvre syndrome and malignant melanoma. Dermatology. 2009;219(2):187–8.

Das S, Nath T, Ghosal A, et al. Papillon-Lefèvre syndrome-like presentation in chronic arsenicosis: a rare mimicry. Indian J Occup Environ Med. 2012;16(3):145–8.

De Vree H, Steenackers K, De Boever J. Periodontal treatment of rapid progressive periodontitis in 2 siblings with Papillon-Lefèvre syndrome: 15year followup. J Clin Periodontol. 2000;27(5):354–60.

Hart T, Hart P. Genetic studies of craniofacial anomalies: clinical implications and applications. Orthod Craniofac Res. 2009; https://doi.org/10.1111/j.1601-6343.2009.01455.x.

Hart T, Bowden D, Ghaffar K, et al. Sublocalization of the Papillon-Lefèvre syndrome locus on 11q14q21. Am J Med Genet. 1998;79(2):134–9.

Hart T, Hart P, Bowden D, et al. Mutations of the cathepsin C gene are responsible for Papillon-Lefèvre syndrome. J Med Genet. 1999;36(12):881–7.

Hart T, Hart P, Michalec M, et al. Localisation of a gene for prepubertal periodontitis to chromosome 11q14 and identification of a cathepsin C gene mutation. J Med Genet. 2000;37:95–101.

Hewitt C, Wu C, Hattab F, et al. Coinheritance of two rare genodermatoses (Papillon-Lefèvre syndrome and oculocutaneous albinism type 1) in two families: a genetic study. Br J Dermatol. 2004;151(6):1261–5.

Kanthimathinathan H, Browne F, Ramirez R, et al. Multiple cerebral abscesses in Papillon-Lefèvre syndrome. Childs Nerv Syst. 2013;29(8):1227–9.

Khan FY, Jan SM, Mushtaq M. Papillon-Lefèvre syndrome (PLS) without cathepsin C mutation: a rare early onset partially penetrant variant of PLS. Saudi Dent J. 2014;26(1):25–8.

Lee M, Wong L, Fischer G. Papillon-Lefèvre syndrome treated with acitretin. Australas J Dermatol. 2005;46(3):199–201.

Lundgren T, Parhar R, Renvert S, et al. Impaired cytotoxicity in Papillon-Lefèvre syndrome. J Dent Res. 2005;84(5):414–7.

Meyle J, Gonzales J. Influences of systemic diseases on periodontitis in children and adolescents. Periodontol 2000. 2001;26:92–112.

Morgan R, Hannon E, Lakhoo K. Renal abscess in Papillon-Lefèvre syndrome. Pediatr Surg Int. 2011;27(12):1381–3.

Muppa R, Prameela B, Duddu M, et al. Papillon-Lefèvre syndrome: a combined approach from the dermatologist and dentist – a clinical presentation. Indian J Dermatol. 2011;56(6):740–3.

Murthy R, Honavar S, Vemuganti G, et al. Ocular surface squamous neoplasia in Papillon-Lefèvre syndrome. Am J Ophthalmol. 2004;139(1):207–9.

Nagy N, Valyi P, Csoma Z, et al. CTSC and Papillon-Lefèvre syndrome; detection of recurrent mutations in Hungarian patients, a review of published variants and database update. Mol Genet Genomic Med. 2014;2(3):217–28.

Nickles K, Schacher B, RatkaKruger P, et al. Longterm results after treatment of periodontitis in patients with Papillon-Lefèvre syndrome: success and failure. J Clin Periodontol. 2013;40(8):789–98.

NIH. Papillon-Lefèvre syndrome. Genetic and Rare Diseases Information Center. 2018. https://rarediseases.info.nih.gov/diseases/3100/papillon-lefevre-syndrome. Accessed 19 Jan 2018.

Pacheco J, Coelho C, Salazar F, et al. Treatment of Papillon-Lefèvre syndrome periodontitis. J Clin Periodontol. 2002;29(4):370–4.

Papillon M, Lefèvre P. 2 cases of symmetrically, familiarly palmar and plantar hyperkeratosis (Meleda disease) within brother and sister combined with severe dental alterations in both cases. Soc Franc Dermat Syph. 1924;31:82–4.

Posteraro A. Papillon-Lefèvre syndrome. J Ala Dent Assoc. 1992;76(3):16–9.

Pratchyapruit W, Kullavanijaya P. Papillon-Lefèvre syndrome: a case report. J Dermatol. 2002;29(6):329–35.

Rai R, Thiagarajan S, Mohandas S, et al. Haim-Munk syndrome and Papillon-Lefèvre syndrome – allelic mutations in cathepsin C with variation in phenotype. Int J Dermatol. 2010;49(5):541–3.

Steijlen P, Neumann H, der Kinderen D, et al. Congenital atrichia, palmoplantar hyperkeratosis, mental retardation, and early loss of teeth in four siblings: a new syndrome? J Am Acad Dermatol. 1994;30(5 Pt 2):893–8.

Van Steensel M, Van Geel M, Steijlen P. New syndrome of hypotrhichosis, striate palmoplantar keratoderma, acroosteolysis and periodontitis not due to mutations in cathepsin C. Br J Dermatol. 2002;147(3):575–81.

Chapter 6
Interdisciplinary Care Model: Cardiovascular Diseases and Oral Health

Neel Shimpi, Richard Dart, Peter Umukoro, and Amit Acharya

6.1 Definition and Prevalence

Cardiovascular diseases (CVDs) have been defined as a group of circulatory system disorders involving impairment of heart and blood vessels (WHO 2018). It is estimated that about 17.7 million people globally died in 2015 from CVDs (WHO 2017). This represented about 31% of total global deaths. The American Heart Association (AHA) report stated that about 40.5% men and 35.5% women between the ages of 40 and 59 years suffered some form of CVD (Writing Group Members et al. 2016). The most recent AHA report states that about 92.1 million American adults suffer from some form of the CVD and 2,200 Americans die of CVD each day (AHA 2017). The World Health Organization (WHO) categorizes the CVDs into six types: coronary heart disease (CHD), cerebrovascular disease (CeVD), peripheral arterial disease (PAD), congenital heart disease, deep vein thrombosis, and pulmonary embolism (WHO 2018). Figure 6.1 illustrates the WHO classification of cardiovascular diseases.

This chapter focuses on CHD that affect the blood vessels that supply the heart muscle, CeVD that disrupts the blood supply to the brain causing strokes (hemorrhagic or ischemic), and PAD that causes disruption of blood vessels supplying arms and legs. Although the pathogenesis of these diseases is not fully understood because of its complexity, a present working hypothesis of the role of infection in

N. Shimpi · A. Acharya (✉)
Center for Oral and Systemic Health, Marshfield Clinic Research Institute, Marshfield, WI, USA
e-mail: shimpi.neel@marshfieldresearch.org; acharya.amit@marshfieldresearch.org

R. Dart
Center for Human Genetics, Marshfield Clinic Research Institute, Marshfield, WI, USA
e-mail: dart.richard@marshfieldresearch.org

P. Umukoro
Department of Internal Medicine, Marshfield Clinic, Marshfield, WI, USA
e-mail: umukoro.peter@marshfieldclinic.org

A. Acharya et al. (eds.), *Integration of Medical and Dental Care and Patient Data*, Health Informatics, https://doi.org/10.1007/978-3-319-98298-4_6

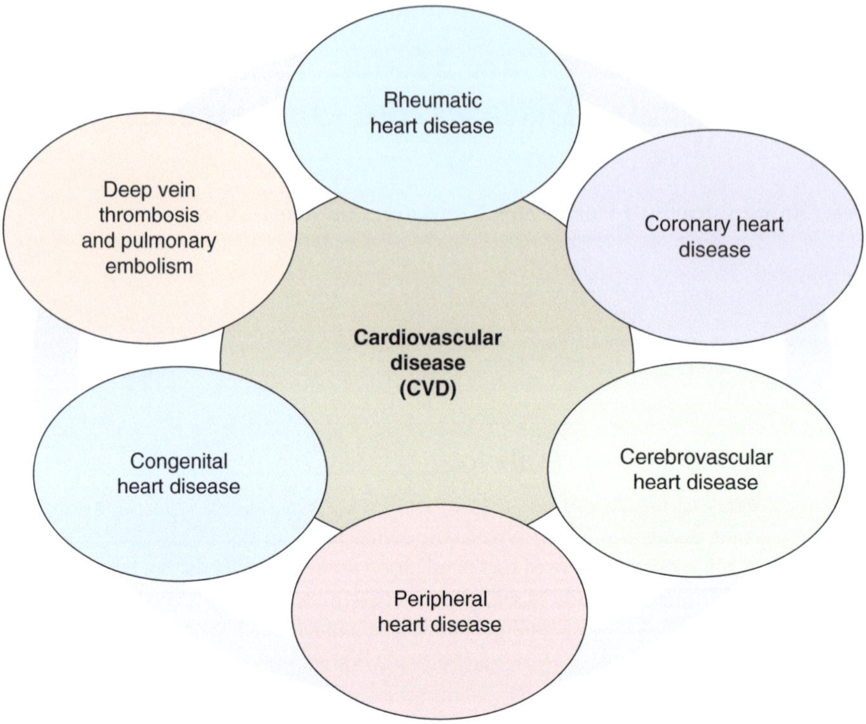

Fig. 6.1 WHO classification of cardiovascular diseases

CVDs has been proposed, in which infection increases the levels of inflammation leading to increased CVDs and CVD-related events (Dinakaran 2017; Rezaee-Zavareh et al. 2016; Zebrack and Anderson 2003).

6.2 Systemic Manifestations of Cardiovascular Diseases

Risk factors well established that are associated with CVD, especially cardiovascular and peripheral vascular forms, include: hypertension, hyperlipidemia, smoking, diabetes, and obesity. CVD and related end-organ damage may be initially asymptomatic but can manifest with findings on clinical examination such as hypertensive retinopathy, xanthoma in corneas and inner canthi of eyes due to hyperlipidemia and hypercholesterolemia, eruptive xanthomas on back, elbows, knees, and buttocks due to hypertriglyceridemia, and palmar xanthomas due to dysbetalipoproteinemia (Brewer et al. 1983; Saksena 2007). Additionally, elevated blood pressure, and such things as bruits heard over critical arterial beds, can lead to the clinical diagnosis of CVD, while clinical symptoms may be absent or subclinical in presentation. Usual symptoms may include shortness of breath or chest pain (angina) on exertion, or leg cramps induced with exercise. On the other hand, CeVD may manifest with signs and symptoms such as severe headache, hemiplegia, hemiparesis, confusion, loss of half vision, loss of balance, and loss of consciousness (Burchell et al. 1951; Kreutzer et al. 2011; Ohlsson et al. 2017).

More recently, the role of the metabolic syndrome has been associated with an increased risk for CVDs and Type 2 diabetes mellitus (Isomaa et al. 2001; Preil et al. 2017; Tortosa-Caparrós et al. 2017; Wilson et al. 1998).

6.3 Oral Manifestations

Oral manifestations can be indicative of underlying systemic diseases. Although the causative association between CVDs and oral health is not yet established, studies have associated some of the commonest forms of periodontal disease (PD) with CVDs (Goulart et al. 2017; Pihlstrom et al. 2005; St Sauver et al. 2017). The results of a study that determined the frequency and nature of oral manifestations secondary to CVDs revealed about 14% of patients manifested xerostomia followed by approximately 4% with lichenoid lesions such as lichen planus and 2% with dysgeusia (Habbab et al. 2010).

Patients receiving treatment of angiotensin converting enzyme inhibitors (ACEI) such as captopril or enalapril and diuretics such as furosemide may present with lichenoid reactions, loss of sensation, burning mouth sensation, loss of taste sensation, and xerostomia respectively (Cruz-Pamplona et al. 2011). Studies have shown that calcium channel blockers can increase the incidence of gingival hyperplasia (Critchlow 2017; Ikeda 2017).

6.4 Oral-Systemic (Cardiovascular) Connection

There are studies that have associated poor oral health with an increase in cardio metabolic risk factors, atherothrombotic/sclerotic disease, and mortality (Dietrich et al. 2017; González Navarro et al. 2017; Hatahira et al. 2017; Ionel et al. 2016; Joshy et al. 2016; Morita et al. 2010; Sanchez et al. 2017). Similarly, a Finnish study has described a lower risk of cardiovascular mortality for patients with filled teeth—a marker for better oral care (Meurman et al. 2004). Studies are being conducted to explore the underlying mechanisms and impact of oral health on CVDs (Dietrich et al. 2017; Ma et al. 2017; St Sauver et al. 2017; Vogtmann et al. 2017). Although there is considerable uncertainty regarding oral health and CVDs, some studies hypothesize that chronic infections and pro-inflammatory markers such as C-reactive protein and tumor necrosis factor may contribute to the pathogenesis of periodontal disease as well as CVDs (Beck et al. 2001; Marshe et al. 2017; Sara et al. 2017). The JUPITER trial exploring the role of high sensitivity C-reactive protein (hsCRP) in the association between inflammation and CVDs failed to show a major role of hsCRP (Ridker et al. 2003). However, an ongoing low-dose methotrexate trial to see if mild anti-inflammatory effects will reduce cardiovascular diseases is underway (Ridker 2013).

The oral microbiome has been shown to play an important role in altering the balance between health and disease (Sampaio-Maia et al. 2016). Interestingly, a study that characterized and compared the oral microbiome of patients with dental caries who had symptoms from coronary artery diseases (CADs) and those who did not show a bacterial diversity between the two cohorts. Out of 31 phyla that were found in all the samples, *Firmicutes*, *Proteobacteria*, *Fusobacteria*, *Bacteroidetes*, *Actinobacteria* and *Candidatus saccharibacteria* (*TM7*) constituted about 46% and 39%, 18% and 10%, 13% and 18%, 12% and 23%, 8% and 8%, and 2% and 3% among those with symptomatic CAD versus those who were asymptomatic respectively (Menon et al. 2017). The results of a recent cross sectional study showed that patients with peripheral arterial disease suffered from PD and loss of teeth (Aoyama et al. 2017). Another cross sectional study evaluated the relationship of tooth loss and periodontitis to prevalent coronary heart disease showing that patients with CVD had a greater incidence of periodontal attachment loss and eventually tooth loss (Elter et al. 2004; Holmstrup et al. 2017). In addition, the correlation was observed to be greater amongst patients who had missing teeth or who were edentulous (Okoro et al. 2005; Watt et al. 2012).

A recent study of patients exploring the relationship between maintenance of good oral health and patients developing infective endocarditis in patients with severe rheumatic heart disease showed that the plaque and gingival index scores were poor in about half of the patients (n = 44) (Maharaj and Vayej 2012). Several longitudinal studies have demonstrated that poor periodontal health can lead to cardiovascular events (DeStefano et al. 1993; Joshipura 2002; Lee et al. 2017; Mattila et al. 1995; Morrison et al. 1999). Amongst these longitudinal studies, one utilized a national sample of American adults (n = 9760) reporting that patients who had periodontitis had a 25% increased risk for coronary artery disease. This same study also showed that poor oral hygiene defined by the presence of dental debris and calculus was also associated with an increased risk of developing CHD (DeStefano et al. 1993). Another study that conducted a prospective follow-up of 214 participants showed that dental health along with the presence of diabetes, number of previous myocardial infarctions, and body mass index were significant predictors of cardiac events (Mattila et al. 1995).

6.5 Diagnostic Codes

Cardiovascular diagnostic ICD9 and ICD 10 codes are listed in Table 6.1. It is important to note the many classifications of the CVD subtypes.

A diagnostic code that includes periodontal disease (ICD9-523.8/ICD10-K05.6), edentulism (ICD9-525.50/ICD10-K08.109) and missing teeth (ICD9-525.10/ICD10-K08.409) as a complication of cardiovascular disease can be introduced.

6.6 Risk Assessment

There are now, several clinical tools which incorporate various risk factors associated with or causal to the development of CVDs (Bertoluci and Rocha 2017; Breunig et al. 2018; D'Agostino et al. 2008; DeFilippis et al. 2016; del Sol et al. 2001;

Table 6.1 ICD9/10 CM Codes for cardiovascular diseases

Diagnostic Codes	Codes	Description
ICD 9 CM	390–392	Acute rheumatic fever
ICD 10 CM	I00–I02	Acute rheumatic fever
ICD 9 CM	410	Acute myocardial infarction includes cardiac infarction, coronary embolism/occlusion/rupture/thrombosis
ICD 10 CM	I21	Acute myocardial infarction includes cardiac infarction, coronary embolism/occlusion/rupture/thrombosis
ICD 10 CM	I24	Other acute ischemic heart diseases
ICD 9 CM	414	Coronary atherosclerosis, aneurysms
ICD 10 CM	I25.1	Atherosclerotic heart disease
ICD 9 CM	421	Acute and subacute endocarditis
ICD 10 CM	I33	Acute and subacute endocarditis
ICD 9 CM	430–438	Cerebrovascular disease (Stroke of various types included here)
ICD 10 CM	I60–I69	Cerebrovascular disease (Stroke of various types included here)
ICD 9 CM	443	Peripheral vascular disease
ICD 10 CM	I73	Peripheral vascular disease
ICD 9 CM	440.21	Intermittent claudication
ICD 10 CM	I70.211	Intermittent claudication

Karmali et al. 2017; Collins and Altman 2012; Sarrafzadegan et al. 2017; Nambi et al. 2010; Nojiri and Daida 2017; Novo et al. 2017; Rajanandh et al. 2018; Richtering et al. 2017; Studziński et al. 2017; Vuruskan et al. 2017).

The "Framingham Risk Score" is valuable for use in primary care settings to estimate the risk of CVD events and for preventive care guidance. The risk assessment tool predicts a person's risk for developing CVD in the next 10 years (Wilson 2008). A general cardiovascular risk profile was developed by D'Agostino et al. using the 8491 Framingham study participants between the ages of 30 and 74 years (D'Agostino et al. 2008). The study used multivariate analysis by incorporating variables such as age, total cholesterol, high density lipids, systolic blood pressure, treatment for hypertension, smoking, and present status of diabetes. The algorithm developed was compared with the Framingham risk score and showed a good calibration and discrimination.

A subsequent study prospectively followed the Framingham Offspring cohort between the ages of 20 and 59 years to develop a 30-year prediction risk tool (Pencina et al. 2009). The results of the study showed that additional risk burden information was offered by the 30-year risk prediction that complemented the 10-year risk function tool.

Another study utilized a scoring system similar to the Framingham Score, and carotid intima-media thickness to predict the risk of developing future coronary heart disease and CVD (del Sol et al. 2001). A total of eight independent factors including previous myocardial infarction, stroke, diabetes mellitus, smoking, systolic and diastolic blood pressure, total cholesterol, and HDL levels were used. When the study used two variables such as age and gender the Receiver Operating Curve (ROC) was 0.65 (95% CI, 0.62–0.69) and it increased to 0.72 (95% CI, 0.69–0.75) after incorporating the eight factors displaying a correct prediction for 17% of the total study participants. When the variable carotid intima-media thickness was added to age and gender the ROC markedly increased to 0.71 (95% CI, 0.68–0.74) and 14% of all the study participants were predicted correctly (del Sol et al. 2001).

The Quebec Cardiovascular study was conducted to investigate the association between large and small low-density lipoproteins and long term ischemic heart disease. The study observed that the large LDL subfraction was not associated with an increased risk of Ischemic Heart Disease (IHD) in men and that the cardiovascular risk attributable to variations in the LDL size phenotype was largely related to markers of a preferential accumulation of small dense LDL particles (Després et al. 2000).

Studies have shown that the risk of developing coronary heart disease increases five- to eightfold in women with systemic lupus erythematosus (SLE) (Bruce et al. 2003; Manzi et al. 1997). Bruce et al. conducted a case control study in women with SLE and assessed the CHD risk factors in that cohort (Bruce et al. 2003). A total number of 250 cases (ages 44.8 ± 12) and an equal number of controls (44.3 ± 15) were included in the study. The authors concluded that women with SLE display a range of detectable CHD risk factors such as hypertension, diabetes, high low density lipids, high total triglycerides, and homocysteine levels.

6.7 Systems Biology: Genomics, Proteomics, Microbiomics, Phenotypes

Several genes associated with CVDs have been identified (O'Donnell and Nabel 2008, 2011). These have varied patterns of inheritance. Studies have assembled the various cardiovascular variants using genotyping arrays, statistical methods, and haplotype maps showing the polygenic nature of CVDs (C. J. O'Donnell and Nabel 2008). Many genome wide association studies (GWAS) have reported genetic variants of CVDs in the form of peripheral arterial disease, myocardial infarction, stroke, and atrial fibrillation (Manolio et al. 2008). The meta-analysis involving 14 studies and 22,233 cases (patients suffering from coronary artery disease (CAD)) and 64,762 controls identified 13 loci associated with CADs. This study also reported ABO and ADAMTS7 were associated with coronary atherosclerosis (Schunkert et al. 2011). Another study showed that mutations in DNMT3A, TET2, ASXL1 and JAK2 were associated with coronary heart disease and the presence of clonal hematopoiesis of indeterminate potential that doubled the risk of CVD (Jaiswal et al. 2017). It is evident that CVD is strongly associated with multiple genomic risk factors. Mendelian randomization studies have shown a causal association between low density lipid and CADs (Linsel-Nitschke et al. 2008).

Studies have shown that proteomes of cardiac muscle reflect the various CVDs (Arrell et al. 2006). Studies have attempted to create databases of 2-D gels with an inventory of proteins that help in obtaining information for the proteomic studies (Corbett et al. 1995; Li et al. 1999). The polygenic nature of CVDs adds to the complex nature of the many co-variables often seen in these populations. Much remains to be defined as to their respective roles in the development of CVDs.

6.8 Treatment

Identifying patients with an increased risk of cardiovascular events is vital. The resultant complications of CVDs still remain the principal cause of global deaths (Fuster and Kelly 2010; Gaziano et al. 2006; Jung and Choi 2014; Low Wang et al. 2016).

According to the National Heart, Lung, and Blood Institute the main goal of treatment is to reduce the risk of CVDs events. These include preventing myocardial infarctions, reducing atherosclerosis, adopting healthy eating behaviors, maintaining healthy weight, participating in physical activities, and quitting. The main focus of treatment for CVDs is directed towards emergency antithrombotic therapy and stroke treatment (NHLBI 2018). The Centers for Disease Control and Prevention recommends reducing the risk of CVDS by adopting healthy lifestyle changes (CDC 2018).

Because it has been demonstrated that periodontal disease may be an independent risk factor for CVD, alteration in the oral bacterial level by incorporating good oral hygiene behavior may help in reducing the risk of developing CVDs (Karnoutsos et al. 2008; Lang et al. 1973; Zhang et al. 2017).

6.9 Interdisciplinary Care Team

The complex nature of CVD prevention implies a team-based approach to patient care management and may include primary care physicians, cardiologists, general dentists, periodontists, clinic nurse specialists, physician assistants, occupational therapists, mental health professionals, social workers and case managers, dieticians, dental hygienists, exercise physiologists, nurse practitioners, pharmacists, nutritionists and medical assistants. Each can play a direct/indirect role in case management of patients with oral hygiene issues and CVDs.

6.10 Guidelines

The American Heart Association (AHA) has laid down some guidelines on assessment of cardiovascular risk that provide clear recommendations for estimating the heart disease risk (ACCF/AHA 2010; AHA 2018; Demmer and Desvarieux 2006; Goff et al. 2014; Goldstein et al. 2006). Epidemiological evidence shows that periodontitis may increase the risk for future CVDs suggesting periodontal treatment as a preventive measure for developing CVDs (Demmer and Desvarieux 2006; Dietrich et al. 2017; Merchant and Virani 2017; Tonetti et al. 2013). The AHA recommends greater emphasis on improved access to dental care and oral health in patients with underlying cardiac conditions (Fuster and Kelly 2010; Fuster 2011; Lamster and Eaves 2011; U.S. Department of Health and Human Services Oral Health Coordinating Committee 2016; Wilson et al. 2007).

6.11 Existing Gaps and Recommendations

The exact role and mechanisms involved in oral/systemic health, here specifically focusing on CVDs, requires more research around the pathogenesis and the role of oral diseases in the development of CVDs. Although evidence shows an association between oral health and CVDs, the exact cause and effect, if any, remains to be clarified. If the presence of dental diseases becomes a proven risk factor, there will be the need to redefine CVDs that include 'oral hygiene' as one of the clinical components in CVD preventive measures. Until a proven direct connection is found, oral hygiene remains an important part of general overall hygienic practices.

6.12 Technology Implications

The role of technology is certain to improve and aid in clinical decision making through a variety of decision support systems, educational brochures, and web applications which should help in improving decision making quality and enhancing shared decision making. Alterations in present CVD prevention guidelines in which oral hygiene becomes a recognized component should also lead to better risk assessment tools used to predict the risk to a patient for CVDs.

6.12.1 Electronic Health Records

Apart from maintaining the electronic version of patients' medical clinical data, the EHRs support care-related activity directly or indirectly including evidence-based decision support, quality management, and outcomes reporting (Capó-Lugo et al. 2017; Faiola and Holden 2017; Kern et al. 2013). Having CVDs and periodontal registries will help the care team to track the number of interventions and clinical parameters important in the management of CVDs. This will improve the disease management process and increase the quality of care.

Implementing data quality measures for healthcare delivery by developing dashboards for the healthcare providers will enable healthcare providers to instantly quantify treatment outcomes, patient's perceptions, population health, and efficient use of health care resources (Hegde et al. 2017). Using computer assisted applications, more personalized and tailored information can be made available for the end users.

6.13 Ontology

Ontology in healthcare has facilitated the development of knowledge representation applications such as ontology driven decision support tools for chest pain risk assessment (Farooq et al. 2012). CVDs are diseases of a subdivision of the hemolymphoid system (MGI 2018). Study results that examined alterations in cardiac gene expression patterns in the rat model (Zucker Diabetic Fatty rats) showed significant upregulation of 36 genes and down-regulation of 49 genes, thus, demonstrating that the metabolic syndrome significantly alters cardiac gene expression (Sárközy et al. 2013).

6.14 Care Plan

There needs to be awareness among healthcare providers of the association of CVDs and oral health. The dental and medical providers play an active and an important role in communicating clinical management of oral and systemic health. A proper referral mechanism will play a significant role in delivering this interdisciplinary care.

Dental providers should check for oral health and look for the symptoms of CVDs. Dental providers should screen for patients who are at a risk of developing CVD events (Glick and Greenberg 2005). Medical providers should evaluate the patient's oral cavity for their oral status. Oral health education should be provided to all the patients.

6.15 Recommendations on Dental Diagnosis of CVDs

- Dental care providers need to be aware of the connection that may exist between CVDs and oral health. They may wish to consider incorporating patient education surrounding oral and systemic health including CVDs during their dental practice.
- To aid in the awareness of the oral and CVD connection, guidelines for dental providers will serve as a tool to promote consistent, comprehensive, and preventive CVD care that includes oral health.
- Educating patients about oral and systemic health involving CVDs should be a part of the dental provider's training process.

References

ACCF/AHA. Guideline for assessment of cardiovascular risk in asymptomatic adults. American College of Cardiology Foundation, (November), 11–24; 2010. doi:https://doi.org/10.2214/ajr.11.6758

AHA. The American Heart Association's diet and lifestyle recommendations. 2018. http://www.heart.org/HEARTORG/HealthyLiving/HealthyEating/Nutrition/The-American-Heart-Associations-Diet-and-Lifestyle-Recommendations_UCM_305855_Article.jsp#.Wzbe4K2Wxok. Accessed 29 June 2018.

American Heart Association (AHA). Heart disease and stroke statistics 2017 at-a-glance. AHA; 2017. https://healthmetrics.heart.org/wp-content/uploads/2017/06/Heart-Disease-and-Stroke-Statistics-2017-ucm_491265.pdf

Aoyama N, Suzuki J, Kobayashi N, Hanatani T, Ashigaki N, Yoshida A, et al. Periodontitis deteriorates peripheral arterial disease in Japanese population via enhanced systemic inflammation. Heart Vessels. 2017;32(11):1314–9. https://doi.org/10.1007/s00380-017-1003-6.
Arrell K, Neverova I, Van Eyk J. Cardiovascular proteomics. Circulation. 2006:65–74. https://doi.org/10.1007/0-387-23329-6_3.
Beck JD, Elter JR, Heiss G, Couper D, Mauriello SM, Offenbacher S. Relationship of periodontal disease to carotid artery intima-media wall thickness: the atherosclerosis risk in communities (ARIC) study. Arterioscler Thromb Vasc Biol. 2001;21(11):1816–22. http://www.ncbi.nlm.nih.gov/pubmed/11701471
Bertoluci M, Rocha V. Cardiovascular risk assessment in patients with diabetes. Diabetol Metab Syndr. 2017;9:25. https://doi.org/10.1186/s13098-017-0225-1.
Breunig M, Kleinert S, Lehmann S, Kneitz C, Feuchtenberger M, Tony H, et al. Simple screening tools predict death and cardiovascular events in patients with rheumatic disease. Scand J Rheumatol. 2018;47(2):102–9. https://doi.org/10.1080/03009742.2017.1337924.
Brewer H, Zech L, Gregg R, Schwartz D, Schaefer E. NIH conference. Type III hyperlipoproteinemia: diagnosis, molecular defects, pathology, and treatment. Ann Intern Med. 1983;98(5 Pt 1):623–40. http://www.ncbi.nlm.nih.gov/pubmed/6846977
Bruce I, Urowitz M, Gladman D, Ibañez D, Steiner G. Risk factors for coronary heart disease in women with systemic lupus erythematosus: the Toronto Risk Factor Study. Arthritis Rheum. 2003;48(11):3159–67. https://doi.org/10.1002/art.11296.
Burchell H, Allen E, Moersch F. Clinical manifestations of arteriosclerosis. JAMA. 1951;147(16):1511. https://doi.org/10.1001/jama.1951.03670330003002.
Capó-Lugo C, Kho A, O'Dwyer L, Rosenman M. Data sharing and data registries in physical medicine and rehabilitation. PM&R. 2017;9(5):S59–74. https://doi.org/10.1016/j.pmrj.2017.04.003.
CDC. CDC - DHDSP - Heart Disease Prevention: What you can do. 2018. https://www.cdc.gov/heartdisease/what_you_can_do.htm. Accessed 29 June 2018.
Collins G, Altman D. Predicting the 10 year risk of cardiovascular disease in the United Kingdom: independent and external validation of an updated version of QRISK2. BMJ. 2012;344:e4181. https://doi.org/10.1136/BMJ.E4181.
Corbett J, Wheeler C, Dunn M. Coelectrophoresis of cardiac tissue from human, dog, rat and mouse: towards the establishment of an integrated two-dimensional protein database. Electrophoresis. 1995;16(1):1524–9. https://doi.org/10.1002/elps.11501601252.
Critchlow D. Part 3: Impact of systemic conditions and medications on oral health. Br J Commun Nurs. 2017;22(4):181–90. https://doi.org/10.12968/bjcn.2017.22.4.181.
Cruz-Pamplona M, Jimenez-Soriano Y, Sarrion-Perez M. Dental considerations in patients with heart disease. J Clin Exp Dent. 2011;3(2):e97–105. https://doi.org/10.4317/jced.3.e97.
D'Agostino R, Vasan R, Pencina M, Wolf P, Cobain M, Massaro J, Kannel W. General cardiovascular risk profile for use in primary care: the Framingham Heart Study. Circulation. 2008;117(6):743–53. https://doi.org/10.1161/CIRCULATIONAHA.107.699579.
DeFilippis A, Young R, McEvoy J, Michos E, Sandfort V, Kronmal R, et al. Risk score overestimation: the impact of individual cardiovascular risk factors and preventive therapies on the performance of the American Heart Association-American College of Cardiology-Atherosclerotic Cardiovascular Disease risk score in a modern multi-ethnic cohort. Eur Heart J. 2016;38(8):ehw301. https://doi.org/10.1093/eurheartj/ehw301.
del Sol A, Moons K, Hollander M, Hofman A, Koudstaal P, Grobbee D, et al. Is carotid intima-media thickness useful in cardiovascular disease risk assessment? The Rotterdam Study. Stroke. 2001;32(7):1532–8. http://www.ncbi.nlm.nih.gov/pubmed/11441197
Demmer R, Desvarieux M. Periodontal infections and cardiovascular disease: the heart of the matter. J Am Dent Assoc. 2006;137(Suppl):14S–20S; quiz 38S. http://www.ncbi.nlm.nih.gov/pubmed/17012731
Després J, Lemieux I, Dagenais G, Cantin B, Lamarche B. HDL-cholesterol as a marker of coronary heart disease risk: the Québec cardiovascular study. Atherosclerosis. 2000;153(2):263–72. http://www.ncbi.nlm.nih.gov/pubmed/11164415
DeStefano F, Anda R, Kahn H, Williamson D, Russell C. Dental disease and risk of coronary heart disease and mortality. BMJ. 1993;306(6879):688–91. http://www.ncbi.nlm.nih.gov/pubmed/8471920

Dietrich T, Webb I, Stenhouse L, Pattni A, Ready D, Wanyonyi K, et al. Evidence summary: the relationship between oral and cardiovascular disease. Br Dent J. 2017;222(5):381–5. https://doi.org/10.1038/sj.bdj.2017.224.

Dinakaran V. Microbial translocation in the pathogenesis of cardiovascular diseases: a microbiome perspective. J Cardiol Curr Res. 2017;8(6) https://doi.org/10.15406/jccr.2017.08.00305.

Elter J, Champagne C, Offenbacher S, Beck J. Relationship of periodontal disease and tooth loss to prevalence of coronary heart disease. J Periodontol. 2004;75(6):782–90. https://doi.org/10.1902/jop.2004.75.6.782.

Faiola A, Holden R. Consumer health informatics: empowering healthy-living-seekers through mHealth. Prog Cardiovasc Dis. 2017;59(5):479–86. https://doi.org/10.1016/j.pcad.2016.12.006.

Farooq K, Hussain A, Leslie S, Eckl C, MacRae C, Slack W. An ontology driven and Bayesian network based cardiovascular decision support framework. Berlin: Springer; 2012. p. 31–41. https://doi.org/10.1007/978-3-642-31561-9_4.

Fuster V. AHA guidelines and scientific statements handbook. 1st ed. Chichester: Wiley; 2011. https://books.google.com/books?id=w5VHKxCO6CMC&pg=PT16&lpg=PT16&dq=Aha+guidelines+and+scientific+statements+handbook+(1st+edition).&source=bl&ots=OuPchiJ7nl&sig=aWSYYLkoLQ1HXRAan5FqhJEC350&hl=en&sa=X&ved=0ahUKEwjfp8jeoPrbAhVwtlkKHc19AhgQ6AEIXDAH#v=onepage

Fuster V, Kelly B. Epidemiology of cardiovascular disease - promoting cardiovascular health in the developing world - NCBI Bookshelf. Washington, DC: National Academies Press (US); 2010. https://www.ncbi.nlm.nih.gov/books/NBK45688/

Gaziano T, Reddy K, Paccaud F, Horton S, Chaturvedi V. Cardiovascular disease. Disease control priorities in developing countries. The International Bank for Reconstruction and Development/The World Bank; 2006. http://www.ncbi.nlm.nih.gov/pubmed/21250342

Glick M, Greenberg B. The potential role of dentists in identifying patients' risk of experiencing coronary heart disease events. J Am Dent Assoc. 2005;136(11):1541–6. https://doi.org/10.14219/JADA.ARCHIVE.2005.0084.

Goff D, Lloyd-Jones D, Bennett G, Coady S, D'Agostino R, Gibbons R, et al. 2013 ACC/AHA guideline on the assessment of cardiovascular risk: a report of the American College of Cardiology/American Heart Association Task Force on Practice Guidelines. Circulation. 2014;129(25 Suppl 2):S49–73. https://doi.org/10.1161/01.cir.0000437741.48606.98.

Goldstein L, Adams R, Alberts M, Appel L, Brass L, Bushnell CD, et al. Primary prevention of ischemic stroke: a guideline from the American Heart Association/American Stroke Association Stroke Council: Cosponsored by the Atherosclerotic Peripheral Vascular Disease Interdisciplinary Working Group; Cardiovascular Nursing Council; Clinical Cardiology Council; Nutrition, Physical Activity, and Metabolism Council; and the Quality of Care and Outcomes Research Interdisciplinary Working Group: The American Academy of Neurology affirms the value of this guideline. Stroke. 2006;37(6):1583–633. https://doi.org/10.1161/01.STR.0000223048.70103.F1.

González Navarro B, Pintó Sala X, Jané Salas E. Relación entre la enfermedad cardiovascular y la afección dental. Revisión sistemática. Med Clin. 2017;149(5):211–6. https://doi.org/10.1016/j.medcli.2017.05.010.

Goulart A, Armani F, Arap A, Nejm T, Andrade J, Bufarah HB, Dezen D. Relationship between periodontal disease and cardiovascular risk factors among young and middle-aged Brazilians. Cross-sectional study. Sao Paulo Med J. 2017;135(3):226–33. https://doi.org/10.1590/1516-3180.2016.0357300117.

Habbab K, Moles D, Porter S. Potential oral manifestations of cardiovascular drugs. Oral Dis. 2010;16(8):769–73. https://doi.org/10.1111/j.1601-0825.2010.01686.x.

Hatahira H, Abe J, Hane Y, Matsui T, Sasaoka S, Motooka Y, et al. Drug-induced gingival hyperplasia: a retrospective study using spontaneous reporting system databases. J Pharm Health Care Sci. 2017;3:19. https://doi.org/10.1186/s40780-017-0088-5.

Hegde H, Steinmetz A, Theisen J, Koralkar R, Finnamore J, Halstead S, et al. Dental quality analytics: dental measures and provider performance dashboard. J Dent Res. 2017;96:566.

Holmstrup P, Damgaard C, Olsen I, Klinge B, Flyvbjerg A, Nielsen C, Hansen P. Comorbidity of periodontal disease: two sides of the same coin? An introduction for the clinician. J Oral Microbiol. 2017;9(1):1332710. https://doi.org/10.1080/20002297.2017.1332710.

Ikeda K. Drug-induced oral complications. Atlas Oral Maxillofac Surg Clin North Am. 2017;25(2):127–32. https://doi.org/10.1016/j.cxom.2017.04.005.

Ionel A, Lucaciu O, Bondor C, Moga M, Ilea A, Feurdean C, et al. Assessment of the relationship between periodontal disease and cardiovascular disorders: a questionnaire-based study. Clujul Med (1957). 2016;89(4):534–41. https://doi.org/10.15386/cjmed-639.

Isomaa B, Almgren P, Tuomi T, Forsén B, Lahti K, Nissén M, et al. Cardiovascular morbidity and mortality associated with the metabolic syndrome. Diabetes Care. 2001;24(4):683–9. http://www.ncbi.nlm.nih.gov/pubmed/11315831

Jaiswal S, Natarajan P, Silver A, Gibson C, Bick A, Shvartz E, et al. Clonal hematopoiesis and risk of atherosclerotic cardiovascular disease. N Engl J Med. 2017;377(2):111–21. https://doi.org/10.1056/NEJMoa1701719.

Joshipura K. The relationship between oral conditions and ischemic stroke and peripheral vascular disease. J Am Dent Assoc. 2002;133(Suppl):23S–30S. https://doi.org/10.14219/JADA.ARCHIVE.2002.0373.

Joshy G, Arora M, Korda R, Chalmers J, Banks E. Is poor oral health a risk marker for incident cardiovascular disease hospitalisation and all-cause mortality? Findings from 172 630 participants from the prospective 45 and Up Study. BMJ Open. 2016;6(8):e012386. https://doi.org/10.1136/bmjopen-2016-012386.

Jung U, Choi M. Obesity and its metabolic complications: the role of adipokines and the relationship between obesity, inflammation, insulin resistance, dyslipidemia and nonalcoholic fatty liver disease. Int J Mol Sci. 2014;15(4):6184–223. https://doi.org/10.3390/ijms15046184.

Karmali K, Persell S, Perel P, Lloyd-Jones D, Berendsen M, Huffman M. Risk scoring for the primary prevention of cardiovascular disease. Cochrane Database Syst Rev. 2017;3:CD006887. https://doi.org/10.1002/14651858.CD006887.pub4.

Karnoutsos K, Papastergiou P, Stefanidis S, Vakaloudi A. Periodontitis as a risk factor for cardiovascular disease: the role of anti-phosphorylcholine and anti-cardiolipin antibodies. Hippokratia. 2008;12(3):144–9. http://www.ncbi.nlm.nih.gov/pubmed/18923669

Kern L, Barrón Y, Dhopeshwarkar R, Edwards A, Kaushal R, HITEC Investigators. Electronic health records and ambulatory quality of care. J Gen Intern Med. 2013;28(4):496–503. https://doi.org/10.1007/s11606-012-2237-8.

Kreutzer J, Caplan B, DeLuca J. Encyclopedia of clinical neuropsychology. New York: Springer; 2011.

Lamster I, Eaves K. A model for dental practice in the 21st century. Am J Public Health. 2011;101(10):1825–30. https://doi.org/10.2105/AJPH.2011.300234.

Lang N, Cumming B, Löe H. Toothbrushing frequency as it relates to plaque development and gingival health. J Periodontol. 1973;44(7):396–405. https://doi.org/10.1902/jop.1973.44.7.396.

Lee J, Oh J, Youk T, Jeong S, Kim Y, Choi S. Association between periodontal disease and non-communicable diseases: a 12-year longitudinal health-examinee cohort study in South Korea. Medicine. 2017;96(26):e7398. https://doi.org/10.1097/MD.0000000000007398.

Li X, Pleißner K, Scheler C, Regitz-Zagrosek V, Salnikow J, Jungblut P. A two-dimensional electrophoresis database of rat heart proteins. Electrophoresis. 1999;20(4–5):891–7. https://doi.org/10.1002/(SICI)1522-2683(19990101)20:4/5<891::AID-ELPS891>3.0.CO;2-2.

Linsel-Nitschke P, Götz A, Erdmann J, Braenne I, Braund P, Hengstenberg C, et al. Lifelong reduction of LDL-cholesterol related to a common variant in the LDL-receptor gene decreases the risk of coronary artery disease—a Mendelian randomisation study. PLoS One. 2008;3(8):e2986. https://doi.org/10.1371/journal.pone.0002986.

Low Wang C, Hess C, Hiatt W, Goldfine A. Clinical update: Cardiovascular disease in diabetes mellitus: atherosclerotic cardiovascular disease and heart failure in Type 2 diabetes mellitus - mechanisms, management, and clinical considerations. Circulation. 2016;133(24):2459–502. https://doi.org/10.1161/CIRCULATIONAHA.116.022194.

Ma Y, Huang T, Lin M, Chen P, Chen M. Early detection of oral health status and cardiometabolic risk factors among reproductive-aged women in rural areas: a cross-sectional study. Eur J Cardiovasc Nurs. 2017;16(6):484–91. https://doi.org/10.1177/1474515116688386.

Maharaj B, Vayej A. Oral health of patients with severe rheumatic heart disease. Cardiovasc J Afr. 2012;23(6):336–9. https://doi.org/10.5830/CVJA-2012-009.
Manolio T, Brooks L, Collins F. A HapMap harvest of insights into the genetics of common disease. J Clin Investig. 2008;118(5):1590–605. https://doi.org/10.1172/JCI34772.
Manzi S, Meilahn E, Rairie J, Conte C, Medsger T, Jansen-McWilliams L, et al. Age-specific incidence rates of myocardial infarction and angina in women with systemic lupus erythematosus: comparison with the Framingham Study. Am J Epidemiol. 1997;145(5):408–15. http://www.ncbi.nlm.nih.gov/pubmed/9048514
Marshe V, Pira S, Mantere O, Bosche B, Looper K, Herrmann N, et al. C-reactive protein and cardiovascular risk in bipolar disorder patients: a systematic review. Prog Neuropsychopharmacol Biol Psychiatry. 2017;79(Pt B):442–51. https://doi.org/10.1016/j.pnpbp.2017.07.026.
Mattila K, Valtonen V, Nieminen M, Huttunen J. Dental infection and the risk of new coronary events: prospective study of patients with documented coronary artery disease. Clin Infect Dis. 1995;20(3):588–92. http://www.ncbi.nlm.nih.gov/pubmed/7756480
Menon T, Gopalakrishnan S, Balasubramanian R, Justin S. Characterisation of the human oral microbiome in patients with coronary artery disease using next-generation sequencing of 16SrRNA amplicons. Indian J Med Microbiol. 2017;35(1):101. https://doi.org/10.4103/ijmm.IJMM_16_370.
Merchant A, Virani S. Evaluating periodontal treatment to prevent cardiovascular disease: challenges and possible solutions. Curr Atheroscler Rep. 2017;19(1):4. https://doi.org/10.1007/s11883-017-0640-7.
Meurman J, Sanz M, Janket S. Oral health, atherosclerosis, and cardiovascular disease. Crit Rev Oral Biol Med. 2004;15(6):403–13. http://www.ncbi.nlm.nih.gov/pubmed/15574681
MGI. Cardiovascular system disease Disease Ontology Browser - DOID:1287. 2018. http://www.informatics.jax.org/disease/DOID:1287. Accessed 29 June 2018.
Morita T, Yamazaki Y, Mita A, Takada K, Seto M, Nishinoue N, et al. A cohort study on the association between periodontal disease and the development of metabolic syndrome. J Periodontol. 2010;81(4):512–9. https://doi.org/10.1902/jop.2010.090594.
Morrison H, Ellison L, Taylor G. Periodontal disease and risk of fatal coronary heart and cerebrovascular diseases. J Cardiovasc Risk. 1999;6(1):7–11. http://www.ncbi.nlm.nih.gov/pubmed/10197286
Nambi V, Chambless L, Folsom A, He M, Hu Y, Mosley T, et al. Carotid intima-media thickness and presence or absence of plaque improves prediction of coronary heart disease risk. J Am Coll Cardiol. 2010;55(15):1600–7. https://doi.org/10.1016/j.jacc.2009.11.075.
NHLBI. Coronary heart disease. National Heart, Lung, and Blood Institute (NHLBI); 2018. https://www.nhlbi.nih.gov/health-topics/coronary-heart-disease. Accessed 30 June 2018.
Nojiri S, Daida H. Atherosclerotic cardiovascular risk in Japan. Jpn Clin Med. 2017;8:117906601771271. https://doi.org/10.1177/1179066017712713.
Novo J, Hermida A, Ortega M, Barreira N, Penedo M, López J, Calvo C. Hydra: a web-based system for cardiovascular analysis, diagnosis and treatment. Comput Methods Programs Biomed. 2017;139(C):61–81. https://doi.org/10.1016/j.cmpb.2016.10.019.
O'Donnell C, Nabel E. Cardiovascular genomics, personalized medicine, and the National Heart, Lung, and Blood Institute: Part I: The beginning of an era. Circ Cardiovasc Genet. 2008;1(1):51–7. https://doi.org/10.1161/CIRCGENETICS.108.813337.
O'Donnell C, Nabel E. Genomics of cardiovascular disease. N Engl J Med. 2011;365:2098–109. https://www.nejm.org/doi/pdf/10.1056/NEJMra1105239
Ohlsson C, Bygdell M, Sondén A, Jern C, Rosengren A, Kindblom J. BMI increase through puberty and adolescence is associated with risk of adult stroke. Neurology. 2017;89(4):363–9. https://doi.org/10.1212/WNL.0000000000004158.
Okoro C, Balluz L, Eke P, Ajani U, Strine T, Town M, et al. Tooth loss and heart disease. Am J Prev Med. 2005;29(5):50–6. https://doi.org/10.1016/j.amepre.2005.07.006.
Pencina M, D'Agostino R, Larson M, Massaro J, Vasan R. Predicting the 30-year risk of cardiovascular disease: the Framingham Heart Study. Circulation. 2009;119(24):3078–84. https://doi.org/10.1161/CIRCULATIONAHA.108.816694.

Pihlstrom B, Michalowicz B, Johnson N. Periodontal diseases. Lancet. 2005;366(9499):1809–20. https://doi.org/10.1016/S0140-6736(05)67728-8.
Preil S, Thorsen A, Christiansen A, Poulsen M, Karsdal M, Leeming D, Rasmussen L. Is cardiovascular disease in patients with diabetes associated with serum levels of MMP-2, LOX, and the elastin degradation products ELM and ELM-2? Scand J Clin Lab Invest. 2017;77(7):493–7. https://doi.org/10.1080/00365513.2017.1346822.
Rajanandh M, Suresh S, Manobala K, Nandhakumar R, Jaswanthi G, Neha S. Prediction of cardiovascular risk in cancer patients of South India using WHO/ISH risk prediction charts and Framingham score – a prospective study. J Oncol Pharm Pract. 2018;24(5):354–8. https://doi.org/10.1177/1078155217707334.
Rezaee-Zavareh M, Tohidi M, Sabouri A, Ramezani-Binabaj M, Sadeghi-Ghahrodi M, Einollahi B. Infectious and coronary artery disease. ARYA Atherosclerosis. 2016;12(1):41–9. http://www.ncbi.nlm.nih.gov/pubmed/27114736
Richtering S, Hyun K, Neubeck L, Coorey G, Chalmers J, Usherwood T, et al. eHealth literacy: predictors in a population with moderate-to-high cardiovascular risk. JMIR Human Factors. 2017;4(1):e4. https://doi.org/10.2196/humanfactors.6217.
Ridker P. Moving beyond JUPITER: will inhibiting inflammation reduce vascular event rates? Curr Atheroscler Rep. 2013;15(1):295. https://doi.org/10.1007/s11883-012-0295-3.
Ridker P, Buring J, Cook N, Rifai N. C-reactive protein, the metabolic syndrome, and risk of incident cardiovascular events: an 8-year follow-up of 14 719 initially healthy American women. Circulation. 2003;107(3):391–7. http://www.ncbi.nlm.nih.gov/pubmed/12551861
Saksena F. Local and systemic manifestations of cardiovascular disease. In: Ranganathan N, Sivaciyan V, Saksena FB, editors. The art and science of cardiac physical examination, vol. 1; 2007. p. 361–95. https://doi.org/10.1007/978-1-59745-023-2_11.
Sampaio-Maia B, Caldas I, Pereira M, Pérez-Mongiovi D, Araujo R. The oral microbiome in health and its implication in oral and systemic diseases. Adv Appl Microbiol. 2016;97:171–210. https://doi.org/10.1016/bs.aambs.2016.08.002.
Sanchez P, Everett B, Salamonson Y, Ajwani S, Bhole S, Bishop J, et al. Oral health and cardiovascular care: perceptions of people with cardiovascular disease. PLoS One. 2017;12(7):e0181189. https://doi.org/10.1371/journal.pone.0181189.
Sara J, Prasad M, Zhang M, Lennon R, Herrmann J, Lerman LO, Lerman A. High-sensitivity C-reactive protein is an independent marker of abnormal coronary vasoreactivity in patients with non-obstructive coronary artery disease. Am Heart J. 2017;190:1–11. https://doi.org/10.1016/j.ahj.2017.02.035.
Sárközy M, Zvara A, Gyémánt N, Fekete V, Kocsis G, Pipis J, et al. Metabolic syndrome influences cardiac gene expression pattern at the transcript level in male ZDF rats. Cardiovasc Diabetol. 2013;12:16. https://doi.org/10.1186/1475-2840-12-16.
Sarrafzadegan N, Hassannejad R, Marateb H, Talaei M, Sadeghi M, Roohafza H, et al. PARS risk charts: a 10-year study of risk assessment for cardiovascular diseases in Eastern Mediterranean Region. PLoS One. 2017;12(12):e0189389. https://doi.org/10.1371/journal.pone.0189389.
Schunkert H, König IR, Kathiresan S, Reilly MP, Assimes T, Holm H, et al. Large-scale association analysis identifies 13 new susceptibility loci for coronary artery disease. Nat Genet. 2011;43(4):333–8. https://doi.org/10.1038/ng.784.
St Sauver J, Carr A, Yawn B, Grossardt B, Bock-Goodner C, Klein L, et al. Linking medical and dental health record data: a partnership with the Rochester Epidemiology Project. BMJ Open. 2017;7(3):e012528. https://doi.org/10.1136/bmjopen-2016-012528.
Studziński K, Tomasik T, Krzyszton J, Jóźwiak J, Windak A. Effect of using cardiovascular risk scoring in routine risk assessment in primary prevention of cardiovascular disease: protocol for an overview of systematic reviews. BMJ Open. 2017;7(3):e014206. https://doi.org/10.1136/bmjopen-2016-014206.
Tonetti M, Van Dyke T, Working Group 1 of the Joint EFP/AAP Workshop. Periodontitis and atherosclerotic cardiovascular disease: consensus report of the Joint EFP/AAP Workshop on Periodontitis and Systemic Diseases. J Periodontol. 2013;84(4 Suppl):S24–9. https://doi.org/10.1902/jop.2013.1340019.

Tortosa-Caparrós E, Navas-Carrillo D, Marín F, Orenes-Piñero E. Anti-inflammatory effects of omega 3 and omega 6 polyunsaturated fatty acids in cardiovascular disease and metabolic syndrome. Crit Rev Food Sci Nutr. 2017;57(16):3421–9. https://doi.org/10.1080/10408398.2015.1126549.

U.S. Department of Health and Human Services Oral Health Coordinating Committee. U.S. Department of Health and Human Services oral health strategic framework, 2014–2017. Public Health Rep. 2016;131(2):242–57. http://www.ncbi.nlm.nih.gov/pubmed/26957659

Vogtmann E, Etemadi A, Kamangar F, Islami F, Roshandel G, Poustchi H, et al. Oral health and mortality in the Golestan Cohort Study. Int J Epidemiol. 2017;46(6):2028–35. https://doi.org/10.1093/ije/dyx056.

Vuruskan E, Saracoglu E, Polat M, Duzen I. Prediction of coronary artery disease severity in lower extremity artery disease patients: a correlation study of TASC II classification, Syntax and Syntax II scores. Cardiol J. 2017;24(5):495–501. https://doi.org/10.5603/CJ.a2017.0033.

Watt R, Tsakos G, de Oliveira C, Hamer M. Tooth loss and cardiovascular disease mortality risk--results from the Scottish Health Survey. PLoS One. 2012;7(2):e30797. https://doi.org/10.1371/journal.pone.0030797.

WHO. Cardiovascular diseases (CVDs). 2017. http://www.who.int/news-room/fact-sheets/detail/cardiovascular-diseases-(cvds). Accessed 30 June 2018.

WHO. Types of cardiovascular disease. 2018. http://www.who.int/cardiovascular_diseases/en/cvd_atlas_01_types.pdf

Wilson P. Cardiovascular risk assessment-where are we going? Prev Cardiol. 2008;11(3):183–4. https://doi.org/10.1111/j.1751-7141.2008.07770.x.

Wilson P, D'Agostino R, Levy D, Belanger A, Silbershatz H, Kannel W. Prediction of coronary heart disease using risk factor categories. Circulation. 1998;97(18):1837–47. https://doi.org/10.1161/01.cir.97.18.1837.

Wilson W, Taubert K, Gewitz M, Lockhart P, Baddour L, Levison M, et al. Prevention of infective endocarditis: guidelines from the American Heart Association: a guideline from the American Heart Association Rheumatic Fever, Endocarditis, and Kawasaki Disease Committee, Council on Cardiovascular Disease in the Young, and the Council on Clinical Cardiology, Council on Cardiovascular Surgery and Anesthesia, and the Quality of Care and Outcomes Research Interdisciplinary Working Group. Circulation. 2007;116(15):1736–54. https://doi.org/10.1161/CIRCULATIONAHA.106.183095.

Writing Group Members, Mozaffarian D, Benjamin E, Go AS, Arnett D, Blaha M, et al. Heart disease and stroke statistics-2016 update: a report from the American Heart Association. Circulation. 2016;133(4):e38–360. https://doi.org/10.1161/CIR.0000000000000350.

Zebrack J, Anderson J. The role of infection in the pathogenesis of cardiovascular disease. Prog Cardiovasc Nurs. 2003;18(1):42–9. http://www.ncbi.nlm.nih.gov/pubmed/12624571

Zhang J, Jiang H, Sun M, Chen J. Association between periodontal disease and mortality in people with CKD: a meta-analysis of cohort studies. BMC Nephrol. 2017;18(1):269. https://doi.org/10.1186/s12882-017-0680-9.

Chapter 7
Interdisciplinary Care Model: Chronic Kidney Disease and Oral Health

Ingrid Glurich, Neel Shimpi, and Amit Acharya

7.1 Definition and Prevalence

The kidney is largely comprised of nephrons which represent discrete filtration units composed of glomeruli comprised of rich capillaries networks for filtering fluids that are subsequently processed by tubules for either re-absorption or excretion as urine. The kidney is responsible for establishing electrolyte balance across the fluid gradient, maintaining pH, and additionally produces hormones which assist with red blood cell production, calcium metabolism, conversion of vitamin D into its active form, and blood pressure control. Figure 7.1 summarizes essential renal physiological functions. The kidney filters and retains approximately 50 gallons of fluid daily, and approximately two quarts are processed into urine to assist with excretion of toxic wastes removed during the filtration process. Renal function is achieved by capillary-rich glomeruli that perform filtration processes within the approximately one million nephrons that comprise the basic renal unit. Tubules within the nephrons reabsorb essential components driven by chemical gradients and physiological needs of the body, while processing toxic materials and excess fluids into urine for excretion.

Because of the important functions performed by the kidney, good renal health is essential to overall health. Kidney health is assessed by monitoring for absence of proteinuria and glomerular filtration rates (GFR), which provide insight into glomerular integrity and functionality.

Development of chronic kidney disease (CKD) is characterized by incremental loss of kidney function over time and may progress in severity to end stage renal disease (ESRD) and renal failure. Renal failure results when damage to glomeruli

I. Glurich · N. Shimpi · A. Acharya (✉)
Center for Oral and Systemic Health, Marshfield Clinic Research Institute, Marshfield, WI, USA
e-mail: glurich.ingrid@marshfieldresearch.org; shimpi.neel@marshfieldresearch.org; acharya.amit@marshfieldresearch.org

A. Acharya et al. (eds.), *Integration of Medical and Dental Care and Patient Data*, Health Informatics, https://doi.org/10.1007/978-3-319-98298-4_7

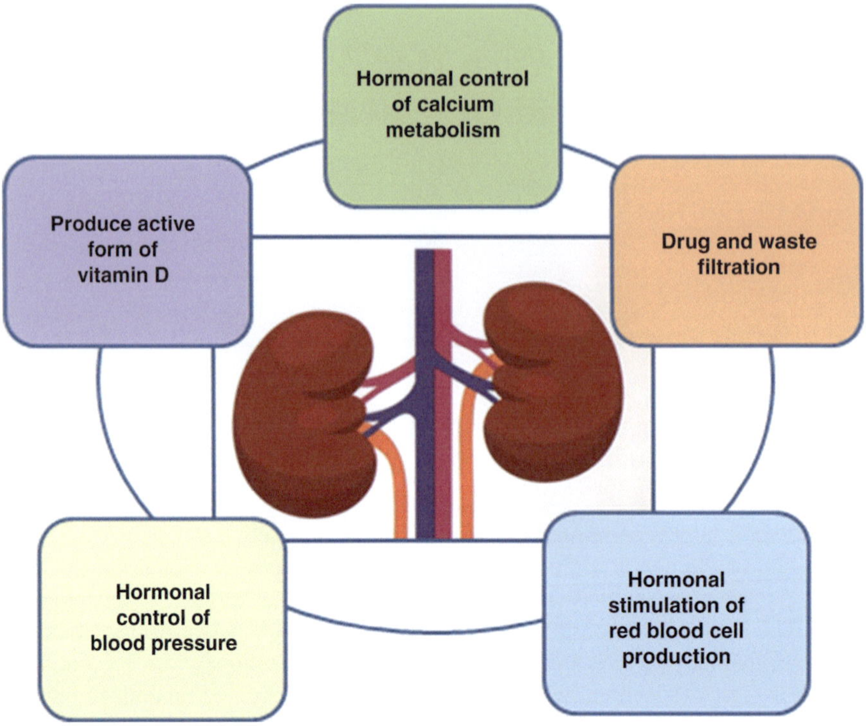

Fig. 7.1 Renal physiological functions: The kidney filters and retains approximately 50 gallons of fluid daily, and approximately two quarts are processed into urine to assist with excretion of toxic wastes removed during the filtration process. Renal function is achieved by capillary-rich glomeruli that perform filtration processes within the approximately one million nephrons that comprise the basic renal unit. Tubules within the nephrons reabsorb essential components driven by chemical gradients and physiological needs of the body, while processing toxic materials and excess fluids into urine for excretion

and/or tubular disorders achieve a critical mass due to other oral-systemic pathophysiological processes that impact on its functionality as described later in this chapter.

Expert renal workgroups have established a globally-accepted definition for staging of renal disease severity based on the extent of decline in glomerular filtration rate (GFR). Diagnosis of moderate CKD is defined by decline in GFR to less than 60 ml/min/1.73 m^2 for at least 3 months, often accompanied by proteinuria. Figure 7.2 provides a graphic depicting CKD staging as defined by KDIGO workgroup for classification of CKD (Levey et al. 2003).

7.1.1 Prevalence of CKD

An estimated 15% of the US adult population (approximately 30 million individuals) has CKD (National Kidney Foundation 2017). Kidney disease ranks 9th among the top 10 leading causes of mortality in the United States, with nearly 50,000

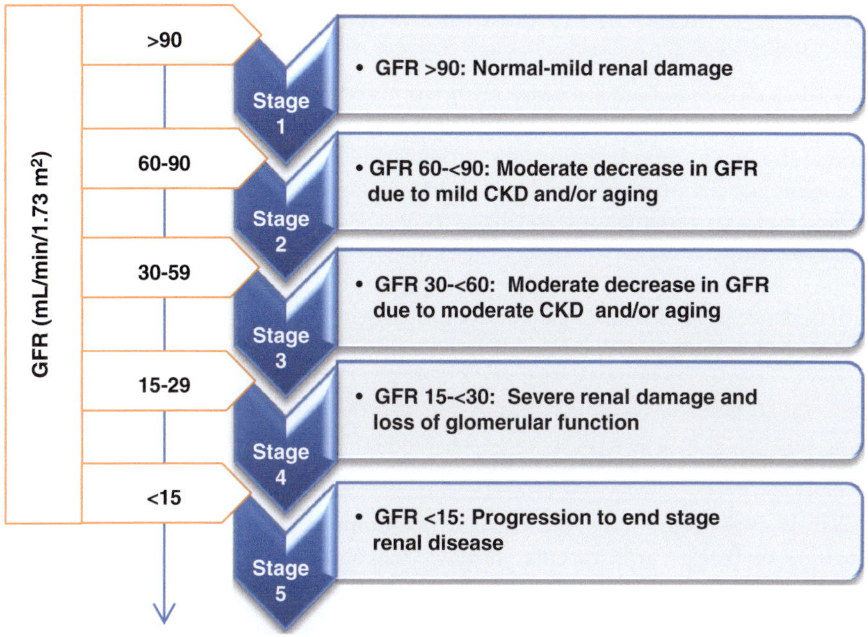

Fig. 7.2 Staging of CKD as a function of decline in GFR

deaths recorded annually and was the 18th leading cause of death globally in 2010. Nearly three out of four incident CKD cases are attributable to comorbid hypertension and diabetes.

Global prevalence of CKD across the five stages is estimated at approximately 13% (range: 12–15%), with 10.6% of cases at CKD Stage 3 or higher. Prevalence of Stage 3 is highest, at 7.6% (Hill et al. 2016). Approximately 50% of the population impacted by CKD stages 3–5 is 60 years of age or older (Glassock et al. 2017). Prevalence of CKD is estimated to be higher in women, impacting 1 in 4 women compared to 1:5 men aged 65–75 years (Jha et al. 2013; National Kidney Foundation 2015).

In the United States, the cost for treatment of Medicare beneficiaries in 2014–2015 for CKD stages 1–4 was estimated between $61 and $64 billion in each year, or approximately $23,000 per individual. Treatment of ESRD in the Medicare population was estimated at an additional $33 and $34 billion during the same years, or approximately $75,000 per individual. Claims associated with treatment of ESRD alone accounted for approximately 7% of Medicare expenditures for paid claims (CDC 2017).

Prevalence of CKD has increased significantly, globally, rising from being ranked 27th among causes for mortality in 1990 to 18th in 2010. Globally, only 20% of patients with ESRD receive treatment for kidney failure due to low treatment availability across 112 developing countries. Eighty percent of patients with ESRD who received treatment were mainly residents of affluent countries. Due to the high cost of treatment, the annual death rate among individuals with ESRD across 112 countries who cannot afford treatment is over one million (National Kidney Foundation 2017).

7.1.2 Prevalence of Periodontal Disease

Prevalence of periodontal disease (PD) worldwide has attained epidemic proportions. Institutions of full mouth surveillance and updated case definitions have corrected the previous underestimation of prevalence. In the US, an estimated 46% of the adult population is affected by PD with prevalence exceeding 50% in Hispanic, Black, and Asian populations, and disparity populations (Eke et al. 2015). Prevalence of PD worldwide varies by country. In Europe, prevalence is estimated at 50%, and approaches rates up to 85% in the elderly greater than 60 years of age (König et al. 2010). Developing low-mid income countries are also experiencing increased prevalence in association with diet and life-style changes (Petersen and Ogawa 2012).

7.2 Systemic Manifestations

CKD is classified among the chronic non-communicable diseases which also include diabetes, cardiovascular disease, osteoporosis, hypertension and some lung conditions, which often occur as co-morbid conditions. Due to the importance of kidney function to overall health, development and progression of CKD impact functionality of nearly all organs in the body. With progression of CKD a variety of physiologic consequences and comorbid conditions may emerge including:

- Hypertension
- Electrolyte imbalances
- Malnutrition and protein-energy wasting syndrome
- Bone disorders
- Muscle weakness
- Peripheral and pulmonary edema
- Anemia
- Increased risk for cardiovascular disease, heart failure, and cardiac-related mortality
- Cognitive impairment
- Reduced efficacy of immune function
- Hyperphosphatemia and hyperparathyroidism

Notably, the risk for premature death in patients diagnosed with CKD is nearly tenfold higher than progression to end stage renal disease and need for dialysis. This increased risk of mortality is associated with increased risk for other chronic conditions with high rates of mortality including cardiovascular disease and diabetes and patients with CKD additionally are at high risk for cancer.

With progression to ESRD in the absence of adequate dialysis, additional emergent systemic symptomology and disorders may include:

- Pericarditis
- Encephalopathy
- Peripheral neuropathy

- Restless leg syndrome
- Gastrointestinal symptomology (loss of appetite, nausea, vomiting, diarrhea)
- Dermatological conditions (dry skin, pruritus, ecchymosis)

7.3 Oral Manifestations

Oral/maxillofacial impact is noted in the context of CKD. Because of the central role of the kidneys in the production of 1-α-hydrolase, the activated form of vitamin D, which is involved in the absorption of calcium by the intestines, declining renal function will impact bone metabolism, including that of oral and craniofacial osseous structures. Progression of CKD is associated with development of renal osteodystrophy which manifests as CKD-Mineral and Bone Disorder (CKD-MBD) syndrome and is attributable to secondary hyperparathyroidism which gives rise to dysregulation of calcium, phosphorus, magnesium, vitamin D metabolism, and parathyroid hormone dysfunction (Ott and Elder 2013). In the oral cavity, excessive parathyroid hormone activity promotes dysregulation of calcium metabolism, osteoporosis, instability and sensitivity of dentition, root calcification, jaw pain, mucositis, changes in flow rates and salivary compositions (Oyetola et al. 2015), and altered dental eruption (Pontes et al. 2018). Grave's disease, calcinosis, osteitis fibrosa/renal osteodystrophy (OF-RO) and brown tumor of hyperparathyroidism (BTH) are further consequences of secondary hyperparathyroidism (Pontes et al. 2018). BTH is characterized by multinucleated giant cells and formation of lesions in jaw bones. OF-RO, a complication of untreated secondary hyperparathyroidism consequential to CKD which impacts an estimated 30% of patients with CKD-MBD, is associated with bone weakness and deformities (Pontes et al. 2018). A manifestation includes Sagliker syndrome, a condition newly defined in 2004, that is associated with gross maxillary and mandibular deformities and abnormalities of the oro-facial complex (Sagliker et al. 2004).

Additional oral conditions arising in the context of CKD (and extent of frequency reported in observational studies systematically reviewed by Ruospo et al. (2014)) include:

- xerostomia (dry mouth) was reported by approximately 48.4% of individuals with stages 1–5 CKD and 69% of patients with Stage 5 CKD and an approximately 48% of these individuals also reported difficulties with swallowing. Xerostomia may be a potentially adverse event associated with pharmaceutical management of patients with CKD and predisposes affected patients to PD and caries consequential to reduced salivary flow.
- The prevalence of PD was 31.6% among patients with CKD stages 1–5, and 56.8% among patients with stage 5 CKD. Rates of missing teeth and edentulism = 42%.
- Moderate to severe dental caries were documented across studies, with an average number of teeth exhibiting decay in stages 1–5 CKD = 2.6, and an average number of filled teeth = 3.8, at stages 1–5 CKD and 20.6% of teeth in studies of Stage 5 CKD.

- Oral mucositis including ulceration affected 8.6% of patients with Stage 5 CKD and oral candidiasis was reported among 19.6% of adults with CKD stages 1–5. Oral pain and burning was documented in 18.7% of patients with Stage 5 CKD.
- Halitosis consequential to increased uremia and a metallic taste have also been documented in patients with CKD.

Causal underpinnings of the increased rates of oral disease among patients with CKD observed in many of the studies and especially at advanced stages of CKD is multi-factorial, with contributing factors including among others, high levels of inflammation, physiological imbalances associated with decline in renal function, malnutrition and metabolic imbalances, poor oral hygiene in a subset of patients, poverty, psycho-social issues, and lack of access to oral/dental care.

7.4 Oral-Systemic Connection

Cardio-renal syndrome is characterized by physiological interaction between advancing renal failure and deleterious impacts on cardiac-related disease, which is estimated to contribute approximately 60% of all-cause mortality in individuals with CKD in the US (NIDDK 2018). Prevalence of cardiovascular disease in individuals >age 65 with CKD is approximately 70%, and nearly double the 35% prevalence rate among individuals in the same age range with no CKD (NIDDK 2018). Notably, a recent meta-analysis of cohort studies examining factors contributing to mortality in individuals with CKD found a statistically significant association between PD and mortality although evidence to support an association between PD and cardiovascular mortality did not achieve statistical significance (Zhang et al. 2017).

Notably, a pooled meta-analysis of observational (n = 22), cohort (n = 4), cross sectional (n = 6) and case studies (n = 12) determined an odds ratio (OR) of 2.02 (95% CI 1.59–2.57) across the studies, indicating increased risk for myocardial infarction in association with presence of periodontitis across approximately 130,000 subjects evaluated in the study. Notably there was high heterogeneity in odds ratio when stratified by study type (Xu et al. 2017). Moreover, a meta-analysis of the association between PD and cerebrovascular disease also reported a relative risk (RR = 1.63; 95% CI 1.25–2.0). Further, a study of approximately 12,000 dentate participants of the US-based third National Health and Nutrition Examination Survey (NHANES) cohort conducted statistical modeling of the association between elevated systolic blood pressure and documented PD in subjects not on hypertensive treatment. The study reported a statistically significant association between the two conditions in their fully adjusted statistical model. Since maintenance of blood pressure homeostasis is a central role of the kidneys, determination of nephropathy and microalbuminuria among variables contributing to hypertensive risk was highly compatible with these observations. Moreover, the study observed a positive linear relationship between PD severity and magnitude of the systolic blood pressure elevation (Tsakos et al. 2010). Additional studies have similarly validated an association between PD and hypertension (reviewed by Macedo Paizan and Vilela-Martin (2014)). Collectively, periodontal inflammation and hypertension contribute to enhancing risk for cardiovascular disease.

High rates of poor oral health and especially presence of PD among patients with advancing CKD have been identified as risk factors for poor prognosis and are associated with malnutrition, protein-energy wasting syndrome, and increased levels of systemic inflammation. Notably, a nationwide retrospective cohort study undertook longitudinal tracking of the emergence of ESRD through insurance record review of a Taiwanese population. The study compared ESRD incidence among greater than 35,000 patients who received surgical management for PD and >141,000 individuals with no equivalent treatment. Investigators reported a significantly lower rate of ESRD in the treated *vs.* the untreated group (4.7 and 7.4 per 10,000 person years, respectively, [$p < 0.01$]) (Lee et al. 2014).

Mechanisms through which PD contributes to CKD and cardiovascular risk include increased local and systemic inflammation, and chronic stimulation of immune response to bacteremia and infectious processes at the level of the periodontium. Systemic inflammation is promoted by several mechanisms in this scenario. White blood cell counts, including numbers of neutrophils, increase incrementally with severity of periodontitis. Local inflammatory response is driven by innate immune mechanisms and increase in levels of proinflammatory cytokines released by white cells or damaged tissue sustaining enzymatic damage consequential to non-specific release of enzymes by neutrophils responding to pathogenic microbial presence. Proinflammatory molecules such as C-reactive protein levels increase incrementally as levels of inflammation increase. Microbial presence in periodontal pockets and shifts in oral microbiome constituency additionally contribute to metabolic alterations which further drive inflammatory processes and chronically stimulate innate and acquired immune responses. Untreated, PD progresses and stimulates systemic inflammatory processes which contribute to oxidative stress. Nitric oxide activity decreases and levels of reactive oxygen species rise, thus driving endothelial dysfunction, increasing vasoconstriction, and establishing a hypertensive state.

Heightened immune response at the level of the arterial walls contributes to arterial plaque deposition. Additional risk factors including dyslipidemia may further enhance formation of foam cells, arterial stiffening, and positive promotion of atherosclerotic processes. Collectively, these processes further contribute to exacerbation of cardio and cerebrovascular disease and renal injury. Progressive vascular damage to glomeruli and renal injury promote metabolic changes associated with establishment of energy imbalances, renal hormonal dysfunction, and inability of kidneys to effectively perform filtration functions. Declining renal function ultimately contributes to uremia and systemic toxicity.

Additional risk factors that may further exacerbate these processes include the presence of genetic susceptibility for comorbid conditions such as diabetes, obesity, and immune dysfunction and may further heighten inflammation. External factors such as smoking and dietary insufficiency, lack of physical activity, poor health literacy, and inadequate access to health and dental care, especially among poor or elderly populations, are secondary drivers of chronic inflammation that interact to promote enhancement of chronic conditions. Complications of CKD include vascular degeneration, promotion of insulin resistance, onset of wasting disease, anemia, and promotion of the immune-mediated cardio-renal syndrome, which ultimately contribute to early mortality.

7.5 Diagnostic Codes

Diagnosis of CKD is made based on a decline in GFR to <60 mL/min/1.73 m^2, for a minimum duration of three months (see Fig. 7.2) and documentation of glomerular sclerosis, tubular atrophy, and interstitial fibrosis on renal biopsy, frequently accompanied by documented proteinuria. Since early stages of CKD are generally asymptomatic, CKD is most frequently diagnosed at Stage 3 when patients first become symptomatic, presenting with anemia, metabolic disturbances, and other consequences attributable to increasing CKD severity. Diagnostic codes for CKD and several associated oral complications are shown in Table 7.1.

7.6 Risk Assessment

CKD at stages below Stage 3 represent silent disease which is infrequently diagnosed at early stages. Emergence of symptomology at Stage 3 is generally associated with risk for disease progression and onset of complications, and increasing risk for morbidity, decline in quality of life, and mortality. Because of high rates of CKD prevalence and deleterious outcomes associated with CKD progression, onset

Table 7.1 Diagnostic Codes for chronic kidney disease

ICD9 Code	ICD10 Code	Description
585.1	N18.1	CKD Stage 1
585.2	N18.2	CKD Stage 2
585.3	N18.3	CKD Stage 3
585.4	N18.4	CKD Stage 4
585.5	N18.5	CKD Stage 5
585.6	N18.6	End-stage renal disease (ESRD)
249.4	E08.22	Diabetes Mellitus due to underlying condition of CKD
528.0	K12.30	Oral mucositis (ulcerative), unspecified
521.0	K02.9	Dental caries, unspecified
523.8	K05.6	Other specified periodontal disease
527.7	R68.2	Xerostomia/Dry Mouth, unspecified

of complications, and high risk for morbidity and mortality, the National Institute of Diabetes, Digestive and Kidney disease (NIDDK) in 1988 launched the United States Renal Data System (USRDS), a national surveillance system for CKD and ESRD. USRDS data can be downloaded from the USRDS website at: https://www.usdrs.org/. A detailed summary of data sources and key findings of their 2017 annual data report including the chapters and executive summary can be found at https://www.usrds.org/adr.aspx.

In 2006, the Centers for Disease Control launched the CDC CKD Surveillance System with priority focus on monitoring early stages of CKD (Saran et al. 2010). An overview of the CDC's surveillance system and data sources is available at: https://nccd.cdc.gov/ckd/default.aspx.

The system tracks and summarizes data on incidence, prevalence, CKD awareness, risk factor burden, consequences to health, quality of care, and health care system capacity and includes a focus on disease burden within special populations including children, transplant population, polycystic disease population and Native Americans. The project also focuses on tracking of risk factors and outcomes including age, diabetes, hypertension, race/ethnicity, and acute kidney injury (CDC 2018).

Bioinformatics approaches to modeling CKD risk have also generated tools with high accuracy for identifying individuals at increased risk. For example, a 2016 study described the use of multivariate models including 'K-nearest neighbor' and 'support vector machine' to predict risk for developing CKD. The regression and classification models utilized clinical data from 386 patients. Study results showed that the overall accuracy achieved by the multivariate models was more than 93%, indicating feasibility of using multimodal models to determine CKD risk (Chen et al. 2016).

Gheewala et al. (2018a) have recently developed and validated QKidney®, a risk assessment tool trained using data from an Australian population and used this tool to assess knowledgeability surrounding CKD in the general population. The mean knowledge score was 10.3 out of a potential maximum score of 24. The authors concluded that improvement of public knowledge surrounding CKD was paramount in achieving improvement of early detection of CKD in their population (Gheewala et al. 2018b). In a follow-up study, these investigators conducted screening of patients (n = 389) of 24 Tasmanian pharmacies in Australia, to further evaluate the QKidney® risk calculator to test the plausibility of using pharmacists to screen for CKD risk in patients between the ages of 50 and 74. Patients whose risk of developing moderate to severe CKD in the next 5 years was 3% or greater (n = 203/389 patients screened) were referred to their general practitioner and follow-up on 126 of referred patients was possible to assess the outcome of the referral over a 9 month period. The study results showed that only 27% (n = 26) of the patients discussed their risk assessment outcomes with their medical provider. However, only 9/26 patients received comprehensive renal health checks and only a subset of patients whose testing showed potential CKD received further testing to confirm their status The authors concluded that there was a need for improvement for assessing risk of early CKD and communicating results of risks with patients (Gheewala et al. 2018a). To date, no studies have reported on implementation of CKD risk assessment in dental settings.

7.7 Systems Biology: Genomics, Proteomics, Microbiomics, Phenotypes

7.7.1 Microbiota, Periodontitis and CKD

Advancing potential for translation of precision medicine approaches to the clinical arena to optimize CKD management across the disease spectrum has the potential to improve CKD detection and outcomes and delineate its potential association with oral health. The evidence based advancing application of omics and systems biology analyses to CKD and PD has grown considerably in the past decade and some important outcomes of these studies are summarized in this section.

Microbiome characterization in subjects with CKD and PD has shown some distinctive alterations relative to constituency of microbial communities. On comparison of individuals with periodontitis and CKD not being managed with dialysis and subjects with periodontitis and no CKD (Artese et al. 2012), reported significantly lower representation of Enterococcus faecalis in patients with CKD ($p < 0.05$), with levels showing reduction in the control group only after periodontal treatment. Notably, these authors reported higher representation of *Actinomyces israelii, Campylobacter rectus, Fusobacterium periodonticum, Peptostreptococcus micra, Prevotella nigrescens, Tannerella forsythia, Neisseria mucosa,* and *Streptococcus anginosus* ($p < 0.05$) in subjects with CKD than in subjects with PD and no CKD. The authors noted that while subgingival microbiota associated with periodontitis was similar across subjects with and without CKD, periodontal pathogens in subjects with CKD persisted at higher levels following scaling and root planing. Notably, the authors also reported persistence of the following periodontal pathogens at sites showing non-responsiveness to treatment compared to responsive treatment sites in subjects with or without CKD: *T. forsythia, Porphyromonas gingivalis, Treponema denticola, Fusobacterium spp., Dialister pneumosintes, E. faecalis and Staphylococcus aureus*; $p < 0.05$) (Artese et al. 2012). Periodontal microbiome analyses in subjects with ESRD and control subjects with PD matched by clinical and demographic parameters but with no CKD found that while taxa associated with PD across cases and controls did not differ, patients with ESRD undergoing dialysis showed lower diversity in their microbiomes especially with respect to decrease in representation of *P denticola* and *Abiotrophia defectiva* (Araújo et al. 2015). A further study which characterized longitudinal analyses of oral and other microbiomes in patients pre- and post-renal transplantation described considerable diversity in oral microbiota cross-sectionally across individuals and in the same individual pre- and post-transplantation. Notably, oral microbiota patterns in patients that did not experience transplant rejection differed when compared to those that experienced transplant rejection. Higher levels of *Fusobacteria leptotrichia, Proteobacter neisseria,* and *Actinobacter* species *coriobacterineae* and *corynebacterineae* were detected in patients with no transplant rejection prior to renal transplantation (Fricke et al. 2014).

7.7.2 'Omics' and CKD

'Omic' approaches to understanding pathogenic mechanisms in the progression of CKD have contributed insights with potentially high clinical relevance. While GWAS studies have contributed to increased understanding of genetic associations underlying CKD, how CKD-associated genes contribute to disease progression remains to be elucidated and translation into clinical care requires further investigation. Because CKD represents an outcome for a spectrum of renal diseases with multiple etiologies, definition of distinct CKD phenotypes will promote opportunities for implementation of precision medicine in facilitating risk assessment and early detection of CKD, disease intervention, prevention of progression and onset of complications, with the goal of improving prognosis.

Whereas monitoring of urinary albumin excretion, creatinine clearance rate and eGFR are reliable measures for detecting decline in renal function, hemoglobin and blood pressure are reliable biomarkers for monitoring progression to later-stage CKD. An important focus for CKD monitoring and management is the definition of biomarkers that could be monitored in early stages of CKD where disease symptomology is largely covert but where intervention would have the greatest probability of stemming CKD progression and onset of complications. One application of proteomics with potential for translation into clinical practice involves proteomic analysis of urinary protein content catalogued in the Human Urine Proteome Database (Mosaiques Diagnostics, Hannover, Germany) in an easily accessible bodily fluid to identify peptides with potential to predict Stage 3 CKD. The proteomic classifier CKD273, represents a composite biomarker based on detection of the presence of 273 urinary peptides that demonstrate strong association to CKD and high potential for use in monitoring at-risk patients for progression to Stage 3 CKD. A clinical trial of capacity of CKD273 to correctly classify subjects with Stage 3 CKD compared to urinary albumin excretion (UAE) rate in $n = 2087$ subjects drawn from six cohorts demonstrated high potential to correctly classify patients with respective specificities of 83% (CDK273) and 82% (UAE) ($p \leq 0.0001$) (Pontillo et al. 2017).

Genome-wide association studies (GWAS) to identify polymorphisms associated with CKD has identified 52 polymorphic loci in 20 of 22 chromosomes in association with 7 phenotypes including CKD, creatinine based eGFR, cisplatin C-based eGFR, ESRD, focal segmental glomerulosclerosis, IgA nephropathy and diabetic nephropathy (Atzler et al. 2014). Further characterization of CKD genomics in large cohorts collectively totaling to nearly 240,000 individuals were stratified into discovery and validation cohorts to identify polymorphisms in genes known to impact renal function (Köttgen et al. 2010a, b; Pattaro et al. 2012). Collectively, loci demonstrated replicable association with eGFR (creatinine production/secretion) or CKD (renal structure/function). Among these, individuals with increased urinary uromodulin levels encoding UMOD SNP rs4293393 had a projected increase in 10-year risk for CKD development exceeding 70% (Köttgen et al. 2010a).

In addition, metabolomic studies have identified metabolites specifically related to CKD ($n = 5$), ESRD ($n = 9$), kidney transplant allograft rejection ($n = 5$), diabetic nephropathy (n = 4), and acute kidney injury (n = 7) and have delineated their associated physiological pathway (Atzler et al. 2014). A study assessing additive value of analyzing both metabolomic and proteomic biomarkers for monitoring of CKD progression and/or prognosis reported no improvement in correlation with eGFR although both approaches independently demonstrated excellent predictive potential (Nkuipou-Kenfack et al. 2014).

A study by Corredor et al. (2015) demonstrated significantly elevated levels of oxidative damage to DNA of both pre-dialysis subjects with various stages of CKD and dialysis patients compared to control subjects. Notably, these authors also demonstrated a positive association between extent of genetic damage and mortality and posited that extent of genomic damage represents a potential predictor of CKD prognosis.

Collectively, the potential biomarkers described above have high translational value for application in precision medicine approaches to renal disease risk prediction in the future. Multi-'omics' approaches and application of systems biology approaches involving mathematical modeling of CKD at a molecular level are being promoted as venues for therapeutic target discovery that may inform development of new interventional pharmaceuticals or other preventive strategies (Cisek et al. 2016). Further, advances in pharmacogenomics which permits assessment of therapeutic response to pharmaceuticals based on profiling drug metabolism capacity at the level of the individual holds further promise in targeting precision medicine approaches to pharmaceutical management of CKD (Schena 2014).

7.7.3 'Omics' of Periodontitis

Periodontitis is posited to be the index oral disease with potential bidirectional ties to renal disease. However despite several decades of 'omics' approaches including microbiome analyses and systems analysis, definition of molecular patterns to aid in the diagnosis or prognosis of PD and potential biomarkers remain elusive and pose the challenge of applying integrated omics approaches for assessing molecular interaction between CKD and periodontitis-associated pathology. Currently diagnosis and treatment of periodontitis remain dependent on evaluation of clinical measures and parameters. However, advances in the oral microbiome arena (as defined in Sect. 7.1 above) have offered new insights into distinctive shifts in constituency patterns among oral microbial communities and molecular signatures in the context of oral health and disease.

Other 'omics' investigation has produced additional insights into the establishment of oral health and disease as illustrated by selected examples presented below. As an early example, investigation of polymorphisms associated with severe PD identified specific mutations in IL1A and IL1B in association with aggressive periodontitis (Kornman et al. 1997) and later, IL1B and TNFα polymorphisms, in association with chronic periodontitis in specific populations (Yang et al. 2013). Generalizability of these findings remains to be demonstrated. GWAS conducted by Teumer et al. in a general German population did not identify definitive specific genomic markers in association with PD, indicating that polygenic contribution likely modulates oral health and disease states (Teumer et al. 2013). A study employing microarray analyses in the context of heightened inflammation associated with periodontitis provided evidence for upregulation of the leukocytic transendothelial pathway in the context of periodontitis and down-regulation of molecules mediating cellular communication including connexin, desmogrein 1, desmocollin 1, and nestin (Abe et al. 2011). Examination of RNA transcripts of inflammatory mediators upregulated during infectious and inflammatory processes associated with periodontitis profiled heightened expression of IL6, CXC ligand 8 and macrophage chemotactic factor 1 (Davanian et al. 2012).

Proteomic and metabolomic analyses of gingival crevicular fluid and saliva profiling protein expression patterns in healthy subjects and those with PD have shown differential expression patterns of structural inflammatory response proteins, inflammatory mediators, and molecules associated with tissue disruption consequential to disease processes (reviewed by Trindade et al. (2014)). These authors also conducted a systematic analysis of currently-available 'omics' data applying informatics tools and defined differential patterns associated with periodontal health and disease. Outcomes of these analyses are available online at: (https://onlinelibrary.wiley.com/action/downloadSupplement?doi=10.1002%2Fprca.201400028&attachmentId=91139099.)

Metagenomic approaches are important research approaches which can give insights not only to alterations in health and disease states but can help to define specific metabolic pathways and genes that are associated with oral health and disease emergence and define metabolic pathways utilized by bacteria in establishment of health or disease states (Xu and Gunsolley 2014). For example, results of a gingival transcriptomic evaluation by Klebschull et al. characterized distinct cluster patterns and clinical profiles with capacity to differentiate between chronic and aggressive PD phenotypes. Statistically significant levels in subgingival cell count were reported for *Porphyromonas gingvalis*, *Tannerella forsythia*, *Prevotella intermedia*, *Micromonas micros*, *Treponema denticola*, *Campylobacter rectus*, and *Actinomyces naeslundii*. Further, statistically significant differences were reported in levels of serum IgG with specificity for the latter three species and infection ratios for the latter two species (Kebschull et al. 2014).

7.8 Treatment

7.8.1 Treatment of Renal Disease

Due to the central role of the kidneys in maintaining overall health, early detection and management of CKD is paramount in preserving renal function, reducing progression and co-morbid exacerbation of other chronic diseases. International collaborative efforts have resulted in the compilation of the KDIGO clinical practice guidelines for management of patients with diagnosis of, or at high risk for, CKD progression, and onset and progression of complications associated with poor health outcomes, decline in quality of life, and early mortality (KDIGO 2018). These guidelines are available at: http://www.kdigo.org/clinical_practice_guidelines/pdf/CKD/KDIGO_2012_CKD_GL.pdf. Notably, a recent workshop was convened to address controversies within the guidelines in the context of management of some of the complications and updates have since been published summarizing recent updates (Davison et al. 2015). Moreover, the guidelines are silent on oral disease assessment and management in the context of oral disease. Considerations for oral health management in the context of CKD are presented below.

7.8.2 *Treatment of Oral Disease*

Oral disease, especially assessment of PD in patients, should be treated with scaling and root planing as the standard of care and current clinical practice guidelines. Patients should receive a care plan to ensure treatment followed by monitoring for disease recurrence. In addition, medication exposures in patients with CKD should be carefully captured and assessment for xerostomia made to minimize the risk for pharmaceutically-induced dry mouth as a contributory factor to emergence of periodontitis due to decrease in salivary flow and reduction in antibacterial activity present in saliva. Patients at risk should be advised to use oral rinses that stimulate restoration of salivary flow. Dental professionals should also screen for symptomology of oral diseases associated with calcium deficiency, hormonal, vitamin, iron or other mineral and/or dietary deficiency. At a minimum, dental practitioners should monitor vital signs, including blood pressure, in patients with CKD and take a thorough medical history, inquiring about diet and nutritional status, calcium and vitamin D intake and supplementation, blood pressure, glycemic status and management, pharmacological exposures, and monitor for the presence of any physical or mental symptomology the patient may be experiencing which may require referral to other medical providers for management. Patients receiving dialysis who experience elevated levels of uremia may be at increased risk for periodontitis and other oral diseases and may require more frequent monitoring due to increased physiological stress associated with the heightened uremic status and increased potential for onset of oral dysbiosis.

7.9 Guidelines

In 2002, current staging of CKD progression was defined and classified jointly by the National Kidney Foundation (NKF) and Kidney Disease Outcomes Quality Initiative (KDOQI) workgroups (Levey et al. 2003) with introduction of some modifications during the creation of an international guideline issued jointly by the Kidney Disease Improving Global Outcomes (KDIGO) and KDOQI workgroups in 2012 (KDIGO workgroup 2013). These guidelines comprehensively define CKD, its classification and staging, and appropriate monitoring and management strategies of renal disease and its complications. Criteria defining CKD include glomerular filtration rate <60 ml/min/1.73 m^2 with a minimum duration of >3 months based on documentation or inference, and demonstration of renal damage as defined by functional structural abnormalities, in addition to decreased GFR status.

The American Dental Association (ADA) convened an expert panel to create an evidence based clinical practice guideline for management of PD in compliance with the ADA's guideline methodology which included a systematic literature review of the current evidence base (Smiley et al. 2015). These guidelines focus on nonsurgical treatment of chronic PD, including conduct of scaling and root planing, follow-up, and recommendations with respect to the use of antimicrobial treatment in these patients (Smiley et al. 2015).

7.10 Existing Gaps and Suggestions

Notably, recent systematic reviews of evidence based research have reported high rates of oral disease and disease associations in PD patients with CKD and a statistically significant association between PD and mortality in the context of CKD (Ruospo et al. 2014; Zhang et al. 2017). Despite the growing body of literature linking association of these conditions, the clinical practice guidelines are silent on oral disease prevention and management in the context of CKD. In the face of this evidence, a need to include recommendations for oral health monitoring in patients with CKD should be considered in future updates to clinical practice guidelines to promote integrated care delivery to these patients.

Interdisciplinary care delivery should include primary care provider involvement in patient management across both medical and dental domains, but such care delivery represents a current gap. As a component of oral care delivery, patients should at a minimum receive an annual assessment of oral health status and prophylactic intervention involving removal of oral biofilms and periodontal plaque to discourage establishment of dysbiosis. If PD is present, patients should receive scaling and root planing intervention and periodicity of dental visits should be adjusted to monitor recurrence of periodontitis. Medical care providers should be attentive to frequency of dental visits by patients with CKD, screen the general health of the oral cavity and refer patients with oral disease to dental care programs commensurate with their insurance status for receipt of care delivery including community health centers that deliver care to or under-insured patients.

7.11 Technology Implications

In the clinical setting, development of point-of-care technologies that leverage electronic health records (EHR) such as clinical decision support tools, patient portals, and disease-specific registries, allow monitoring of patient outcomes and support quality improvement monitoring, thus adding significant value to health care delivery. In addition, harnessing telehealth and tele-dentistry in primary care and dental settings may support patient-centered care delivery.

Biomedical and healthcare informatics approaches may be leveraged for development of risk assessment tools for disease prediction. Mining of data in the EHR and data warehouses which serve as repositories of longitudinally-captured EHR data are invaluable big data resources used by researchers to generate the evidence base that supports establishment of clinical practice guidelines, decision-making on population based screening for undiagnosed diseases, and development of quality indicators surrounding performance and effectiveness of clinical care delivery. All of these activities have high relevance to the management of patients with CKD.

Technology also is indispensable for future translation of precision medicine into clinical practice in the context of CKD. Systems biology and analyses of 'omics' data would be inconceivable without the development of extensive databases that track, capture and catalog all available 'omics' data at the point of discovery for creation of data repositories that can be mined during analysis of big data sets.

7.11.1 Electronic Health Records

EHRs have demonstrated great value in clinical care delivery to patients with CKD (Navaneethan et al. 2013). EHRs are invaluable to the establishment of CKD registries that aggregate patient data and inform on improvement of quality of healthcare delivery while leveraging early identification of CKD patients. EHRs may further incorporate use of automated alerts and referral mechanisms and patient navigator programs (Jolly et al. 2015) to facilitate clinical care delivery and may employ patient portals to engage patients and provide access to their personal data. The use of clinical alerts by the laboratory settings for eGFR values were shown to improve referrals to nephrology departments (Drawz et al. 2015). Implementation of clinical decision support tools along with clinical practice guidelines in the EHR additionally provides provider access to specific recommendations to improve CKD care in clinical settings.

7.12 Ontology

A recent study conducted by (Cole et al. 2018) utilized Ontology Web Language (OWL) to develop ontology for CKD. Categories of all the concepts relevant to CKD (including, among others, diagnosis, treatment, procedure, process of care) were created and organized. Concepts used in the ontology were similar to those delineated in Improving Global Outcomes (KDIGO 2013). The ontology is available online at: http://bioportal.bioontology.org/ontologies/CKDO.

7.13 Care Plan

Emerging evidence from recent systematic reviews indicating increased risk for mortality in patients with CKD and PD strongly promotes the need for interdisciplinary care delivery in management of patients with CKD. As defined in Sect. 7.3

of this chapter, the presence of CKD and especially the emergence of complications including anemia, calcium imbalance, onset of energy imbalances, wasting disease and malnutrition, sources of increased systemic inflammation, and uncontrolled hypertension all may promote oral disease, while other shared risk factors between CKD and PD promote bidirectional exacerbation of oral disease and CKD. Progression and establishment of chronicity of PD in the context of CKD in turn, drive physiological processes that promote CKD progression.

Interdisciplinary care team planning should therefore ultimately strive to provide the CKD patient with a medical home and include team members who can address prevention or management of emergent complications. Based on the range of potential complications the integrated care team should be multi-disciplinary and include the following medical and dental primary care practitioners: medical primary care physicians, nurse practitioners, medical assistants, physician assistants, and primary dental providers (including dentists and dental hygienists) who triage patients, as required, to health educators, pharmacists, dieticians and relevant medical, mental health, and palliative care specialists.

The integrated care team should contribute to the definition of an interdisciplinary care plan document that ensures patients with CKD are properly evaluated across all health domains and educated about their condition. The executive summary defining considerations for quality care delivery in the context of management of patients with CKD emanating from the KDIGO Controversies Conference on Supportive Care in Chronic Kidney Disease (Davison et al. 2015), among other resources, offers a resource to inform thorough consideration of patient care needs, essential care team members, and considerations in care plan development. At a minimum, patients with CKD should be offered nutritional counseling by a dietician, monitored for adequacy of calcium, vitamin D intake, the presence of anemia, and should be assessed for osteoporosis, which may impact the integrity of craniofacial bone structure. Inclusion of referral to specialists including an endocrinologist to monitor risk for hormonal imbalance, nephrologist to monitor renal integrity, and mental health support, as required, should be considered to educate and support the patient. The care plan should be shared with the patient to optimally motivate the patient to become an active, engaged participant in the preservation of renal function and prevention of complications with a high potential to decrease the patient's quality of life.

7.14 Recommendations

Dental practitioners should be included as members of the healthcare team delivering care to patients with CKD. Dental practitioners (dentists and hygienists) should monitor patients for CKD diagnosis and be informed of symptomology associated with CKD in order to monitor for signs of disease. In patients diagnosed with CKD, dental practitioners should also monitor for presence and status of associated co-morbidities that increase risk for CKD progression and are known complications associated with CKD (including diabetic and hypertension status and family history of CKD) since these conditions also increase the risk for oral disease.

Patients at risk for, or diagnosed with, CKD, should be assessed for the presence of potentially-related oral manifestations such as moderate to severe PD, oral mucositis, dental caries, xerostomia, and other conditions detailed in Sect. 7.3. Triage to medical care should be offered to patients at perceived risk for exacerbation of medical conditions that interfere with effective management of oral conditions. As a member of the integrated care team addressing healthcare needs of the patient, cross-disciplinary consultation will help to promote quality care delivery and ideally improve compliance with the care plan in order to achieve holistic optimization of patient health outcomes and quality of life. Recognition of the association between oral and renal disease is paramount and future versions of clinical practice guidelines on CKD should be inclusive of ascertainment of oral care as a healthcare quality indicator for patients with CKD to ensure holistic healthcare delivery to these patients and improvement in health outcomes and quality of life.

References

Abe D, Kubota T, Morozumi T, Shimizu T, Nakasone N, Itagaki M, Yoshie H. Altered gene expression in leukocyte transendothelial migration and cell communication pathways in periodontitis-affected gingival tissues. J Periodontal Res. 2011;46(3):345–53. https://doi.org/10.1111/j.1600-0765.2011.01349.x.

Araújo M, Hong B, Fava P, Khan S, Burleson J, Fares G, et al. End stage renal disease as a modifier of the periodontal microbiome. BMC Nephrol. 2015;16(1):80. https://doi.org/10.1186/s12882-015-0081-x.

Artese H, Sousa C, Torres M, Silva-Boghossian C, Colombo A. Effect of non-surgical periodontal treatment on the subgingival microbiota of patients with chronic kidney disease. Braz Oral Res. 2012;26(4):366–72. https://doi.org/10.1590/S1806-83242012005000008.

Atzler D, Schwedhelm E, Zeller T. Integrated genomics and metalomics in nephrology. Nephrol Dial Transplant. 2014;29:1467–74. https://doi.org/10.1093/ndt/gft492.

Centers for Disease Control and Prevention. Chronic kidney disease (CKD) surveillance project. 2018. https://nccd.cdc.gov/ckd/default.aspx. Accessed 10 June 2018.

Centers for Disease Control and Prevention. Chronic kidney disease basics. Chronic kidney disease initiative. CDC. 2017. https://www.cdc.gov/kidneydisease/basics.html. Accessed 30 Aug 2018.

Chen Z, Zhang X, Zhang Z. Clinical risk assessment of patients with chronic kidney disease by using clinical data and multivariate models. Int Urol Nephrol. 2016;48(12):2069–75. https://doi.org/10.1007/s11255-016-1346-4.

Cisek K, Krochmal M, Klein J, Mischak H. The application of multi-omics and systems biology to identify therapeutic targets in chronic kidney disease. Nephrol Dial Transplant. 2016;31(12):2003–11. https://doi.org/10.1093/ndt/gfv364.

Cole N, Liyanage H, Suckling R, Swift P, Gallagher H, Byford R, et al. An ontological approach to identifying cases of chronic kidney disease from routine primary care data: a cross-sectional study. BMC Nephrol. 2018;19(1):85. https://doi.org/10.1186/s12882-018-0882-9.

Corredor Z, Stoyanova E, Rodriguez-Ribera L, Coll E, Silva I, Diaz J, et al. Genomic damage as a biomarker of chronic kidney disease status. Environ Mol Mutagen. 2015;56:301–12. https://doi.org/10.1002/em.21911.

Davanian H, Stranneheim H, Båge T, Lagervall M, Jansson L, Lundeberg J, Yucel-Lindberg T. Gene expression profiles in paired gingival biopsies from periodontitis-affected and healthy tissues revealed by massively parallel sequencing. PLoS One. 2012;7(9):e46440. https://doi.org/10.1371/journal.pone.0046440.

Davison S, Levin A, Moss AH, Jha V, Brown E, Brennan F, et al. Executive summary of the KDIGO Controversies Conference on Supportive Care in Chronic Kidney Disease: developing a roadmap to improving quality care. Kidney Int. 2015;88(3):447–59. https://doi.org/10.1038/ki.2015.110.

Drawz P, Archdeacon P, McDonald C, Powe N, Smith K, Norton J, et al. CKD as a model for improving chronic disease care through electronic health records. Clin J Am Soc Nephrol. 2015;10(8):1488–99. https://doi.org/10.2215/CJN.00940115.

Eke P, Dye B, Wei L, Slade G, Thornton-Evans G, Borgnakke W, et al. Update on prevalence of periodontitis in adults in the United States: NHANES 2009 to 2012. J Periodontol. 2015;86(5):611–22. https://doi.org/10.1902/jop.2015.140520.

Fricke W, Maddox C, Song Y, Bromberg J. Human microbiota characterization in the course of renal transplantation. Am J Transplant. 2014;14(2):416–27. https://doi.org/10.1111/ajt.12588.

Gheewala P, Peterson G, Zaidi S, Jose M, Castelino R. Evaluation of a chronic kidney disease risk assessment service in community pharmacies. Nephrology. 2018a; https://doi.org/10.1111/nep.13247.

Gheewala P, Peterson G, Zaidi S, Jose M, Castelino R. Public knowledge of chronic kidney disease evaluated using a validated questionnaire: a cross-sectional study. BMC Public Health. 2018b;18(1):371. https://doi.org/10.1186/s12889-018-5301-4.

Glassock R, Warnock D, Delanaye P. The global burden of chronic kidney disease: estimates, variability and pitfalls. Nat Rev Nephrol. 2017;13(2):104–14. https://doi.org/10.1038/nrneph.2016.163.

Hill N, Fatoba S, Oke J, Hirst J, O'Callaghan C, Lasserson D, Hobbs F. Global prevalence of chronic kidney disease – a systematic review and meta-analysis. PLoS One. 2016;11(7):e0158765. https://doi.org/10.1371/journal.pone.0158765.

Jha V, Garcia-Garcia G, Iseki K, Li Z, Naicker S, Plattner B, et al. Chronic kidney disease: global dimension and perspectives. Lancet. 2013;382(9888):260–72. https://doi.org/10.1016/S0140-6736(13)60687-X.

Jolly S, Navaneethan S, Schold J, Arrigain S, Konig V, Burrucker YK, et al. Development of a chronic kidney disease patient navigator program. BMC Nephrol. 2015;16(1):69. https://doi.org/10.1186/s12882-015-0060-2.

KDIGO Workgroup. KDIGO 2012 clinical practice guideline for the evaluation and management of chronic kidney disease. Kidney Int Suppl. 2013;3(1):1–150.

KDIGO. Guidelines. KDIGO; 2018. https://kdigo.org/guidelines/. Accessed 9 June 2018.

Kebschull M, Demmer R, Grün B, Guarnieri P, Pavlidis P, Papapanou PN. Gingival tissue transcriptomes identify distinct periodontitis phenotypes. J Dent Res. 2014;93(5):459–68. https://doi.org/10.1177/0022034514527288.

König J, Holtfreter B, Kocher T. Periodontal health in Europe: future trends based on treatment needs and the provision of periodontal services - position paper 1. Eur J Dent Educ. 2010;14:4–24. https://doi.org/10.1111/j.1600-0579.2010.00620.x.

Kornman K, Crane A, Wang H, di Giovine F, Newman M, Pirk F, et al. The interleukin-1 genotype as a severity factor in adult periodontal disease. J Clin Periodontol. 1997;24(1):72–7. http://www.ncbi.nlm.nih.gov/pubmed/9049801

Köttgen A, Hwang S-J, Larson MG, Van Eyk JE, Fu Q, Benjamin EJ, et al. Uromodulin levels associate with a common UMOD variant and risk for incident CKD. J Am Soc Nephrol. 2010a;21(2):337–44. https://doi.org/10.1681/ASN.2009070725.

Köttgen A, Pattaro C, Böger C, Fuchsberger C, Olden M, Glazer N, et al. New loci associated with kidney function and chronic kidney disease. Nat Genet. 2010b;42(5):376–84. https://doi.org/10.1038/ng.568.

Lee C, Lin C, Lin M, Lin S, Sung F, Kao C. Surgical treatment for patients with periodontal disease reduces risk of end-stage renal disease: a nationwide population-based retrospective cohort study. J Periodontol. 2014;85(1):50–6. https://doi.org/10.1902/jop.2013.130015.

Levey A, Coresh J, Balk E, Kausz A, Levin A, Steffes M, et al. National Kidney Foundation practice guidelines for chronic kidney disease: evaluation, classification, and stratification. Ann Intern Med. 2003;139(2):137–47. http://www.ncbi.nlm.nih.gov/pubmed/12859163

Macedo Paizan M, Vilela-Martin J. Is there an association between periodontitis and hypertension? Curr Cardiol Rev. 2014;10(4):355–61. https://doi.org/10.2174/1573403X10666140416094901.

National Kidney Foundation. Global facts: about kidney disease. National Kidney Foundation; 2015. https://www.kidney.org/kidneydisease/global-facts-about-kidney-disease. Accessed 9 June 2018.

National Kidney Foundation. Global facts: about kidney disease. 2017. https://www.kidney.org/kidneydisease/global-facts-about-kidney-disease#_ENREF_3. Accessed 30 Aug 2018.

Navaneethan S, Schold J, Kirwan J, Arrigain S, Jolly S, Poggio ED, et al. Metabolic syndrome, ESRD, and death in CKD. Clin J Am Soc Nephrol. 2013;8(6):945–52. https://doi.org/10.2215/CJN.09870912.

NIDDK. Kidney disease statistics for the United States. NIDDK; 2018. https://www.niddk.nih.gov/health-information/health-statistics/kidney-disease. Accessed 9 June 2018.

Nkuipou-Kenfack E, Duranton F, Gayrard N, Argilés À, Lundin U, Weinberger K, et al. Assessment of metabolomic and proteomic biomarkers in detection and prognosis of progression of renal function in chronic kidney disease. PLoS One. 2014;9(5):e96955. https://doi.org/10.1371/journal.pone.0096955.

Ott SM, Elder G. Osteoporosis associated with chronic kidney disease. In: Osteoporosis. Amsterdan: Elsevier; 2013. p. 1387–424. https://doi.org/10.1016/B978-0-12-415853-5.00058-3.

Oyetola E, Owotade F, Agbelusi G, Fatusi O, Sanusi A. Oral findings in chronic kidney disease: implications for management in developing countries. BMC Oral Health. 2015;15(1):24. https://doi.org/10.1186/s12903-015-0004-z.

Pattaro C, Köttgen A, Teumer A, Garnaas M, Böger C, Fuchsberger C, et al. Genome-wide association and functional follow-up reveals new loci for kidney function. PLoS Genet. 2012;8(3):e1002584. https://doi.org/10.1371/journal.pgen.1002584.

Petersen P, Ogawa H. The global burden of periodontal disease: towards integration with chronic disease prevention and control. Periodontol 2000. 2012;60(1):15–39. https://doi.org/10.1111/j.1600-0757.2011.00425.x.

Pontes F, Lopes M, de Souza L, dos Santos da Mata Rezende D, Santos-Silva A, Jorge J, et al. Oral and maxillofacial manifestations of chronic kidney disease–mineral and bone disorder: a multicenter retrospective study. Oral Surg Oral Med Oral Pathol Oral Radiol. 2018;125(1):31–43. https://doi.org/10.1016/j.oooo.2017.09.011.

Pontillo C, Zhang Z, Schanstra J, Jacobs L, Zürbig P, Thijs L, et al. Prediction of chronic kidney disease stage 3 by CKD273, a urinary proteomic biomarker. Kidney Int Rep. 2017;2(6):1066–75. https://doi.org/10.1016/j.ekir.2017.06.004.

Ruospo M, Palmer S, Craig J, Gentile G, Johnson D, Ford P, et al. Prevalence and severity of oral disease in adults with chronic kidney disease: a systematic review of observational studies. Nephrol Dial Transplant. 2014;29(2):364–75. https://doi.org/10.1093/ndt/gft401.

Sagliker Y, Balal M, Sagliker Ozkaynak P, Paydas S, Sagliker C, Sabit Sagliker H, et al. Sagliker syndrome: uglifying human face appearance in late and severe secondary hyperparathyroidism in chronic renal failure. Semin Nephrol. 2004;24(5):449–55. http://www.ncbi.nlm.nih.gov/pubmed/15490409

Saran R, Hedgeman E, Plantinga L, Burrows N, Gillespie B, Young E, et al. Establishing a national chronic kidney disease surveillance system for the United States. Clin J Am Soc Nephrol. 2010;5(1):152–61. https://doi.org/10.2215/CJN.05480809.

Schena F. Biomarkers and personalized therapy in chronic kidney diseases. Expert Opin Investig Drugs. 2014;23(8):1051–4. https://doi.org/10.1517/13543784.2014.922953.

Smiley C, Tracy S, Abt E, Michalowicz B, John M, Gunsolley J, et al. Evidence-based clinical practice guideline on the nonsurgical treatment of chronic periodontitis by means of scaling and root planing with or without adjuncts. J Am Dent Assoc. 2015;146(7):525–35. https://doi.org/10.1016/j.adaj.2015.01.026.

Teumer A, Holtfreter B, Völker U, Petersmann A, Nauck M, Biffar R, et al. Genome-wide association study of chronic periodontitis in a general German population. J Clin Periodontol. 2013;40(11):977–85. https://doi.org/10.1111/jcpe.12154.

Trindade F, Oppenheim F, Helmerhorst E, Amado F, Gomes PS, Vitorino R. Uncovering the molecular networks in periodontitis. Proteomics Clin Appl. 2014;8(9–10):748–61. https://doi.org/10.1002/prca.201400028.

Tsakos G, Sabbah W, Hingorani A, Netuveli G, Donos N, Watt R, D'Aiuto F. Is periodontal inflammation associated with raised blood pressure? Evidence from a National US survey. J Hypertens. 2010;28(12):1. https://doi.org/10.1097/HJH.0b013e32833e0fe1.

Xu P, Gunsolley J. Application of metagenomics in understanding oral health and disease. Virulence. 2014;5(3):424–32. https://doi.org/10.4161/viru.28532.

Xu S, Song M, Xiong Y, Liu X, He Y, Qin Z. The association between periodontal disease and the risk of myocardial infarction: a pooled analysis of observational studies. BMC Cardiovasc Disord. 2017;17(1):50. https://doi.org/10.1186/s12872-017-0480-y.

Yang W, Jia Y, Wu H. Four tumor necrosis factor alpha genes polymorphisms and periodontitis risk in a Chinese population. Hum Immunol. 2013;74(12):1684–7. https://doi.org/10.1016/j.humimm.2013.08.009.

Zhang J, Jiang H, Sun M, Chen J. Association between periodontal disease and mortality in people with CKD: a meta-analysis of cohort studies. BMC Nephrol. 2017;18(1):269. https://doi.org/10.1186/s12882-017-0680-9.

Chapter 8
Interdisciplinary Care Model: Odontogenic Infections and Systemic Complications

Jayanth Kumar Medam and Thankam Paul Thyvalikakath

8.1 Odontogenic Infections and Prevalence

Odontogenic infections are infections that arise due to dental caries and periodontal disease that progress to periapical tissues through the apex of the teeth (Bahl et al. 2014). They can spread to adjacent orofacial regions and distant regions of the body and have a mortality of 10–40% among affected patients (Bali et al. 2015; Moghimi et al. 2013). The signs and symptoms of the resultant infections vary based on the region and severity of the spreading odontogenic infections. Common signs and symptoms include tenderness, swelling filled with purulent material, erythema, discomfort, dysphagia and fever. (Bali et al. 2015; Igoumenakis et al. 2014; Lypka and

J. K. Medam
Dental Informatics Core, Department of Cariology, Operative Dentistry & Dental Public Health, Indiana University School of Dentistry, IUPUI, Indianapolis, IN, USA

School of Informatics and Computing, IUPUI, Indianapolis, IN, USA
e-mail: jaymedam@iu.edu

T. P. Thyvalikakath (✉)
Dental Informatics Core, Department of Cariology, Operative Dentistry & Dental Public Health, Indiana University School of Dentistry, IUPUI, Indianapolis, IN, USA

School of Informatics and Computing, IUPUI, Indianapolis, IN, USA

Centre for Biomedical Informatics, Regenstrief Institute, Indianapolis, IN, USA
e-mail: tpt@iu.edu

A. Acharya et al. (eds.), *Integration of Medical and Dental Care and Patient Data*, Health Informatics, https://doi.org/10.1007/978-3-319-98298-4_8

Table 8.1 ICD 9, 10-CM Diagnostic codes for oral and systemic infections of odontogenic origin

ICD-9 CM codes	Description
522.7	Periapical abscess with sinus
522.5	Periapical abscess without sinus
478.21	Cellulitis of pharynx
682.9	Cellulitis otherwise not specified
787.20	Dysphagia otherwise not specified
787.23	Dysphagia pharyngeal phase
ICD-10 CM codes	**Description**
B95	Streptococcus, Staphylococcus, and Enterococcus as the cause of diseases classified elsewhere
B96	Other bacterial agents as the cause of diseases classified elsewhere
B97	Viral agents as the cause of diseases classified elsewhere
G08	Intracranial and intraspinal phlebitis and thrombophlebitis
I38	Endocarditis otherwise not specified
I33.0	Infective endocarditis
I33.9	Subacute bacterial endocarditis
J85.3	Diseases of mediastinum, not elsewhere classified
J01.00	Maxillary sinusitis acute type
J01.01	Maxillary sinusitis acute recurrent type
J02.9	Pharyngitis otherwise not specified
J32.09	Maxillary sinusitis chronic type
K04.6–K04.7	Periapical abscess
K05.21	Periodontal abscess
K12.2	Abscess of oral tissue otherwise not specified
K12.2	Abscess of buccal cavity, floor of the mouth, submandibular region, sublingual region, palate, and cheek
K12.2	Cellulitis of the buccal cavity, floor of the mouth, sublingual region, submandibular region, Ludwig's angina
R13.13	Pharyngeal dysphagia

Hammoudeh 2011; Moghimi et al. 2013). The International Classification of Disease (ICD) codes for various oral and systemic infections of odontogenic origin are enlisted in the Table 8.1.

8.2 Systemic Manifestations

Odontogenic infections that spread to adjacent tissues and oro-fascial spaces result in systemic manifestations such as odontogenic maxillary sinusitis, para- and retropharyngeal infections secondary to odontogenic infections, cavernous sinus thrombosis, descending necrotizing mediastinitis, and infective endocarditis secondary to odontogenic infections. In the sections below, we describe each condition in detail.

8.3 Odontogenic Maxillary Sinusitis (OMS)/ Odontorhinosinusitis

OMS is caused by infective or non-infective odontogenic conditions of the maxillary first and second molar teeth due to their proximity to the floor of the maxillary sinus (Abubaker 1999). Approximately 10–12% of maxillary sinusitis are of odontogenic origin (Maloney and Doku 1968; Vallo et al. 2010). OMS is predominantly anaerobic in nature, whereas non-odontogenic maxillary sinusitis is predominantly aerobic (Vidal et al. 2017; Yuvaraj et al. 2012; Taschieri et al. 2015). The acute form of OMS spreads to adjacent tissues, and patients typically present with pain over the maxillary sinus region of the face and nasal discharge (Bali et al. 2015). Patients with the chronic form have a longer disease history with signs and symptoms that include gnawing dental pain, purulent foul smelling nasal discharge and bleeding gums of the affected region. The noninfectious causes of OMS are odontogenic cysts and tumors (Alias Ramesh Colbert and Sankar 2014; Simuntis et al. 2014). The occipito-mental or Waters view and orthopantomogram (OPG) are the routine radiographic examinations performed in a dental setting to assess the maxillary sinus for OMS. Computed tomography (CT) and diagnostic nasal endoscopy are the advanced diagnostic tools used to visualize the maxillary sinus. Maxillary sinuses with two-third fluid opacity and mucosal thickening of a moderate level, have an 86% chance of a dental source of infection (Bomeli et al. 2009). Penicillin or clindamycin (Moenning et al. 1989) along with drainage of the pus from the maxillary sinus are suggestive treatments for OMS (Alias Ramesh Colbert and Sankar 2014). The dental source of infection is managed by endodontic therapy, periodontal management (in cases of localized or generalized periodontal disease) or surgical treatment (for antrally placed or displaced implant or even peri-implantitis, cysts or tumors leading to OMS) to prevent the recurrence of OMS.

8.4 Para- and Retropharyngeal Space Infections Secondary to Odontogenic Infection

Parapharyngeal spaces are lateral to the oral cavity and medial to the parotid gland; the prevertebral space is anterior and in close proximity to the vertebral column extending from the skull base to coccyx and the retropharyngeal space is between the prevertebral space and alar fascia extending from the skull base to the upper mediastinum (Debnam et al. 2012). Danger space lies in between the retropharyngeal and prevertebral space. Established odontogenic infections, mainly originating from the posterior teeth region spread to the parapharyngeal spaces and extend to the retropharyngeal space (Blomquist and Bayer 1988) and mediastinal region. The symptoms include stiffness of the neck, difficulty in breathing and swallowing, fever and other systemic septic manifestations (Herzon and Martin 2006). Parapharyngeal or a retropharyngeal suppurative abscess is also seen in some cases. Carotid artery erosion and vagus nerve involvement can be the complications leading to death. CT or ultrasound guided needle aspiration for pus extraction and examination has been widely advocated (Herzon and Martin 2006). This life threatening condition can be managed only by guided surgical drainage, intensive medical management with intravenous antimicrobial therapy and treating the origin of infection.

8.5 Cavernous Sinus Thrombosis

Cavernous sinus thrombosis is a septic condition of the cavernous sinus which drains the blood from the brain tissue and "7% of all the cavernous sinus infections are of dental origin" (Kiddee et al. 2010). Major veins of the facial region which have communication with the dural venous sinuses, act as channels for the spread of palatal infections from anterior maxillary teeth. Cranial nerves, namely the oculomotor, ophthalmic, trochlear, maxillary, and the trigeminal ganglion are affected. Ptosis, restricted eye movement with exophthalmos, poor eye sight, chemosis, and in few case scenarios, seizures and altered sensorium are observed (Feldman et al. 2000). CT of the cranial region without contrast in toxic conditions is suggested and magnetic resonance imaging (MRI) stands out as the standard protocol (Le et al. 2017). Controlled anticoagulation and intracranial pressure maintenance should be attempted promptly, with inclusion of antimicrobial therapy. The origin of the odontogenic infection should be treated to control further damage.

8.6 Descending Necrotizing Mediastinitis (DNM)

Descending necrotizing mediastinitis is a life threatening infectious condition with a high mortality rate of nearly 60% (Wei et al. 2017). It is defined as the secondary infection of the mediastinal region caused by the downward spread of odontogenic, oropharyngeal, or parapharyngeal space infection. Odontogenic infections, middle ear infections (otitis media), epiglottitis, and mastoiditis are the common causes of DNM, however 50% are due to odontogenic infections (Palma et al. 2016; Sakamoto et al. 2000). Symptoms and signs observed include pain in the upper chest region, fever, difficulty in breathing and swallowing, crepitation on auscultation of the chest and suppuration in the cervical region, upper thoracic region, or in the oral cavity (Novakov et al. 2010). Signs of odontogenic origin include raised floor of the mouth, raised tongue, and trismus.

A diagnosis of DNM is confirmed based on the criteria published in 1983 by Estrera and coworkers (Estrera et al. 1983) as listed below:

1. Clinical evidence of severe infection
2. Characteristic radiographic evidence of features of mediastinitis such as mediastinal widening, mediastinal emphysema, mediastinal fluid collection with bubbles or abscesses with air fluid level
3. Intraoperative and or post mortem documentation of DNM
4. A clearly established evidence of the spread of oropharyngeal infection causing the DNM.

CT and MRI are the most important diagnostic tools in the confirmation of DNM (Foroulis and Sileli 2011). Ultrasonography is also used in guided fine needle aspiration of pus from the infected region and laboratory analysis of the sample would help in the determination of the bacteria (Edlich et al. 2010). Increase in white blood cell (WBC) count and C-reactive protein are the two main features of the complete blood picture (CBP) in DNM patients (Ishinaga et al. 2013). DNM is classified based on the spread of infection detected using CT scans (Endo et al. 1999):

1. **Localized descending necrotizing mediastinitis-Type I**, where the infection spread is localized to the upper mediastinum and above the tracheal bifurcation.
2. **Diffuse descending necrotizing mediastinitis-Type IIA**, here the infection is spread to the lower anterior mediastinum.
3. **Diffuse descending necrotizing mediastinitis-Type IIB**, where the infection extends to both the anterior and posterior lower mediastinum.

Edlich et al. (2010) have supported the use of MRI, because it is a safe multiplanar imaging modality that uses no ionizing radiation or contrast. Maintenance of patent airway with tracheotomy is the foremost step in the treatment of DNM, as the edema fluid constricts the larynx. Intravenous antibiotics such as Penicillin, Clindamycin, and Piperacillin are prescribed until the specific microorganism is detected through microbial culture. Upon confirmation, targeted antimicrobial treatment is started. In case of resistant strains, Meropenem-Vancomycin or Doripenem is suggested (Fukuchi et al. 2015; Prado-Calleros et al. 2016; Sakamoto et al. 2000). Surgical management varies based on the type of DNM. The Type-I is treated by cervicotomy and transcervical drainage, whereas the Type-IIA is treated by median sternotomy and necrotic tissue debridement. The posterior mediastinal infection in the Type-IIB DNM can be accessed by uni- or bilateral thoracotomy or VATS (video-assisted thoracoscopic surgery) (Abu-Omar et al. 2017).

8.7 Infective Endocarditis Secondary to Odontogenic Infection

Bacteremia following odontogenic infections can lead to Infective Endocarditis (IE) (Kiefer and Bashore 2012). IE is defined as an "infection of a heart valve or other cardiac structure or even cardiac devices at a site of endothelial damage" (Kiefer and Bashore 2012). Increased turbulence in blood flow damages the endothelial lining of the heart and leads to fibrin clot formation by the activity of tissue factors and cytokines. At this stage, it is referred as nonbacterial thrombotic endocarditis. The bacterial involvement of these fibrin clots from the bacteremia results in infective endocarditis (Taubert and Wilson 2017). Bor et al. (2013) analysis on the 1998–2009 Agency for Healthcare Research and Quality's Nationwide Inpatient Sample (NIS) data showed 2.4% increase in the unique admissions of endocarditis with *Staphylococcus aureus* (28.7%) as the most common causative organism of IE. In the past, medical providers prescribed antibiotic prophylaxis for dental patients with cardiac conditions according to the American Heart Association (AHA) guidelines for antibiotic prophylaxis for IE (Wilson et al. 2007). However, recently, AHA and the European Society of Cardiology (ESC) proposed the use of antibiotic prophylaxis only in high risk cardiac patients undergoing dental treatment (Taubert and Wilson 2017).

8.8 Oral Manifestations of Odontogenic Infections

Acute odontogenic infections or exacerbation of chronic odontogenic infections breach the periapical bone and traverse either through the buccal or the lingual/palatal cortical bony plates. Subsequently, they spread to single or multiple fascial spaces of the oral cavity, depending on the anatomical location of the tooth. It could lead to fascial space infections, which primarily affect the following fascial spaces: submandibular, buccal, submental, palatal, lateral pharyngeal, and pterygomaxillary spaces. For example, Ludwig's angina is a fascial space infection that includes the submandibular, sublingual, and submental spaces (Carlson and Pfadt 2011). Pus-filled erythematous edema, raised floor of the mouth associated with fever and chills, obstructed laryngeal and pharyngeal spaces leading to dysphagia and hypopnea have been reported extensively as signs and symptoms. CT is the diagnostic tool of choice to observe the spread and locate the origin of infection. Orthopantomogram in the dental setting can be used to locate the infection origin. Total blood and white blood cell (WBC) counts and pus exudate examinations for microbial strains have to be performed simultaneously. Ultrasonography guided needle aspiration has been advocated for collection of pus as it reduces the risk of discomfort due to multiple needle entries (Mukhi and Mahindra 2012). Most recently, the importance of C-reactive protein and serum prealbumin level evaluation have been emphasized for estimating the severity and prognosis of the fascial space infections (Bagul et al. 2017; Sharma et al. 2014). Fascial space infections can deteriorate to life threatening conditions and have a high mortality rate due to the rapid progress of adverse events. Intubation by tracheostomy, in severe cases, is the first step in the treatment protocol. Drainage of pus and irrigation of the wound, and control of infection by antibiotic therapy prevent further sepsis. Analgesics play an important role in reducing the discomfort due to pain and anxiety associated with the severity of the condition.

8.9 Risk Assessment

Patients with chronic medical and dental diseases are increasing in the United States (CDC 2013). Coordination of care between dental and medical care providers has the potential to assess a patient's risk status and prevent the initiation and progression of chronic diseases such as diabetes, coronary artery disease, and periodontal disease. Recent studies also reported a bidirectional relationship between diabetes, and periodontal disease. For instance, the prevalence of odontogenic infections in patients with diabetes was higher compared to non-diabetics (Ko et al. 2017). Studies showed that diabetic patients are immuno-compromised leading to increased risk of odontogenic infections and eventual hospitalization (Huang et al. 2005). In these medically compromised patients, typically, the dentist requires a medical consultation while planning dental treatment. Also, assessing the overall risk of medical and dental conditions before proceeding with dental treatment helps reduce complications.

8.10 Systems Biology: Genomics, Proteomics, Microbiomics, Phenotypes

According to the study by Moenning et al. (1989) unlike specific infections of other organs of the body, majority of the odontogenic infections are polymicrobial in nature with multiple strains of aerobic and anaerobic bacteria. Bacteroides, Fusobacterium, Peptococcus, Peptostreptococcus and few other facultative anaerobes are the most common anaerobes found in these infections (Gill and Scully 1990). Storoe et al. (2001) conducted a retrospective study of dental and microbiology records and concluded that changes in the nomenclature, identification protocols, and isolation techniques have led to changes in the bacteria identified as causative organisms of the odontogenic infections.

8.11 Treatment

Odontogenic infections are treated by managing systemic complications through therapeutic and surgical interventions and by treating the dental cause of infection. Moenning et al. (1989) found that 51% of the infections produced beta-lactamase enzyme and therefore, suggested the use of beta-lactamase inhibitors such as ampicillin-sulbactam combinations (Yuvaraj et al. 2012). Increasingly, methicillin-resistant *Staphylococcus aureus* is found as the causative organism of the established spread of infection. In such cases, Vancomycin is the antibiotic of choice along with rigid sterile protocols (Bali et al. 2015).

8.12 Prognosis

Prognosis of complications due to odontogenic infections is good with prompt detection and treatment. If undetected, odontogenic infection can turn fatal due to spread of infection to adjacent fascial spaces and to distant regions of the human body. In recent times, serum C-reactive protein along with pre albumin levels have been proposed for monitoring the prognosis of treatment in patients with complications due to odontogenic infections (Bagul et al. 2017; Sharma et al. 2014).

8.13 Interdisciplinary Care Team

8.13.1 Medical Providers

Primary care physician, medical radiologist, otorhinolaryngologist, emergency physician, cardiologist and cardiothoracic surgeon, neurosurgeon, nurse practitioner.

8.13.2 Dental Providers

General dentists, dental specialists, dental radiologists, oral health educators, dental hygienists.

8.14 Guidelines

As of year 2018, no evidence-based guidelines exist to prevent systemic complications due to odontogenic infections except for the antibiotic prophylaxis guidelines developed to prevent infective endocarditis. According to the 2017 American Heart

Association (AHA) and American College of Cardiology (A.C.C.) guidelines, patients with conditions listed below who undergo "dental procedures that involve manipulation of gingival tissue or the periapical region of teeth or perforation of the oral mucosa" require antibiotic prophylaxis: (Antibiotic prophylaxis and ADA 2017; Nishimura et al. 2017).

1. Prosthetic cardiac valves, including transcatheter-implanted prostheses and homografts.
2. Prosthetic material used for cardiac valve repair, such as annuloplasty rings and chords.
3. Previous episode of infective endocarditis.
4. Unrepaired cyanotic congenital heart disease or repaired congenital heart disease, with residual shunt or valvular regurgitation at the site of or adjacent to the site of a prosthetic patch or prosthetic device.
5. Cardiac transplant with valve regurgitation due to structurally abnormal valve.

8.15 Existing Gaps in Care and Role of Informatics to Improve Care

Due to the current fragmented medical and dental care, it is challenging to share patient information and coordinate care between dental and medical professionals. To prevent complications following acute odontogenic infections, it is important to establish an interdisciplinary care between medical and dental specialties. In cases of extensive fascial space infections, proper case evaluation by oral and maxillofacial surgeon and/or emergency physician, with access to updated electronic medical and dental records is invaluable. For example, while treating maxillary sinusitis, the otolaryngologist diagnosing recurring maxillary sinusitis with otherwise no specific etiology should consult the oral and maxillofacial surgeon or the dental team. Many instances have been noted where otolaryngologists overlooked the dental cause of the maxillary sinusitis and failed in treating the condition (Longhini et al. 2012). An oral examination and periapical radiograph of the specific oral region in doubt is of great value in diagnosing the reason for maxillary sinusitis. Such clinical scenarios increase the importance of patient information exchange between dental and medical providers.

Informatics can play an important role to achieve this objective. Future work should focus on determining the relevant information that needs to be shared between medical and dental care providers to improve patient care, developing a framework that facilitates information exchange between providers who practice in large and small healthcare settings, and implementing standards and terminology to document and exchange information in a seamless manner. Recent progress in developing dental diagnostic terminologies and making it a subset of SNOMED-CT, which is a comprehensive vocabulary of medical findings and diagnoses are steps in the right direction (https://www.ada.org/en/member-center/member-benefits/practice-resources/dental-informatics/snodent). Although technology is there, further work is warranted to determine how it could be leveraged to facilitate exchange of information between medical and dental providers effectively (refer to Chapter on Standards and terminologies for details).

8.16 Summary

Since odontogenic infections require multidisciplinary care, the care team includes the patient, patient's guardian, and dental and medical providers. Discussions related to treatment planning must include a reconciled medication list, clinical and psychological concerns related to the patient and health related interventions, which may affect the overall outcome of the treatment. Also, medically compromised patients require such multidisciplinary care for treatment planning as well as for prevention of disease initiation and progress. Such approaches would reduce the overall risk in terms of adverse events and enhance outcomes by enhancing the quality of treatment. Regular and coordinated medical and dental care can help in reducing these events and also in reducing the cost of health care.

Large health care systems with both medical and dental care providers are already benefitting from integrating medical and dental care (Acharya 2016). An integrated EHR that includes medical and dental care data of a patient, unlike the existing standalone medical and dental records have played a crucial role to achieve this integrated care. This unified approach supports the patient's critical information exchange among providers of different departments and facilities within the health care system. This would also enhance the care in cases of medically compromised dental patients by providing the dentists with updated medical information. However, such models of integrated care need to be expanded to small healthcare settings where medical and dental providers currently work in siloes and where majority of the population receive care.

References

Abubaker AO. Applied anatomy of the maxillary sinus. Oral Maxillofac Surg Clin North Am. 1999;11:1–14.

Abu-Omar Y, Kocher GJ, Bosco P, Barbero C, Waller D, Gudbjartsson T, Cardillo G. European Association for Cardio-Thoracic Surgery expert consensus statement on the prevention and management of mediastinitis. Eur J Cardiothorac Surg. 2017;51(1):10–29. https://academic.oup.com/ejcts/article/51/1/10/2670570/European-Association-for-Cardio-Thoracic-Surgery.

Acharya A. Marshfield clinic health system: integrated care case study. J Calif Dent Assoc. 2016;44(3):177–81.

Alias Ramesh Colbert K, Sankar R. Odontogenic maxillary sinusitis – need for multidisciplinary approach—a review. J Dent Med Sci. 2014;13:2279–861. Retrieved from www.iosrjournals.org

Antibiotic Prophylaxis Prior to Dental Procedures. 2017, Sept 14. http://www.ada.org/en/member-center/oral-health-topics/antibiotic-prophylaxis. Retrieved 26 Oct 2017.

Bagul R, Chandan S, Sane VD, Patil S, Yadav D. Comparative evaluation of C-reactive protein and WBC count in fascial space infections of odontogenic origin. J Maxillofac Oral Surg. 2017;16(2):238–42.

Bahl R, Sandhu S, Sahai N, Gupta M, Singh K. Odontogenic infections: microbiology and management. Contemp Clin Dent. 2014;5(3):307. https://doi.org/10.4103/0976-237X.137921.

Bali R, Sharma P, Gaba S, Kaur A, Ghanghas P. A review of complications of odontogenic infections. Natl J Maxillofac Surg. 2015;6(2):136. https://doi.org/10.4103/0975-5950.183867.

Blomquist IK, Bayer AS. Life-threatening deep fascial space infections of the head and neck. Infect Dis Clin N Am. 1988;2(1):237–64.

Bomeli SR, Branstetter BF, Ferguson BJ. Frequency of a dental source for acute maxillary sinusitis. Laryngoscope. 2009;119(3):580–4. https://doi.org/10.1002/lary.20095.

Bor DH, Woolhandler S, Nardin R, Brusch J, Himmelstein DU. Infective endocarditis In the U.S., 1998–2009: a nationwide study. PLoS One. 2013;8(3):e60033.

Carlson DS, Pfadt E. Vincent and Ludwig angina: two damaging oral infections. Nursing. 2011;41(2):55–8.

Centers for Disease Control and Prevention. The state of aging and health in America 2013. Atlanta, GA: Centers for Disease Control and Prevention, US Department of Health and Human Services; 2013.

Debnam JM, Guha-Thakurta N. Retropharyngeal and prevertebral spaces: anatomic imaging and diagnosis. Otolaryngol Clin North Am. 2012;45(6):1293–310.

Edlich RF, Cross CL, Dahlstrom JJ, Long WB. Modern concepts of the diagnosis and treatment of necrotizing fasciitis. J Emerg Med. 2010;39(2):261–5.

Endo S, Murayama F, Hasegawa T, Yamamoto S, Yamaguchi T, Sohara Y, Nishino H. Guideline of surgical management based on diffusion of descending necrotizing mediastinitis. Jpn J Thorac Cardiovasc Surg. 1999;47(1):14–9.

Estrera AS, Landay MJ, Grisham JM, Sinn DP, Platt MR. Descending necrotizing mediastinitis. Surg Gynecol Obstet. 1983;157(6):545–52.

Feldman DP, Picerno NA, Porubsky ES. Cavernous sinus thrombosis complicating odontogenic parapharyngeal space neck abscess: a case report and discussion. Otolaryngol Head Neck Surg. 2000;123(6):744–5.

Foroulis CN, Sileli MN. Descending necrotizing mediastinitis: review of the literature and controversies in management. Open Surg J. 2011;5:12–8.

Fukuchi M, Suzuki O, Nasu D, Koizumi K, Muta Y, Imaizumi H, Ishida H. Descending necrotizing mediastinitis treated with tooth extractions following mediastinal and cervical drainage. Case Rep Gastroenterol. 2015;9(3):311–6.

Gill Y, Scully C. Orofacial odontogenic infections: review of microbiology and current treatment. Oral Surg Oral Med Oral Pathol. 1990;70(2):155–8.

Herzon FS, Martin AD. Medical and surgical treatment of peritonsillar, retropharyngeal, and parapharyngeal abscesses. Curr Infect Dis Rep. 2006;8(3):196–202. https://doi.org/10.1007/s11908-006-0059-8.

Huang TT, Tseng FY, Liu TC, Hsu CJ, Chen YS. Deep neck infection in diabetic patients: comparison of clinical picture and outcomes with nondiabetic patients. Otolaryngol Head Neck Surg. 2005;132(6):943–7.

Igoumenakis D, Gkinis G, Kostakis G, Mezitis M, Rallis G. Severe odontogenic infections: causes of spread and their management. Surg Infect. 2014;15(1):64–8.

Ishinaga H, Otsu K, Sakaida H, Miyamura T, Nakamura S, Kitano M, Takeuchi K. Descending necrotizing mediastinitis from deep neck infection. Eur Arch Otorhinolaryngol. 2013;270(4):1463–6.

Kiddee W, Preechawai P, Hirunpat S. Bilateral septic cavernous sinus thrombosis following the masticator and parapharyngeal space infection from the odontogenic origin: a case report. J Med Assoc Thai. 2010;93(9):1107.

Kiefer TL, Bashore TM. Infective endocarditis: a comprehensive overview. Rev Cardiovasc Med. 2012;13(2–3):e105–20.

Ko HH, Chien WC, Lin YH, Chung CH, Cheng SJ. Examining the correlation between diabetes and odontogenic infection: a nationwide, retrospective, matched-cohort study in Taiwan. PLoS One. 2017;12(6):e0178941.

Le H, Prejean S, Heck M. Septic cerebral venosinus thrombosis secondary to an odontogenic infection. J La State Med Soc. 2017;169(2):33.

Longhini AB, Branstetter BF, Ferguson BJ. Otolaryngologists' perceptions of odontogenic maxillary sinusitis. Laryngoscope. 2012;122(9):1910–4.

Lypka M, Hammoudeh J. Dentoalveolar infections. Oral Maxillofac Surg Clin North Am. 2011;23(3):415–24.

Maloney PL, Doku HC. Maxillary sinusitis of odontogenic origin. J Can Dent Assoc. 1968;34(11):591. https://doi.org/10.1016/0278-2391(89)90383-2.

Moenning JE, Nelson CL, Kohler RB. The microbiology and chemotherapy of odontogenic infections. J Oral Maxillofac Surg. 1989;47(9):976–85. https://doi.org/10.1016/0278-2391(89)90383-2.

Moghimi M, Baart JA, Karagozoglu KH, Forouzanfar T. Spread of odontogenic infections: a retrospective analysis and review of the literature. Quintessence Int. 2013;44(4):351–61.

Mukhi PU, Mahindra UR. The use of ultrasonography in diagnosis and management of superficial fascial space infections. Indian J Dent Res. 2012;23(3):313–9.

Nishimura RA, Otto CM, Bonow RO, Carabello BA, Erwin JP, Fleisher LA, et al. 2017 AHA/ACC focused update of the 2014 AHA/ACC guideline for the management of patients with valvular heart disease: a report of the American College of Cardiology/American Heart Association Task Force on Clinical Practice Guidelines. Circulation. 2017;135(25):e1159–95.

Novakov I, Safev G, Peicheva S. Descending necrotizing mediastinitis of odontogenic origin-personal experience and literature review. Folia Med. 2010;52(3):13–20.

Palma DM, Giuliano S, Cracchiolo AN, Falcone M, Ceccarelli G, Tetamo R, Venditti M. Clinical features and outcome of patients with descending necrotizing mediastinitis: prospective analysis of 34 cases. Infection. 2016;44(1):77–84.

Prado–Calleros HM, Jiménez–Fuentes E, Jiménez–Escobar I. Descending necrotizing mediastinitis: systematic review on its treatment in the last 6 years, 75 years after its description. Head Neck. 2016;38(S1):E2275–83.

Sakamoto H, Aoki T, Kise Y, Watanabe D, Sasaki J. Descending necrotizing mediastinitis due to odontogenic infections. Oral Surg Oral Med Oral Pathol Oral Radiol Endod. 2000;89(4):412–9.

Sharma A, Giraddi G, Krishnan G, Shahi AK. Efficacy of serum prealbumin and CRP levels as monitoring tools for patients with fascial space infections of odontogenic origin: a clinicobiochemical study. J Maxillofac Oral Surg. 2014;13(1):1–9.

Simuntis R, Kubilius R, Vaitkus S. Odontogenic maxillary sinusitis: a review. Stomatologija. 2014;16(2):39–43.

Storoe W, Haug RH, Lillich TT. The changing face of odontogenic infections. J Oral Maxillofac Surg. 2001;59(7):739–48. https://www.ncbi.nlm.nih.gov/pubmed/11429732.

Taschieri S, Torretta S, Corbella S, Del Fabbro M, Francetti L, Lolato A, Capaccio P. Pathophysiology of sinusitis of odontogenic origin. J Investig Clin Dent. 2015:1–7. https://doi.org/10.1111/jicd.12202.

Taubert KA, Wilson W. Is endocarditis prophylaxis for dental procedures necessary? Heart Asia. 2017;9(1):63–7.

Vidal F, Coutinho TM, Carvalho Ferreira DD, Souza RCD, Gonçalves LS. Odontogenic sinusitis: a comprehensive review. Acta Odontol Scand. 2017;75(8):623–33.

Vallo J, Suominen-Taipale L, Huumonen S, Soikkonen K, Norblad A. Prevalence of mucosal abnormalities of the maxillary sinus and their relationship to dental disease in panoramic radiography: results from the Health 2000 Health Examination Survey. Oral Surg Oral Med Oral Pathol Oral Radiol Endod. 2010;109(3):e80–7.

Wei D, Bi L, Zhu H, He J, Wang H. Less invasive management of deep neck infection and descending necrotizing mediastinitis. Medicine. 2017;96(15):e6590. https://doi.org/10.1097/MD.0000000000006590.

Wilson W, Taubert KA, Gewitz M, Lockhart PB, Baddour LM, Levison M, et al. Prevention of infective endocarditis: guidelines from the American heart association: a guideline from the American heart association rheumatic fever, endocarditis, and Kawasaki disease committee, council on cardiovascular disease in the young, and the council on clinical cardiology, council on cardiovascular surgery and anesthesia, and the quality of care and outcomes research interdisciplinary working group. Circulation. 2007;116(15):1736–54.

Yuvaraj V, Alexander M, Pasupathy S. Microflora in maxillofacial infections—a changing scenario? J Oral Maxillofac Surg. 2012;70(1):119–25. https://doi.org/10.1016/j.joms.2011.02.006.

Chapter 9
Interdisciplinary Care Model: Pneumonia and Oral Health

Ingrid Glurich, Neel Shimpi, Frank Scannapieco, Jayanth Vedre, and Amit Acharya

9.1 Definition, Classification, and Epidemiology

9.1.1 Definition

Pneumonia is a respiratory infection due to lower pulmonary microbial infection, or mechanical introduction of pulmonary pathogens into the pulmonary space as a consequence of aspiration of oropharyngeal secretions or intubation (Madhi et al. 2004). A broad spectrum of microbial species may be causal, ranging from established pulmonary pathogens to commensal organisms, including those that colonize the oral cavity, which may emerge as opportunistic pathogens under favorable conditions. Many pulmonary pathogens are anaerobes or facultative anaerobes.

I. Glurich · N. Shimpi · A. Acharya (✉)
Center for Oral and Systemic Health, Marshfield Clinic Research Institute, Marshfield, WI, USA
e-mail: glurich.ingrid@marshfieldresearch.org; shimpi.neel@marshfieldresearch.org; acharya.amit@marshfieldresearch.org

F. Scannapieco
Department of Oral Biology, School of Dental Medicine, State University of New York at Buffalo, Buffalo, NY, USA
e-mail: fas1@buffalo.edu

J. Vedre
Medical Intensive Care Unit, Marshfield Clinic, Marshfield, WI, USA
e-mail: vedre.jayanth@marshfieldclinic.org

A. Acharya et al. (eds.), *Integration of Medical and Dental Care and Patient Data*, Health Informatics, https://doi.org/10.1007/978-3-319-98298-4_9

9.1.2 Classification

Classification of pneumonia is generally based on causal organism and the setting where the infection was acquired. Pneumonia classification is currently defined by the following subtypes.

9.1.3 Pneumonia Subtypes

Pneumonia acquired in various settings shows clinical variability relative to predominant causal pathogens and antibiotic resistance patterns. These characteristics form the basis for stratification of pneumonia into pneumonia subtypes including:

1. community acquired pneumonia (CAP)
2. health care acquired pneumonia (HCAP)
3. hospital-acquired pneumonia (HAP), which includes late onset subtype (LOP), aspiration-associated (AAP), and ventilator-acquired pneumonia (VAP) subtypes. (Evans 2014; Ewig et al. 2012; Kalil et al. 2016; Klompas 2015).

9.1.3.1 Community Acquired Pneumonia (CAP)

This type of pneumonia generally develops independent of exposures to healthcare settings. Emergence of CAP is generally associated with physiological and local environmental changes to the respiratory tract, especially following viral or mycoplasma infection. In combination with compromised host immune response, the altered environment facilitates infection by known pulmonary pathogens or opportunistic commensals which have colonized the oral cavity. While more than 100 microbial species have been identified as causal, the five most frequently documented pathogens causing CAP in adults include *S. pneumoniae*, occurring at nearly three times the frequency of all other bacterial species, with a mean etiological fraction (MEF) of 23%, viral pathogens (including respiratory syncytial virus (RSV), rhinovirus, adenovirus, and influenza: (combined MEF = 19%), *Chlamydia* species (combined MEF = 15%), *Mycoplasma pneumoniae* (MEF = 7%) *and Haemophlus influenza* (MEF = 6%) (Drijkoningen and Rohde 2014). Notably, CAP-associated methicillin-resistant *Staphylococcus aureus* (MRSA) has recently emerged as a causal pathogen (Durrington and Summers 2008). While *S. pneumoniae* is also a common causal agent in young patients (Walker et al. 2013), other pathogens that may also be encountered include: Group B streptococci, gram negative enteric pathogens, viral, and fungal pathogens (DeAntonio et al. 2016; Evans 2014).

9.1.3.2 Health Care Acquired Pneumonia (HCAP)

This pneumonia subtype develops due to exposures in healthcare settings outside of the hospital setting. Examples include residence in a nursing home or rehabilitation center, hospitalization in the preceding 90 days, outpatient treatment including intravenous therapy or dialysis. Originally classified as a subtype of HAP due to the perception of a higher prevalence of multi-drug resistant (MDR) organisms reported with HCAP compared to other categories of pneumonia, HCAP has recently been excluded from HAP guidelines and reclassified as CAP due to updated documentation of lower rates of multi-drug resistance than had been previously reported (Chalmers et al. 2014; Kalil et al. 2016) Justification for this subclassification of pneumonia remains controversial (Ewig et al. 2012).

9.1.3.3 Hospital Acquired (i.e. Nosocomial) Pneumonia (HAP)

HAP pneumonia emerges either following hospitalization or post-discharge and in the absence of exposures to other healthcare settings. Classification parameters include incidence following hospitalization ≥2 days, within 90 days of disease onset. Pathogens frequently seen with HAP include *S. aureus*, *Klebsiella*, and *Actinobacter* species. High rates of antibiotic resistance with HAP include respectively: methicillin-resistant *S. aureus* (MRSA) (50%), ceftazidime- and cefepime-resistant *Klebsiella* species (30%) and carbapenem-resistant *Actinobacter* species (60%) (Klompas 2015).

Late-ONSET PNEUMONIA (LOP)

LOP represents a HAP subtype classified based on emergence >96 h following hospital admission. LOP is associated with poorer outcomes, often occurring in physically debilitated patients with lower capacity to clear oral secretions or immunocompromised patients. Frequently encountered pathogens seen with LOP include *P. aeruginosa*, *K. pneumoniae*, *Actinobacter* species, and MRSA (Evans 2014).

Ventilator-Associated Pneumonia (VAP)

VAP is a subset of HAP, however, may also arise as a result of intubation, or emerge as a nosocomial infection in intubated patients who were hospitalized following trauma experienced in a community setting, or following surgery. VAP commonly emerges >48 h following ventilator placement. Clinical findings in these patients are reminiscent of those noted with HAP and may present with symptomology of congestive heart failure, pulmonary embolization, or hemorrhage.

Aspiration Pneumonia

Aspiration pneumonia is most commonly caused by oral anaerobic bacteria present in oropharyngeal fluids which may become aspirated into the lungs especially in patients with dysphagia or semi-consciousness or who have compromised capacity for clearing respiratory secretions. This type of pneumonia is more frequently encountered in nursing home residents or the elderly and is highly associated with sub-optimal oral hygiene. Common pathogens associated with aspiration pneumonia include *Staphylococcus aureus*, *Pseudomonas aeruginosa*, *Klebsiella pneumonia*, and *Enterobacter cloacae* (Scannapieco 2014).

9.1.4 Epidemiology

Based on 2014 national mortality data for the USA, pneumonia contributed to 15.9 deaths per 100,000 population (National Center for Health Statistics 2017). Pneumonia is implicated in 50% of cases of septic shock as the single most common cause. Prevalence of pneumonia has remained relatively constant over time with little change in mortality rates over the past 50 years. (American Thoracic Society 2015). Attributable mortality rates associated with pneumonia range from 27% to 50% (Tedja and Gordon 2013), depending on acquisitional setting and pneumonia subtype.

9.1.4.1 CAP

Impacting persons of all ages, pneumonia represents a significant global health issue. Individuals at highest risk include the elderly, immuno-compromised, those suffering from malnutrition, hospitalized, institutionalized, bedridden, or intubated, and those with co-morbid burden.

While CAP is not a reportable disease, global CAP incidence rates have been tentatively estimated at 5–6 cases per 1000 person years on average, although rates vary widely by country with higher incidence noted based on risk contributed by gender (male > female), race (Blacks > Caucasians) and advancing age (Van Dyke and Sheilesh 2005). An increase in rate to 18.2 cases/1000 person years was estimated in patients 65–69 years of age, and 52.3 cases/1000 person years in patients ≥85 years of age (Scannapieco 2014).

Globally, between 120–156 million cases of acute lower respiratory infections are reported in children <5 years of age, contribute to an estimated 1.4 million CAP-associated deaths annually, accounting for 15% of childhood mortality, with a disproportionate 81% of cases impacting children under the age of 2 years. The highest pneumonia-associated mortality rates were reported for Southeast Asia and Africa, accounting for >50% of the global rate of pneumonia-associated deaths in children (DeAntonio et al. 2016; Walker et al. 2013).

While nearly four million cases of CAP are documented in the USA, approximately one million hospitalizations are attributed to pneumonia annually, rendering pneumonia the second highest cause of hospitalization (Scannapieco 2014). High overall mortality rates of 17/100,000 population and 3.3/100 discharges have remained stable over the past 50 years (National Center for Health Statistics 2017). The average length of hospital stay for pneumonia in the USA is 5.2 days. Excluding work and productivity loss, the medical cost associated with pneumonia-associated hospitalization in the USA was estimated at $10.6 billion in 2011 for 1.1 million hospital stays, including incremental costs attributable to antibiotic resistance of causal pathogens (American Thoracic Society 2015; Reynolds et al. 2014; Shea et al. 2014).

9.1.4.2 HAP and VAP

Globally, HAP incidence ranks among the most commonly-documented nosocomial infections. In the USA, HAP represents the most prevalent nosocomial infection in medical and ICUs with incidence estimated at 5–15 cases per 1000 hospital admissions, generally extending length of stay. As the second most common nosocomial infection, overall, HAP represents approximately 15% of all hospital acquired infections. HAP may increase length of stay by 7–9 days, with an attributable estimated cost per patient of >$40,000 per event (Tedja and Gordon 2013). Mortality rates associated with HAP range from 30–70% (Tedja and Gordon 2013).

As the most common nosocomial infection among critically ill patients VAP represents approximately 3% of all healthcare-associated infections and the strongest risk factor for incident HAP, increasing risk by as much as 21-fold following intubation (Tedja and Gordon 2013). Following consumer price index adjustments for healthcare costs associated with VAP in 2007, Scott projected the cost of hospital stay associated with incident VAP at $19,600–$28,500 per event (Scott II 2009). An estimated 25% of patients admitted to the ICU experience HAP, with 70–80% of these cases representing VAP (Torres and Cilloniz 2015). In a meta-analysis, mortality attributable to VAP was reported to be 13%, notably with highest risk reported for surgical patients with mid-range severity scores (APACHE or SAPS 2) on admission compared to trauma or medical patients with low or high severity scores (Melsen et al. 2013).

9.2 Systemic Manifestations of Pneumonia

The diagnosis of pneumonia is ascertained based on an assessment of six clinical parameters. The Clinical Pulmonary Infection Score is a decision support tool that is used to assess the possibility of pneumonia and assist in determining the need for treatment in ventilator assisted patients. A score of >6 based on an assessment of the first five parameters is suggestive of pneumonia. Parameters include:

1. Body temperature: >36.5–<38.4 (0 points); >38.5–<38.9 (1 point); <36 or >39 °C (2 points).
2. White cell counts/mm^3: ≥4000–<11,000 (0 points), <4000 or >11,000 (no band forms) (1 point); >11,000 with band forms (2 points).
3. Tracheal secretions: absent (0 points); non-purulent (1 point); purulent (2 points).
4. Oxygenation based on PaO_2/FiO_2 assessment: >240 or acute respiratory distress syndrome (0 points); <230 and no acute respiratory syndrome (2 points).
5. Chest radiograph: no infiltrate (0 points); diffuse or patchy infiltrates (1 point); localized infiltrates (2 points).
6. Tracheal aspirate culture: negative (0 points); positive (2 points).

Other symptomology that may be variably associated with pneumonia that is monitored in the clinical setting includes:

1. Presence of heart rate greater than 100 beats/min.
2. Rapid respiratory rate: 24–30 breaths/min.
3. Decreased systolic blood pressure (<90 mmHg) or diastolic blood pressure <60.
4. O_2 saturation <90% or PaO_2 <60.
5. Vomiting.
6. Confusion.
7. BUN >20.

This symptomology is especially worrisome in patients >65 years of age who may be at higher risk for pneumonia, especially if these patients present with underlying risk factors including comorbid conditions such as cardiac disease, diabetes, or evidence of poor oral health practices. Additional clinical characteristics that may be present pointing to a potential pneumonia diagnosis include enlarged lymph nodes, cough, sore throat, chest pain, and bluish nail coloration related to poor oxygenation in the extremities (Bunting 2014).

To define improved surveillance guidelines, the CDC implemented three categories of VAP in 2011 based on distinct symptomatic presentation.

(a) VAP was defined as radiographic evidence of new or progressive/persistent infiltrates and two of the following symptoms: white count <4000 or >12,000, fever or hypothermia, purulent sputum, or reduced respiratory capacity.
(b) Ventilator-associated condition (VAC) was differentiated by: increased positive end respiratory pressure >3 or increased daily minimum FiO_2 >0.2 for ≥2 days in a patient who had a demonstrated baseline improvement in these measures for 2 days.
(c) Infection-related ventilator-associated condition (IVAC): was defined as an episode of VAC within 2 days of the VAC initiation and >4 days following new antibiotic exposure (Evans 2014).

9.3 Oral Manifestations of Pneumonia

The major impact of oral health on the development of pneumonia is a decline in oral hygiene, e.g. the absence of intervention in the clinical setting or by caregivers of outpatients. If illness sufficiently hinders the patient from performing essential oral hygiene, resident microbes rapidly form oral biofilms on teeth and oral cavity surfaces, placing the patient at increased risk for infection of mucosal surfaces even in the presence of antibiotic exposures associated with pneumonia treatment. Pre-existent oral disease may predispose patients to pneumonia. Shifts in microbiome constituency in the presence of oral disease may also be associated with environmental changes that support colonization by potential pathogens. For example, studies have shown that an increase in the number of decayed teeth associated with cariogenic processes was significantly related to the incidence of aspirational pneumonia (Terpenning et al. 2001).

9.4 Oral-Pneumonia Connection

Many pneumonia-associated pathogens colonize oral biofilms, facilitating pathogen access to the respiratory tract. Access may be gained through aspiration of pathogens already colonizing the oral cavity, inhalation of airborne pathogens, during bacteremia events, during mechanical ventilation, or due to increased dental plaque formation due to restricted capacity of patients to clear oral secretions. Several systematic reviews have demonstrated oral-systemic associations surrounding pneumonia emergence (Azarpazhooh and Leake 2006; Chan et al. 2007). Notably, pathogens isolated from the lungs of patients with VAP were genetically identical to oral cavity isolates collected from the same patient (Heo et al. 2008; Sands et al. 2016, 2017). Applying multivariate modeling, another study demonstrated that risk for pneumonia-associated hospitalization was increased nearly 30% in individuals with dental caries (Laurence et al. 2015). Periodontal pathogens have also been implicated as causal agents of pneumonia. Moreover recent study by Marino et al. (2017) demonstrated highly similar profiles of organisms on analysis of dental plaque, bronchial lavage specimens, and endotracheal tube cultures obtained from mechanically ventilated patients. Organisms present in each of the specimens included both pneumonia pathogens and oral flora.

Moreover, aspiration of periodontal organisms and oral communal bacteria have been identified as causal agents in aspiration pneumonia. (Scannapieco 1999). A systematic review of studies exploring oral health and nosocomial pneumonia identified evidence-based support for increased risk for incident pneumonia based on higher rates of colonization of the oral cavity by potential respiratory pathogens and demonstrated a clinically significant reduction in nosocomial pneumonia incidence following improvement of oral hygiene in the hospital setting (Scannapieco et al. 2003; Hua et al. 2016; Labeau et al. 2011; Li et al. 2015; Richards 2013; Shi et al. 2013).

9.5 Diagnostic Codes

The International Classification of Disease (ICD) ICD-10 coding for pneumonia has maintained historical definitions for pneumonia classification largely by causal agent not by classification of type based on emergence setting (Table 9.1). Thus, no specific codes are assigned to CAP or HCAP which are coded as J18.9: *Pneumonia, unspecified*, while VAP carries the ICD-10 code: J95.851. While there is a code for

Table 9.1 ICD-10 pneumonia codes

	ICD10 code
Pneumonia due to the following specified organisms:	
Due to *Streptococcus pneumoniae*	J13
Haemophilus influenza	J14
Klebsiella pneumoniae	J15.0
Pseudomonas	J15.1
Staphylococcus	J15.2
Streptococcus, group B	J15.3
Other streptococci	JJ15.4
Escherichia coli	J15.6
Pneumonia due to the following Gram negative bacteria:	
Mycoplasma pneumoniae	J15.7
Other bacterial pneumonia	J15.8
Bacterial pneumonia, unspecified	J15.9
Pneumonia due to other specified infectious organisms	J16.8
Pneumonia in bacterial diseases specified elsewhere	J17.0
Pneumonia in mycoses	J17.2
Pneumonia in parasitic diseases	J17.3
Pneumonia in bacterial diseases classified elsewhere	J17.8
Additional clinical findings:	
Bronchopneumonia, unspecified organism	J18.0
Lobar pneumonia, unspecified organism	J18.1
Hypostatic pneumonia, unspecified organism	J18.2
Other pneumonia, unspecified organism	J18.8
Pneumonia, unspecified	J18.9
Ventilator-associated pneumonia	J95.851
Positive sputum culture:	
Viral pneumonia	J12.0–J12.9
Bacterial pneumonia	J13–J17

aspiration pneumonitis, this condition is distinct from aspiration pneumonia and is not be applied to aspiration pneumonia (Scannapieco 2014).

SNODENT CT (National Center for BioMedical Ontology SNOMED CT 2017) coding for pneumonia (Table 9.2) in the dental setting is distinct and supports coding by the environment where the pneumonia emerged.

9.6 Risk Assessment

Significantly, aspiration pneumonias have been strongly associated with poor oral hygiene. Logistic regression modeling of parameters which displayed a significant association with the emergence of aspiration pneumonia included: requiring assistance with eating ($p < 0.001$), underlying comorbid conditions including chronic obstructive pulmonary disease ($p = 0.006$), diabetes mellitus ($p = 0.020$), the presence of *S. aureus* ($p = 0.006$), *P. gingivalis* ($p = 0.004$), *S. sobrinus* ($p = 0.016$), the

Table 9.2 SNODENT CT pneumonia codes

Abscess of lung with pneumonia[a]
Acute mucous pneumonia
Aspiration pneumonia[a]
Bilateral pneumonia[a]
Bronchopneumonia[a]
Catarrhal pneumonia
Cavitary pneumonia
Chronic pneumonia[a]
Community acquired pneumonia
Confluent pneumonia
Congenital pneumonia[a]
Focal pneumonia
Gangrenous pneumonia
Granulomatous pneumonia
Hemorrhagic pneumonia
Hypostatic pneumonia[a]
Infective pneumonia[a]
Interstitial pneumonia[a]
Lobar pneumonia[a]
Lobular pneumonia
Neonatal pneumonia[a]

[a]First level entry-expandable to other sub-levels. To access sublevels, click on link provided as instructed

number of decayed teeth ($p = 0.007$), and the number of paired natural or prosthetic teeth that make contact during chewing ($p = 0.023$) (Terpenning et al. 2001). Methods are being evaluated for developing risk assessment tools for pneumonia. An intelligible model based on generalized additive models with pairwise interactions demonstrated higher accuracy in predicting pneumonia risk and hospital 20 day readmissions (Caruana et al. 2015).

Another study utilized the Rankprop method to rank pneumonia patients according to their probability of mortality (Caruana et al. 1995). A total of 30 risk factors collected in medical settings were utilized along with 35 laboratory factors to train the model. However this model could not be applied in practice because it takes into account the results of future lab tests. Other probabilistic methods have been used to determine the pneumonia risk development (Kawaler et al. 2012; Morillo et al. 2013).

9.7 Systems Biology: Microbiomics and Phenotypes

Microbiome studies focused on the lower respiratory tract have revealed that the lungs are not a sterile environment but harbor a distinct microbiome both in healthy and diseased states. When in equilibrium (healthy microbiome phenotype), the microbiome actively contributes to lung health by regulating nutrient absorption, contributing to vitamin synthesis, xenobiotic metabolism, immune regulation. In contrast, dysbiosis contributes to establishment of disease-associated microbiome phenotypes (Cho and Blaser 2012). Notably, microbiome studies have revealed that establishment of pneumonia is not merely attributable to induction of pathology by an invasive pathogen, but also equilibrium disruption of the resident microbiome leading to dysbiosis and inflammatory activity in the microbial environment which facilitate establishment of disease (Dickson et al. 2013). A study by Flannigan explored the microbiome of VAP in patients with pulmonary colonization by *Pseudomonas aeruginosa* and described a reduction in pulmonary microbiome diversity in conjunction with broad spectrum and anti-pseudomonal antibiotic treatment, followed by re-emergence of Pseudomonas as the predominant organism (Flanagan et al. 2007). Pulmonary microbiome characterization further revealed increased susceptibility to severe pneumonia onset in patients with chronic obstructive pulmonary disease (COPD) following exposure to inhaled corticosteroids. Subsequently shifts in microbiota composition were observed during the temporal frame circumscribing both disease status and drug exposure. These data suggested that inhaled drug exposure may negatively impact microbiome equilibrium (Singh et al. 2009).

Clinical phenotyping of individuals at increased risk for pneumonia, especially CAP which is large treated on an outpatient basis, and prediction of clinical outcome to inform clinical decision support has been actively undertaken through application of logistic regression modeling with the aim of reducing morbidity and mortality. Several tools developed in various countries have been adopted into clinical practice including pneumonia severity index calculator (PSI) (Fine et al. 1997), mBTS severity assessment tool (Neill et al. 1996), Curb 65 (Lim et al. 2003), SMART-COP (Charles et al. 2008) (link to tool): https://lifeinthefastlane.com/wp-content/uploads/2010/07/etg-smartcop.pdf (Therapeutic Guidelines Limited 2010), for assessing severity of CAP, among others.

9.8 Treatment

Per guidelines by the American Lung Association (2017) and CDC, treatment for pneumonia is based on diagnostic workup which includes documentation of physical symptomology, blood count, arterial blood gases assessment, cultures of sputum and pleural fluid if fluid is present, pulse oximetry measures to determine oxygenation and chest X-ray. CAP is generally treated in the outpatient setting if the patient is assessed to be low risk for complications. Patients who may be hospitalized include the elderly, children, those with other serious co-morbidities, those who require assistance with care, or are not responding to antibiotics. Hospitalized patients and those not responding to antibiotic treatment usually undergo a bronchoscopy. Based on microbial culture results, macrolide antibiotics may be initiated per established guidelines to target suspected pathogen. If the infection is of viral origin, anti-viral agents may be administered. If hospitalization is indicated, symptom management is emphasized including control of fever with non-steroidal anti-inflammatory medications or acetaminophen. The patient is kept well hydrated via oral intake of fluids and intravenous (iv) fluids may be administered to hospitalized patients along with iv antibiotics. Oxygen therapy and breathing treatments may also be administered to ease lung function and cough is treated based on severity.

Antibiotics are administered per specified protocols surrounding infectious agent to reduce risk of emergence of antibiotic resistance and dosing is adjusted based on presence of other underlying comorbidities.

Oral health care is emphasized in hospitalized patients especially in intubated patients who cannot clear secretions. Meta—analyses and systematic reviews have determined effectiveness of mechanical removal of oral biofilms and rinsing with anti-microbial antiseptic rinses such as iodopovidone or chlorohexidine in reducing incidence of pneumonia in intubated patients in the ICU (Hua et al. 2016; Labeau et al. 2011; Li et al. 2015; Richards 2013, Scannapieco et al. 2003; Shi et al. 2013).

9.9 Prognosis

Prognosis is generally based on the general health of the patient and is generally good in younger patients with no serious comorbid conditions. Risk of death increases with age and 50% of deaths from pneumonia are associated with sepsis and septic shock arising from bacteremia. In the USA, hospitalization for pneumonia impacts approximately one million adults and with an overall mortality rate of 50,000 individuals. Requirements for mechanical ventilation, ICU stays and nosocomial infection with antibiotic resistant bacterial strains represent serious complications and are associated with increased risk of morbidity and mortality. Globally, 15% of deaths in children under the age of 5 years are attributed to pneumonia and remains the top cause for hospitalization of pediatric patients.

Oral health intervention by the patient and profession has shown effectiveness in preventing onset of pneumonia. Oral prophylaxis of hospitalized patients and institutionalized individuals is especially emphasized to prevent onset of pneumonia in the elderly, persons with immune-deficiencies, serious comorbidities, or of diminished capacity for self-care (Scannapieco 2014).

9.10 Interdisciplinary Care Team

Interdisciplinary care teams are recommended for optimal management of patients with pneumonia. Team members may include: Primary Care Physicians, General Dentists, Periodontists, Hospitalists, Certified registered nurse practitioners, Registered Nurses, Respiratory therapists, Physical therapists, Occupational therapists, Pharmacists, Case managers, Dietitians, Dental hygienists and Medical assistants.

9.11 Guidelines for Management

The CDC has provided links to the Guidelines for management of pneumonia at its website:

https://www.cdc.gov/pneumococcal/clinicians/diagnosis-medical-mgmt.html.

9.11.1 Community-Acquired Pneumonia (CAP)

- IDSA and ATS Consensus Guidelines on the Management of Community-Acquired Pneumonia in Adults, 2007 (Mandel et al. 2007).
- PIDS and IDSA Clinical Practice Guidelines on the Management of Community-Acquired Pneumonia in Infants and Children Older Than 3 Months of Age, 2011 (Bradley et al. 2011).

9.11.2 Hospital Acquired and Ventilator-Associated Pneumonia

- SHEA and IDSA Strategies to Prevent Ventilator-Associated Pneumonia in Acute Care Hospitals, 2008 (Coffin et al. 2008).
- Kalil et al. (2016). "Management of Adults With Hospital-Acquired and Ventilator-Associated Pneumonia: 2016 Clinical Practice Guidelines by the Infectious Diseases Society of America and the American Thoracic Society." *Clinical Infectious Diseases* 63(5):e61–111.
- Yokoe et al. (2014) "A compendium of strategies to prevent healthcare-associated infections in acute care hospitals: 2014 updates. Infect Control Hosp Epidemiol 35; 967–977.

Clinical guidelines for oral hygiene in vulnerable patients and hospitalized patients have been defined by Berry et al. (2011) and are summarized in Fig. 9.1 and scoring based on level of evidence and grade. Figure 9.2 provides the key to which underlies definitions of level of evidence and grade assigned to each recommendation.

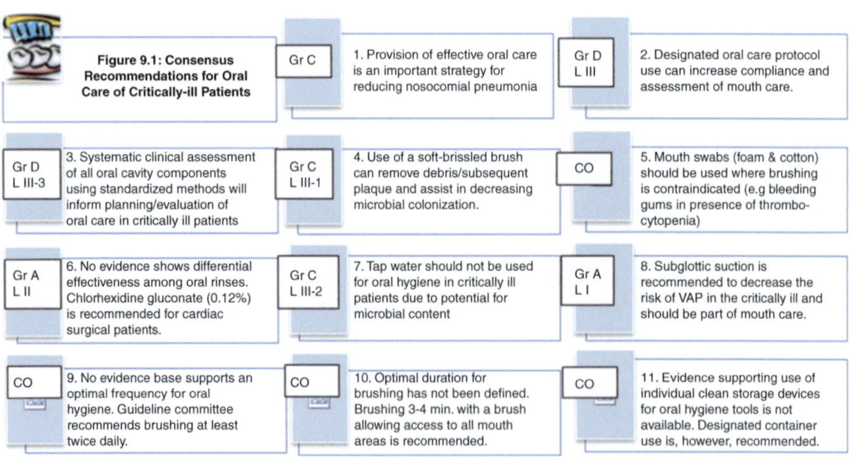

Fig. 9.1 Consensus recommendations for oral care of critically ill patients

Level of Evidence	
I:	Systematic review: randomized controlled trial(s) (RCT)
II:	RCT(s)
III-1:	Pseudo-RCT (applied alternate allocation or method)
III-2:	Comparative study with concurrent controls • Non-randomized trial • Cohort study • Case-control study • Interrupted time series with control group
IV:	Case series with pre/post test results

(Figure adapted from Berry et al; 2011; with permissions)

Grade of Recommendation	
A	Body of evidence can be trusted to guide practice
B	Body of evidence can be trusted to guide practice in most situations
C	Body of evidence provides some support, but care should be taken with application
D	Body of evidence is weak: apply recommendation with caution
Consensus Opinion (CO)	Where no evidence applied, CO was developed by: • Formulation of recommendation through discussion • Assignment of agreement of individual participants (Likert 1-9: consensus set at median of 7.)

Fig. 9.2 Level of evidence and grade of recommendation

9.12 Technology Implications

Informatics can help in promoting new solutions to support developing and presenting the data in a standardized manner to healthcare providers. For example, provision of clinical decision support systems developed through derivation of algorithms derived from modeling electronic data extracted from both medical and dental sources will contribute to derivation of a more comprehensive model. Utilizing various data mining techniques within the EHR can help in developing alert/reminder systems, referral systems and risk assessment tools for pneumonia and underlying oral conditions such as periodontal disease which may contribute to pneumonia pathogenesis.

Improving the quality of patient care in terms of reporting (e.g. documenting pneumonia and periodontal disease prevalence), data analysis and modelling can be supported by implementing dashboards within the electronic health record systems. Availability of these data would help healthcare providers to gain insight on performance goals and measures across patient populations.

9.13 Ontology

Intelligent applications that provide a user-centric view of the data based on pneumonia ontology can be developed for data vizualization. For example, the BioPortal ontology browser representing SNOMED CT in depicts the ontology of the

'Parent'nodes and 'Child'nodes for the term 'Pneumonia'. Links to the National Center for Biomedical Ontology's BioPortal Ontology Browser is accessible at: http://bioportal.bioontology.org/ontologies/SNOMEDCT?p=classes&conceptid=233604007#visualization.

9.14 Care Plan

While awareness knowledgeability among medical and dental providers surrounding oral and systemic health has been reported by several studies, these also identified a need for more research survey research surrounding optimal approaches for dissemination of the medical and dental provider education and training (Shimpi et al. 2016; Umeizudike et al. 2016). Continuing education and training of health care providers surrounding best practices and appropriate preventive measures (e.g., oral hygiene interventions, among others) will contribute to reduced incidence of pneumonia and oral diseases such as periodontal disease.

9.15 Recommendations on Dental Diagnoses and Pneumonia

1. Encouraging the integration of medical and dental records will enable the dental and medical providers to access the comprehensive systemic and oral health history of the patients.
2. As an approach to prevention, modifying pneumonia guidelines to include recommendations for monitoring patient compliance with minimal oral interventions, including daily oral hygiene practice and attending dental visits with recommended periodicity recommended for the patient, will contribute to maintenance of oral health and reductions in pathogen colonization of the oral cavity and respiratory passages.
3. Continuing education and dissemination of educational materials to the medical and dental providers to maintain current knowledgeability regarding links between pneumonia and oral health and best practices surrounding prevention and management. Special emphasis should be placed on management and prevention in particularly vulnerable populations including pediatric and geriatric patients, disparity populations and other special needs populations including institutionalized individuals.

References

American Lung Association. Pneumonia. ©2017 American Lung Association. 2017. http://www.lung.org/lung-health-and-diseases/lung-disease-lookup/pneumonia/?referrer=https://www.google.com/. Accessed 5 May 2017.

American Thoracic Society. Top 20 pneumonia facts-2015. 2015. https://www.thoracic.org/patients/patient-resources/resources/top-pneumonia-facts.pdf. Accessed 5 May 2017.

Azarpazhooh A, Leake J. Systematic review of the association between respiratory diseases and oral health. J Periodontol. 2006;77(9):1465–82.
Berry AM, Davidson PM, Nicholson L, Pasqualotto C, Rolls K. Consensus based clinical guideline for oral hygiene in the critically ill. Intensive Crit Care Nurs. 2011;27(4):180–5.
Bradley J, Byington C, Shah S, Alverson B, Carter E, Harrison C, et al. The management of community-acquired pneumonia in infants and children older than 3 months of age: Clinical Practice Guidelines by the Pediatric Infectious Diseases Society and the Infectious Diseases Society of America. Clin Infect Dis. 2011;53(7):e25–76.
Bunting R. ICD-9 to ICD-10: documentation for pneumonia *McKesson*. 2014. http://www.mckesson.com/bps/blog/icd-9-to-icd-10%2D%2Ddocumentation-for-pneumonia/. Accessed 9 June 2017.
Caruana R, Baluja S, Mitchell T. Using the future to sort outthe present: rankprop and multitask learning for medical risk evaluation. 1995. http://ri.cmu.edu/pub_files/pub1/caruana_r_1995_1/caruana_r_1995_1.pdf. Accessed 9 June 2017.
Caruana R, Lou Y, Gehrke J, Koch P, Sturm M, Elhadad N. Intelligible models for healthcare: predicting pneumonia risk and hospital 30-day readmission. In: KDD '15 Proceedings of the 21th ACM SIGKDD international conference on knowledge discovery and data mining (Aug 10–13, 2015), Sydney, NSW, Australia. New York, NY: ACM; 2015. http://people.dbmi.columbia.edu/noemie/papers/15kdd.pdf. Accessed 9 June 2017.
Centers for Disease Control and Prevention: National Center for Health Statistics. 2017 FastStats – pneumonia. 2017. https://www.cdc.gov/nchs/fastats/pneumonia.htm. Accessed 9 June 2017.
Chan E, Ruest A, Meade M, Cook D. Oral decontamination for prevention of pneumonia in mechanically ventilated adults: systematic review and meta-analysis. BMJ. 2007;334(7599):889.
Charles P, Wolfe R, Whitby M, Fine M, Fuller A, et al. SMART-COP: a tool for predicting the need for intensive respiratory or vasopressor support in community-acquired pneumonia. Clin Infect Dis. 2008;47(3):375–84.
Chalmers JD, Rother C, Salih W, Ewig S. Healthcare-associated pneumonia does not accurately identify potentially resistant pathogens: a systematic review and meta-analysis. Clin Infect Dis. 2014;58(3):330–9.
Cho I, Blaser M. The human microbiome: at the interface of health and disease. Nat Rev Genet. 2012;13(4):260–70.
Coffin S, Klompas M, Classen D, Arias K, Podgorny K, Anderson D, et al. Strategies to prevent ventilator-associated pneumonia in actue care hospitals. Infection Control Hosp Epidemiol. 2008;29:S31–40.
DeAntonio R, Yarzabal J, Cruz J, Schmidt J, Kleijnen J. Epidemiology of community-acquired pneumonia and implications for vaccination of children living in developing and newly industrialized countries: a systematic literature review. Hum Vaccin Immunother. 2016;12(9):2422–40.
Dickson R, Erb-Downward J, Huffnagle G. The role of the bacterial microbiome in lung disease. Expert Rev Respir Med. 2013;7(3):245–57.
Drijkoningen J, Rohde C. Pneumococcal infection in adults: burden of disease. Clin Microbiol Infect. 2014;20(Suppl 5):45–51.
Durrington H, Summers C. Recent changes in the management of community acquired pneumonia in adults. BMJ. 2008;336(7658):1429–33.
Evans O. Pneumonia: challenges in definition, diagnosis and management of disease. Surg Clin North Am. 2014;94:1305–17.
Ewig S, Welte T, Torres A. Is healthcare-associated pneumonia a distinct entity needing specific therapy? Curr Opin Infect Dis. 2012;25(2):166–75.
Fine M, Auble T, Yealy D, Hanusa B, Weissfeld L, Singer D, et al. A prediction rule to identify low-risk patients with community-acquired pneumonia. N Engl J Med. 1997;336(4):243–50.
Flanagan J, Brodie E, Weng L, Lynch S, Garcia O, Brown R, et al. Loss of bacterial diversity during antibiotic treatment of intubated patients colonized with Pseudomonas aeruginosa. J Clin Microbiol. 2007;45(6):1954–62.
Heo S, Haase E, Lesse A, Gill S, Scannapieco F. Genetic relationships between respiratory pathogens isolated from dental plaque and bronchoalveolar lavage fluid from patients in the intensive care unit undergoing mechanical ventilation. Clin Infect Dis. 2008;47(12):1562–70.

Hua F, Xie H, Worthington H, Furness S, Zhang Q, Li C. Oral hygiene care for critically ill patients to prevent ventilator-associated pneumonia. Cochrane Database Syst Rev. 2016;(10):CD008367.

Kalil A, Metersky M, Klompas M, Muscedere J, Sweeney D, Palmer L. Management of adults with hospital-acquired and ventilator-associated pneumonia: 2016 Clinical Practice Guidelines by the Infectious Diseases Society of America and the American Thoracic Society. Clin Infect Dis. 2016;63(5):e61–111.

Kawaler E, Cobian A, Peissig P, Cross D, Yale S, Craven M. Learning to predict post-hospitalization VTE risk from EHR data. 2012. https://www.biostat.wisc.edu/~craven/papers/kawaler-amia12.pdf. Accessed 9 June 2017.

Klompas M. Nosocomial pnuemonia. In: Bennett JE, Dolin R, Blaser MJ, editors. Principles and practice of infectious diseases. Philadelphia: Elsevier; 2015. p. 3325–33. https://books.google.com/books?id=BseNCgAAQBAJ&pg=PA1677&lpg=PA1677&dq=Klompas+M.+303.+Nosocomial+pneumonia+IN:+Principles+and+Practice+of+Infectious+Diseases&source=bl&ots=0JOzv9d6SS&sig=Pq1mon9z0qR1HO7QbNoKaJcaNWk&hl=en&sa=X&ved=0ahUKEwjgqaS2_tjTAhUiwYM. Accessed 9 June 2017.

Labeau S, Van de Vyver K, Bursselaers N, Vogelaers D, Blot S. Prevention of ventilator-associated pneumonia with oral antiseptics: a systematic review and meta-analysis. Lancet Infect Dis. 2011;11(11):845–54.

Laurence B, Mould-Millman N, Scannepieco F, Abron A. Hospital admissions for pneumonia more likely with concomitant dental infections. Clin Oral Invest. 2015;19(6):1261–8.

Li L, Ai Z, Li L, Zheng X, Jie L. Can routine oral care with antiseptics prevent ventilator-associated pneumonia in patients receiving mechanical ventilation? An update meta analysis from 17 randomized controlled trials. Int J Clin Exp Med. 2015;8(2):1645–57.

Lim W, van der Eerden M, Laing R, Boersma W, Karalus N, Town G, Lewis S, Macfarlane J. Defining community acquired pneumonia severity on presentation to hospital: an international derivation and validation study. Thorax. 2003;58(5):377–82.

Madhi S, Klugman K, Vaccine Trialist Group. A role for Streptococcus pneumoniae in virus-associated pneumonia. Nat Med. 2004;10(8):811–3.

Mandel L, Wunderink R, Anzueto A, Bartlett J, Campbell G, Dean N, et al. Infectious Disease Society of America/American Thoracic consensus guidelines on the management of community-acquired pneumonia in adults. CID. 2007;44(Suppl 2):S27–72.

Marino PJ, Wise MP, Smith A, Marchesi JR, Riggio MP, Lewis MAO, Williams DW. Community analysis of dental plaque and endotracheal tube biofilms from mechanically ventilated patients. J Crit Care. 2017;39:149–55.

Melsen W, Rovers M, Groenwold R, Bergmans D, Camus C, Bauer T, et al. Attributable mortality of ventilator-associated pneumonia: a meta-analysis of individual patient data from randomised prevention studies. Lancet Infect Dis. 2013;13(8):665–71.

Morillo D, León Jiménez A, Moreno S. Computer-aided diagnosis of pneumonia in patients with chronic obstructive pulmonary disease. J Am Med Inform Assoc. 2013;20(e1):e111–7.

National Center for BioMedical Ontology SNOMED CT – Pneumonia – Classes: NCBO BioPortal. *BioPortal*. © 2005–2017 Board of Trustees of Leland Stanford Junior University. 2017. http://bioportal.bioontology.org/ontologies/SNOMEDCT?p=classes&conceptid=233604007. Accessed 9 June 2017.

Neill A, Martin I, Weir R, Anderson R, Chereshsky A, Epton M, et al. Community acquired pneumonia: aetiology and usefulness of severity criteria on admission. Thorax. 1996;51(10):1010–6.

Reynolds C, Finkelstien J, Ray G, Moore M, Huang S. Attributable healthcare utilization and cost of pneumonia due to drug-resistant Streptococcus pneumonia: a cost analysis. Antimicrob Resist Infect Control. 2014;3(1):16.

Richards D. Oral hygiene regimes for mechanically ventilated patients that use chlorohexidine reduce ventilator-associated pneumonia. Evid Based Dent. 2013;14(3):91–2.

Sands K, Twigg J, Lewis M, Wise M, Marshesi J, Smith A, et al. Microbial profiling of dental plaque from mechanically ventilated patients. J Med Microbiol. 2016;65(2):147–59.

Sands K, Wilson M, Lewis M, Wise M, Palmer N, Hayes A, et al. Respiratory pathogen colonization of dental plaque, the lower airways, and endotracheal tube biofilms during mechanical ventilation. J Crit Care. 2017;37:30–7.

Scannapieco F. Role of oral bacteria in respiratory infection. J Periodontol. 1999;70(7):793–802.

Scannapieco F. Pneumonia and oral pathogens. In: The oral-systemic health connection: a guide to patient care. Hanovar Park, IL: Quintessence Publishing Co, Inc.; 2014. p. 301.

Scannapieco F, Bush R, Paju S. Associations between periodontal disease and risk for nosocomial bacterial pneumonia and chronic obstructive pulmonary disease. A systematic review. Ann Periodontol. 2003;8(1):54–69.

Scott II D. The Direct medical costs of healthcare-associated infections in U.S. hospitals and the benefits of prevention. Mar 2009. https://stacks.cdc.gov/view/cdc/11550. Accessed 9 June 2017.

Shea K, Edelsberg J, Weycker D, Farkouh R, Strutton D, Oelton S. Rates of pneumococcal disease in adults with chronic medical conditions. Open Forum Infect Dis. 2014;1(1):ofu024.

Shi Z, Xie H, Wang P, Zhang Q, Wu Y, Chen E, et al. Oral hygiene for critically ill paitents to prevent ventilator-associated pneumonia. Cochrance Databases Syst Rev. 2013;(8):CD008367.

Shimpi N, Schroeder D, Kilskdonk J, Chyou P, Glurich I, Penniman E, Acharaya A. Medical providers' oral health knowledgeability, attitudes, and practice behaviors: an opportunity for interprofessional collaboration. J Evid Based Dent Pract. 2016;16(1):19–29.

Singh S, Amin A, Loke Y. Long-term use of inhaled corticosteroids and the risk of pneumonia in chronic obstructive pulmonary disease. Arch Intern Med. 2009;169(3):219–29.

Tedja R, Gordon S. Hospital-acquired, healthcare-acquired and ventilator-associated pneumonia. 2013. http://www.clevelandclinicmeded.com/medicalpubs/diseasemanagement/infectious-disease/health-care-associated-pneumonia/. Accessed 16 June 2017.

Terpenning M, Taylor G, Lopatin D, Kerr C, Dominguez L, Loesche W. Aspiration pneumonia: dental and oral risk factors in an older veteran population. J Am Geriatr Soc. 2001;49(5):557–63.

Therapeutic Guidelines Limited. SMART-COP tool for assessing severity of Community-Acquired Pneumonia (CAP) in adults. *eTG*. © Therapeutics Guidelines Ltd. (www.tg.org.au). 2010. https://lifeinthefastlane.com/wp-content/uploads/2010/07/etg-smartcop.pdf. Accessed 9 June 2017.

Torres A, Cilloniz C. Epidemiology, etiology, and risk factors of bacterial pnuemonia. In: Torres A, Cukkiuz C, editors. Clinical management of bacterial pneumonia. Switzerland: Springer International Publishing; 2015. p. 7–28.

Umeizudike K, Iwuala S, Ozoh O, Ayanbadejo P, Fasanmade A. Association between periodontal diseases and systemic illnesses: a survey among internal medicine residents in nigeria. Saudi Dent J. 2016;28(1):24–30.

Van Dyke T, Sheilesh D. Risk factors for periodontitis. J Int Acad Periodontol. 2005;7(1):3–7.

Walker CLF, Rudan I, Liu L, Nair H, Theodoratou E, Bhutta Z, et al. Global burden of childhood pneumonia and diarrhoea. Lancet. 2013;381(9875):1405–16.

Yokoe D, Anderson D, Berenholtz S, Calfee D, Dubberke E, Ellingson K, et al. A compendium of strategies to prevent healthcare-associated infections in acute care hospitals: 2014 updates. Infect Control Hosp Epidemiol. 2014;35:S21–31.

Chapter 10
Interdisciplinary Care Model: Metabolic Syndrome and Oral Health

Neel Shimpi, Ram Pathak, and Amit Acharya

10.1 Definition and Prevalence

The International Diabetes Federation has defined metabolic syndrome (MetS) as cluster of diseases that includes type 2 diabetes mellitus (T2DM) and prediabetes, increased abdominal obesity, high cholesterol and high blood pressure (BP) (IDF 2018). Evidence suggests that these diseases predispose a person to increased risk of cardiovascular disease (CVD) complications leading to increased mortality. Further, insulin resistance and increased body fat distribution have been considered to be significant factors for increased CVD risk (Després 2012; Kaur 2014a, b; Patel and Abate 2013). Although the complexity of the pathogenesis of these diseases is not well understood, clinical practice worldwide considers central obesity and insulin resistance to be the most important causative factor for MetS (Anderson et al. 2001; Mulè et al. 2014; Roberts et al. 2013; Saad et al. 1991).

MetS affects almost 20–25% of world's adult population (Aguilar et al. 2015; Nolan et al. 2017; Saklayen 2018). Based on the WHO report, nearly 1.9 billion of the world's population (18 years and older) were overweight (WHO 2018). Evidence shows that the prevalence of MetS increased from 25.3% between 1988–1994 to 34.2% between 2007–2012 (Moore et al. 2017). In accordance with the 2016 NCHS Data Brief, the prevalence of obesity in the US adults aged between 40–59 years was 39.8% (Hales et al. 2017). Recently, a greater concern has been

N. Shimpi · A. Acharya (✉)
Center for Oral and Systemic Health, Marshfield Clinic Research Institute, Marshfield, WI, USA
e-mail: shimpi.neel@marshfieldresearch.org; acharya.amit@marshfieldresearch.org

R. Pathak
Department of Endocrinology, Marshfield Clinic, Marshfield, WI, USA
e-mail: pathak.ram@marshfieldclinic.org

A. Acharya et al. (eds.), *Integration of Medical and Dental Care and Patient Data*, Health Informatics, https://doi.org/10.1007/978-3-319-98298-4_10

directed towards presence of MetS in children and adolescents (Teixeira et al. 2017; Wittcopp and Conroy 2017). A systemic review of 85 papers describing the prevalence of MetS in children demonstrated a median prevalence of 3.3% of MetS in whole population, 11.9% and 29.2% in overweight and obese children respectively (Friend et al. 2013).

10.2 Systemic Manifestations

Studies have shown that insulin resistance, which is also associated with MetS, shows some cardinal symptoms like increased abdominal obesity, impaired fasting glucose, elevated BP, hypertriglyceridemia and low HDL cholesterol (Roberts et al. 2013). Furthermore a number of studies have also shown that MetS is associated with conditions such as micro albuminuria, fatty liver, endothelial dysfunction, hyperuricemia and systemic inflammation (Li et al. 2016; Lucero et al. 2017; Marsland et al. 2010; Tomiyama et al. 2011; Watz et al. 2009). In a meta-analysis involving 43 cohorts of 172,573 individuals, Gami et al. (2007) reported that MetS conveyed a relative risk for CVD events and CVD related deaths of 1.78.

According to guidelines from the National Heart, Lung and Blood Institute (NHLBI) and the American Heart Association (AHA), MetS is diagnosed when a patient has at least three of the following conditions (Grundy et al. 2005):

1. Fasting glucose ≥100 mg/dl (or receiving drug therapy for hyperglycemia)
2. BP ≥130/85 mm of Hg (or receiving drug therapy for hypertension)
3. Triglycerides ≥150 mg/dl (or receiving drug therapy for hypertriglyceridemia)
4. High Density Lipid-Cholesterol (HDL-C) <40 mg/dl in men or <50 mg/dl in women (or receiving drug therapy for reduced HDL-C)
5. Waist circumference ≥102 cm (40 in.) in men ≥88 cm (35 in.) in women; [≥90 cm (35 in.) in men or ≥80 (32 in.) in women for Asian Americans].

Increased levels of fibrinogen, plasminogen activator inhibitor-1 and other coagulation factors are also seen in patients with MetS (Alessi and Juhan-Vague 2006; Palomo et al. 2009; Phelan and Kerins 2014). However these findings are rare; and in such cases aspirin prophylaxis is desirable. Reviews of studies have shown that MetS shows elevated cytokines such as tumor necrosis factor and interleukin 6 and acute phase reactants such as C-reactive protein (CRP) and fibrinogen. Elevated CRP is suggestive of chronic inflammation (Christiana et al. 2016; Ferreira-Hermosillo et al. 2015; Monteiro and Azevedo 2010; Ridker et al. 2003; Srikanthan et al. 2016). Studies has confirmed that high sensitivity CRP levels are also linked with MetS (Bennett et al. 2014; den Engelsen et al. 2012; Gowdaiah et al. 2016; Ridker et al. 2004; Sah et al. 2016). Figure 10.1 shows the cluster of diseases and their overlapping effects.

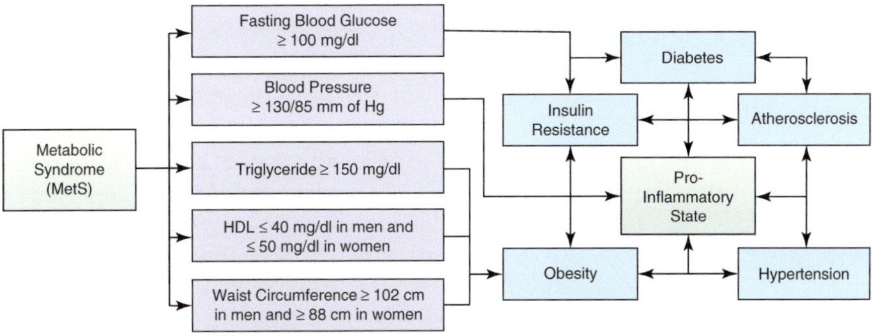

Fig. 10.1 Cluster of diseases and their overlapping effects in MetS

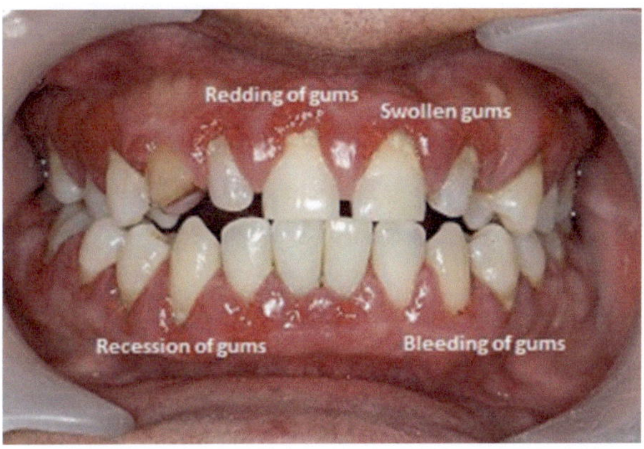

Fig. 10.2 Oral manifestations in MetS

10.3 Oral Manifestations

The exaggerated host response to the local microbial factors associated with MetS appears to be correlated with various inflammatory and soft tissue pathologies in oral cavities (Daudt et al. 2018; Lamster and Pagan 2017; Nibali et al. 2013). This is similar to the observations seen in uncontrolled T2DM and elevated BP. Periodontitis (PD) has been identified as one of the most common oral manifestations of T2DM (Casanova et al. 2014; Mealey 2006). The concomitant manifestation of T2DM also includes fungal and bacterial infections, tooth loss and dental caries (Bascones-Martinez and Matesanz-Perez 2011; Beck et al. 2018; Similä et al. 2018). Figure 10.2 shows the oral manifestations in MetS.

10.4 Oral-Systemic Connection

Studies are being conducted to explore the underlying mechanisms and their associations for MetS and oral health (Beck et al. 2018; D'Aiuto et al. 2008; Koo and Hong 2018; Marchetti et al. 2012; Mealey 2006; Musskopf et al. 2017). Although there is considerable uncertainty regarding oral health and MetS; some studies reveal that both MetS and PD show a common etiopathogenic mechanism (Beck et al. 2018; Iwasaki et al. 2015; Marchetti et al. 2012; Nesbitt et al. 2010). The results of the Third National Health and Nutrition Examination Survey (NHANES III) conducted in 13,170 individuals aged ≥45 years showed a direct relationship between PD and MetS (D'Aiuto et al. 2008). Correspondingly, a study also observed presence of periodontal pockets after 4 years of follow-up of 1023 patients presenting with MetS. In addition, the correlation was observed to be greater amongst elderly individual and more predilections towards males and smokers (Morita et al. 2010).

A longitudinal relationship was studied between MetS and PD among Japanese adults age 70 years or older. The 125 adults selected for the study underwent a full mouth periodontal status examination. The clinical attachment level was recorded at baseline and in follow up examination. The authors in this study found out that the adults with MetS were 2.6 times more likely to develop PD after simultaneous adjustment for other covariates (Iwasaki et al. 2015).

A subsequent study carried out in 2107 Japanese subjects aged 35–60 years over a 5-year period showed significant association between MetS and tooth loss. Evaluation was performed using a logistic regression model between MetS at baseline examination and tooth loss. Data such as gender, obesity, triglycerides, BP, fasting glucose, reduced high-density lipoproteins (HDL), income, and education, smoking status, dental care utilization and brushing frequency were captured. Logistic regression modelling showed that amongst these subjects those with MetS had a higher incidence of tooth loss (Furuta et al. 2016).

10.5 Diagnostic Codes

MetS diagnostic ICD9 and ICD 10 codes are shown in Table 10.1 (International Classification of Diseases Ninth revision 1978).

A diagnostic code that includes PD as a complication of MetS can be introduced.

Table 10.1 Diagnostic codes for MetS

Diagnostic codes	Codes	Description
ICD 9 CM	888.1	Metabolic syndrome
ICD 10 CM	E88.81	Metabolic syndrome

10.6 Risk Assessment

Several methods are being used to estimate 10 year risk for CVD (ACCF/AHA 2010; Grundy et al. 1999; Nojiri and Daida 2017; Pencina et al. 2009). These risk assessment tools incorporate the major risk factors for CVD; cigarette smoking, BP, total cholesterol, HDL, age, gender and sometimes other risk factors such as T2DM (DeBoer and Gurka 2017; Gurka et al. 2017; Toolkit 2018). The State of Missouri uses a MetS screening and monitoring tool that incorporates the vital history such as height, weight, BMI, waist circumference and BP (Missouri 2018). While the other components used are blood glucose levels, lipid panel, and current use of antipsychotic drugs, pregnancy status, smoking status and obesity.

MetS risk assessment tools can be useful in prediction of CVD risks (Kaur 2014b; Motamed et al. 2017; Ofori and Odia 2016; Shillinglaw et al. 2012; Willers and Hahn 2013). A study recruited 120 overweight patients aged 30–60 years for a 12 week weight reduction programme and utilized a diagnostic tool SCORE for CVD risk and MetS. The study results showed that there was decrease in prevalence of MetS and subsequent decrease in SCORE which was highly significant with a p value of <0.001. The study concluded that MetS was more meaningful in determining the risk of CVD events (Willers and Hahn 2013).

The Framingham Heart Study includes abdominal obesity, triglycerides and fasting glucose to calculate a 10 year risk prediction for women for developing CVD (Framingham Heart Study 2018). The Quebec Cardiovascular study was conducted to investigate the association between large and small low-density lipoprotein and long term ischemic heart disease (IHD) (Després et al. 2000). The study observed that the large LDL sub fraction was not associated with an increased risk of IHD in men and that the CVD risk attributable to variations in the low density lipids (LDL) size phenotype was largely related to markers of a preferential accumulation of small dense LDL particles.

The International Task Force for Prevention of Coronary Heart Disease uses a risk assessment tool that includes LDL, HDL, systolic BP, age, triglyceride level, T2DM, MI in family history, fasting blood glucose levels and use of antihypertensive drug (Assmann et al. 1999).

10.7 Systems Biology: Genomics, Proteomics, Microbiomics, Phenotypes

It is evident that MetS is strongly associated with the genomic risk factors (Taylor et al. 2013). The findings of a genome-wide study conducted in Finnish cohorts including 2,637 cases and 7,297 controls for MetS traits suggested that genes from pathways associated with lipid metabolism plays a crucial role in genetic background of MetS (Kristiansson et al. 2012). Studies have shown that the genomic risk factors associated with MetS are also found in development of hypertension and dyslipidemia (Dalal et al. 2012). Evidence also suggests that pathophysiologic mechanisms seen in obesity and T2DM potentially promote pathogenesis and progression of hematologic malignancies in patients with MetS (Berger 2014). The findings of a recent experimental study that used mass spectrometry with two different mouse strains to generate a quantitative proteomic data showed that proteomic data can add a more complementary information similar to the biological functions with respect to MetS (Terfve et al. 2017). Evidence suggests that gut and oral microbiome can have a profound effect in developing MetS (Edlund et al. 2017; Johnson et al. 2017; Mazidi et al. 2016; Sanz et al. 2015).

10.8 Treatment

Prevention and evaluation of MetS is very important in terms of increasing the quality of care. Identifying patients with increased risk of T2DM and CVD events due to excessive weight gain and sedentary lifestyle is imperative. According to the National Institute of Health the main goal of treatment is to reduce the risk of health disease and to prevent the onset of T2DM (Anderson et al. 2001). The main focus of treatment is directed toward managing clinical findings such as increased abdominal circumference, elevated triglycerides, LDL, elevated fasting blood glucose levels and elevated BP (de Toro-Martín et al. 2017; Gierach et al. 2013; National Cholesterol Education Program (NCEP) Expert Panel on Detection, Evaluation, and Treatment of High Blood Cholesterol in Adults (Adult Treatment Panel III) et al. 2002; Peyrol et al. 2017; Sherling et al. 2017; Singh et al. 2015).

The National Institute for Health recommends losing weight to treat abdominal obesity increasing the physical activity and improving healthy food intake (Anderson et al. 2001; Gardner et al. 2018; Villareal et al. 2017). Moreover, the National Heart, Lung and Blood Institute recommend keeping track of lipid panel and blood sugar level to treat MetS (NHLBI 2018). The results of research studies demonstrated the inverse relationship between frequency of tooth brushing and MetS and the study concluded that incorporating good oral hygiene behavior can help in treatment of MetS (Kobayashi et al. 2012; Saito et al. 2018; Tanaka et al. 2018).

10.9 Interdisciplinary Care Team

Care Team includes Primary Care Physicians, General Dentists, Periodontists, Nurses, Endocrinologists, Dieticians, Dental Hygienists, Exercise Physiologist, Nurse Practitioners, Pharmacists, Nutritionist and Medical assistants.

10.10 Guidelines

The American Heart Association has laid down some guidelines to prevent and treat MetS that requires treating several conditions together (AHA 2018; Friedlander et al. 2007). Studies have shown that adopting healthy lifestyle behavior can improve the underlying insulin resistance and prevent progression to MetS (Daskalopoulou et al. 2004; Ebrahimof and Mirmiran 2013; Molavi et al. 2006; VanWormer et al. 2017).

10.11 Existing Gaps and Suggestions

More research needs to be done around the pathogenesis of developing MetS. Although, evidence shows relationship between oral health and MetS, there is a need to redefine MetS that include 'oral hygiene' as one of the clinical components that can lead to increased risk of developing MetS. Emphasizing the importance of oral hygiene is necessary in prevention and treatment of MetS. Currently not much information about the guidelines including oral health is available. With the ongoing refinement of research for oral and MetS, the information should be made easily available. Introducing most predictive models for MetS would be beneficial.

10.12 Technology Implications

Based on current definition of MetS, decision support tools can be developed that predict the risk of a patient for MetS Values such as BP, blood sugar level and others can be easily extracted from electronic health record to know a person's risk of developing MetS.

A study was conducted to determine if unique gene expression profiles are seen with people having metabolic disorders. In the study, peripheral blood was drawn from patients who were suffering from coronary artery disease, T2DM and their precursor, MetS and rheumatoid arthritis and was compared. The results of the study displayed overlapping and non-overlapping patterns of gene expression in patients with MetS that were indicative of unique and underlying immune processes (Grayson et al. 2011).

Another study proposed an analysis called as cross-subspace analysis (CSA) which helps in structuralization of relationships of set of genes by using existing MEDLINE literature (Matsunaga and Muramatsu 2005). Machine learning was used to generate gene objects by retrieving the terms obesity, T2DM, hypertriglyceridemia and hypertension on a 2D plane inferring important concepts from the gene distribution.

10.13 Electronic Health Records

Apart from maintaining the electronic version of patient's medical clinical data, the EHRs support care-related activity directly or indirectly including evidence-based decision support, quality management and outcomes reporting (Kern et al. 2013). Having MetS and periodontal registries will help the care team to track the number of interventions and clinical parameters important in management of MetS. This will improve the disease management process and increase the quality of care.

Implementing data quality measures for healthcare delivery by developing dashboards for the healthcare providers will enable healthcare providers to instantly quantify treatment outcomes, patient's perceptions, population health and efficient use of health care resources.

Use of computer assisted software, a more personalized and tailored information can be made available for the end users. Collecting information on MetS and oral health in electronic health record can help in discovering medical conditions associated with the oral health.

10.14 Ontology

Study results that examined alterations in cardiac gene expression patterns in the rat model (Zucker Diabetic Fatty rats) showed significant upregulation of 36 genes and down-regulation of 49 genes. Thus, demonstrating that MetS significantly alters cardiac gene expression (Sárközy et al. 2013). Another developed a cross-subspace analysis (CSA) method that analyzed gene objects utilizing machine learning methods. Terms such as obesity, T2DM, hypertriglyceridemia and hypertension were retrieved using CSA method by structuralization of relationships of set of genes and validity was checked by comparing the knowledge extracted by ordering with the existing medical knowledge. The results of the study showed that the developed analysis method was able to quantify the relationship among genes by integrating knowledge by computation (Matsunaga and Muramatsu 2005).

10.15 Care Plan

There needs awareness of the bidirectional connection of MetS and oral health between healthcare providers. The dental and medical providers play an active and an important role in communicating clinical management of oral and systemic health. A proper referral mechanism will play a significant role in the delivering this interdisciplinary care.

Dental providers should check for oral health and look for the symptoms MetS. Dental providers should screen for MetS in their dental offices (Friedlander et al. 2007; Gesko et al. 2011). Similarly, patients with MetS should be told about increased risk of PD and other oral health conditions associated with MetS. Medical providers should evaluate patient's oral cavity for the oral status. Oral health education should be provided to all the patients.

10.16 Recommendations on Dental Diagnosis of MetS

1. Dental providers should develop treatment plans to restore the dentition of patients suffering from MetS and consider patient education for MetS.
2. Revisiting and developing guidelines for MetS serve as a tool to support and influence health care provider decision making to promote consistent, comprehensive and preventive MetS care that includes oral health.
3. Educational materials based on association of MetS and oral health should be provided to patients.

References

ACCF/AHA. Guideline for assessment of cardiovascular risk in asymptomatic adults. American College of Cardiology Foundation (November). 2010:11–24. https://doi.org/10.2214/ajr.11.6758

Aguilar M, Bhuket T, Torres S, Liu B, Wong RJ. Prevalence of the metabolic syndrome in the United States, 2003–2012. JAMA. 2015;313(19):1973. https://doi.org/10.1001/jama.2015.4260.

AHA. Prevention and treatment of metabolic syndrome. 2018. http://www.heart.org/HEARTORG/Conditions/More/MetabolicSyndrome/Prevention-and-Treatment-of-Metabolic-Syndrome_UCM_301927_Article.jsp#.Wzg_uq2Wxjo. Retrieved 30 June 2018

Alessi M-C, Juhan-Vague I. PAI-1 and the metabolic syndrome. Arterioscler Thromb Vasc Biol. 2006;26(10):2200–7.

Anderson PJ, Critchley JAJH, Chan JCN, Cockram CS, Lee ZSK, Thomas GN, Tomlinson B. Factor analysis of the metabolic syndrome: obesity vs insulin resistance as the central abnormality. Int J Obes. 2001;25(12):1782–8. https://doi.org/10.1038/sj.ijo.0801837.

Assmann G, Cullen P, Jossa F, Lewis B, Mancini M. Coronary heart disease: reducing the risk: the scientific background to primary and secondary prevention of coronary heart disease. A worldwide view. International task force for the prevention of coronary heart disease. Arterioscler Thromb Vasc Biol. 1999;19(8):1819–24.

Bascones-Martinez A, Matesanz-Perez P. Periodontal disease and diabetes—review of the literature. Med Oral Patol Oral Cir Bucal. 2011;16(6):e722–9.

Beck JD, Moss KL, Morelli T, Offenbacher S. Periodontal profile class is associated with prevalent diabetes, coronary heart disease, stroke, and systemic markers of C-reactive protein and interleukin-6. J Periodontol. 2018;89(2):157–65. https://doi.org/10.1002/JPER.17-0426.

Bennett NR, Ferguson TS, Bennett FI, Tulloch-Reid MK, Younger-Coleman NOM, Jackson MD, et al. High-sensitivity C-reactive protein is related to central obesity and the number of metabolic syndrome components in Jamaican young adults. Front Cardiovasc Med. 2014;1:12. https://doi.org/10.3389/fcvm.2014.00012.

Berger NA. Obesity and cancer pathogenesis. Ann N Y Acad Sci. 2014;1311(1):57–76. https://doi.org/10.1111/nyas.12416.

Casanova L, Hughes FJ, Preshaw PM. Diabetes and periodontal disease: a two-way relationship. BDJ. 2014;217(8):433–7. https://doi.org/10.1038/sj.bdj.2014.907.

Christiana UI, Casimir AE, Nicholas AA, Christian MC, Obiefuna AI. Plasma levels of inflammatory cytokines in adult Nigerians with the metabolic syndrome. Niger Med J. 2016;57(1):64–8. https://doi.org/10.4103/0300-1652.180569.

D'Aiuto F, Sabbah W, Netuveli G, Donos N, Hingorani AD, Deanfield J, Tsakos G. Association of the metabolic syndrome with severe periodontitis in a large U.S. population-based survey. J Clin Endocrinol Metabol. 2008;93(10):3989–94. https://doi.org/10.1210/jc.2007-2522.

Dalal JJ, Padmanabhan TNC, Jain P, Patil S, Vasnawala H, Gulati A. LIPITENSION: interplay between dyslipidemia and hypertension. Indian J Endocrinol Metab. 2012;16(2):240–5. https://doi.org/10.4103/2230-8210.93742.

Daskalopoulou SS, Mikhailidis DP, Elisaf M. Prevention and treatment of the metabolic syndrome. Angiology. 2004;55(6):589–612. https://doi.org/10.1177/000331970405500i601.

Daudt LD, Musskopf ML, Mendez M, Remonti LLR, Leitão CB, Gross JL, et al. Association between metabolic syndrome and periodontitis: a systematic review and meta-analysis. Braz Oral Res. 2018;32:e35. https://doi.org/10.1590/1807-3107bor-2018.vol32.0035.

DeBoer MD, Gurka MJ. Clinical utility of metabolic syndrome severity scores: considerations for practitioners. Diabetes Metab Syndr Obes. 2017;10:65–72. https://doi.org/10.2147/DMSO.S101624.

Després J-P. Body fat distribution and risk of cardiovascular disease: an update. Circulation. 2012;126(10):1301–13. https://doi.org/10.1161/CIRCULATIONAHA.111.067264.

Després JP, Lemieux I, Dagenais GR, Cantin B, Lamarche B. HDL-cholesterol as a marker of coronary heart disease risk: the Québec cardiovascular study. Atherosclerosis. 2000;153(2):263–72. Retrieved from http://www.ncbi.nlm.nih.gov/pubmed/11164415

Ebrahimof S, Mirmiran P. Nutritional approaches for prevantion and treatment of metabolic syndrome in adults. J Paramed Sci. 2013;4(2):123–34.

Edlund A, Garg N, Mohimani H, Gurevich A, He X, Shi W, et al. Metabolic fingerprints from the human oral microbiome reveal a vast knowledge gap of secreted small peptidic molecules. mSystems. 2017;2(4):e00058–17. https://doi.org/10.1128/mSystems.00058-17.

Ferreira-Hermosillo A, Molina-Ayala M, Ramírez-Rentería C, Vargas G, Gonzalez B, Isibasi A, et al. Inflammatory cytokine profile associated with metabolic syndrome in adult patients with type 1 diabetes. J Diabetes Res. 2015;2015:972073. https://doi.org/10.1155/2015/972073.

Framingham Heart Study. Cardiovascular disease | risk | Framingham Heart Study. 2018. Retrieved from https://www.framinghamheartstudy.org/fhs-risk-functions/cardiovascular-disease-10-year-risk/.

Friedlander AH, Weinreb J, Friedlander I, Yagiela JA, Laufer D, Walls A, et al. Metabolic syndrome: pathogenesis, medical care and dental implications. J Am Dent Assoc. 2007;138(2):179–87.; quiz 248. https://doi.org/10.14219/JADA.ARCHIVE.2007.0134.

Friend A, Craig L, Turner S. The prevalence of metabolic syndrome in children: a systematic review of the literature. Metab Syndr Relat Disord. 2013;11(2):71–80. https://doi.org/10.1089/met.2012.0122.

Furuta M, Liu A, Shinagawa T, Takeuchi K, Takeshita T, Shimazaki Y, Yamashita Y. Tooth loss and metabolic syndrome in middle-aged Japanese adults. J Clin Periodontol. 2016;43(6):482–91. https://doi.org/10.1111/jcpe.12523.

Gami AS, Witt BJ, Howard DE, Erwin PJ, Gami LA, Somers VK, Montori VM. Metabolic syndrome and risk of incident cardiovascular events and death. J Am Coll Cardiol. 2007;49(4):403–14. https://doi.org/10.1016/j.jacc.2006.09.032.

Gardner CD, Trepanowski JF, Del Gobbo LC, Hauser ME, Rigdon J, Ioannidis JPA, et al. Effect of low-fat vs low-carbohydrate diet on 12-month weight loss in overweight adults and the association with genotype pattern or insulin secretion. JAMA. 2018;319(7):667. https://doi.org/10.1001/jama.2018.0245.

Gesko DS, Rush WA, Durand EU. The oral-systemic link: an opportunity for collaboration. Diabetes Spectrum. 2011;24(4):187–9. https://doi.org/10.2337/diaspect.24.4.187.

Gierach M, Gierach J, Junik R. Evaluation of lipid profiles in patients with metabolic syndrome according to cardiovascular risk calculated on the basis of the SCORE chart. Endokrynol Pol. 2016;67(3):265–70. https://doi.org/10.5603/EP.a2016.0020.

Gowdaiah PK, Mamatha TR, Nirgude D. High sensitivity C-reactive protein in metabolic syndrome. Int J Adv Med. 2016;3(3):607–10.

Grayson BL, Wang L, Aune TM. Peripheral blood gene expression profiles in metabolic syndrome, coronary artery disease and type 2 diabetes. Genes Immun. 2011;12(5):341–51. https://doi.org/10.1038/gene.2011.13.

Grundy SM, Pasternak R, Greenland P, Smith S, Fuster V. Assessment of cardiovascular risk by use of multiple-risk-factor assessment equations: a statement for healthcare professionals from the American Heart Association and the American College of Cardiology. Circulation. 1999;100(13):1481–92. https://doi.org/10.1161/01.cir.100.13.1481.

Grundy SM, Cleeman JI, Daniels SR, Donato KA, Eckel RH, Franklin BA, et al. Diagnosis and management of the metabolic syndrome. Circulation. 2005;112(17):2735–52.

Gurka MJ, Golden SH, Musani SK, Sims M, Vishnu A, Guo Y, et al. Independent associations between a metabolic syndrome severity score and future diabetes by sex and race: the atherosclerosis risk in communities study and Jackson Heart Study. Diabetologia. 2017;60(7):1261–70. https://doi.org/10.1007/s00125-017-4267-6.

Hales CM, Carroll MD, Fryar CD, Ogden CL. Prevalence of obesity among adults and youth: United States, 2015–2016. NCHS Data Brief. 2017;288(288):1–8. https://doi.org/10.1017/S1368980017000088.

IDF. IDF consensus worldwide definition of the metabolic syndrome. 2018. Retrieved from https://www.idf.org/e-library/consensus-statements/60-idfconsensus-worldwide-definitionof-the-metabolic-syndrome.html.

International Classification of Diseases Ninth revision. Basic tabulation list with alphabetical index. 1978.

Iwasaki M, Sato M, Minagawa K, Manz MC, Yoshihara A, Miyazaki H. Longitudinal relationship between metabolic syndrome and periodontal disease among Japanese adults aged ≥70 years: The Niigata Study. J Periodontol. 2015;86(4):491–8. https://doi.org/10.1902/jop.2015.140398.

Johnson EL, Heaver SL, Walters WA, Ley RE. Microbiome and metabolic disease: revisiting the bacterial phylum bacteroidetes. J Mol Med. 2017;95(1):1–8. https://doi.org/10.1007/s00109-016-1492-2.

Kaur J. A comprehensive review on metabolic syndrome. Cardiol Res Pract. 2014a;2014:943162. https://doi.org/10.1155/2014/943162.

Kaur J. Assessment and screening of the risk factors in metabolic syndrome. Med Sci. 2014b;2(3):140–52. https://doi.org/10.3390/medsci2030140.

Kern LM, Barrón Y, Dhopeshwarkar RV, Edwards A, Kaushal R, HITEC Investigators. Electronic health records and ambulatory quality of care. J Gen Intern Med. 2013;28(4):496–503. https://doi.org/10.1007/s11606-012-2237-8.

Kobayashi Y, Niu K, Guan L, Momma H, Guo H, Cui Y, Nagatomi R. Oral health behavior and metabolic syndrome and its components in adults. J Dent Res. 2012;91(5):479–84. https://doi.org/10.1177/0022034512440707.

Koo HS, Hong SM. Prevalence and risk factors for periodontitis among patients with metabolic syndrome. Metab Syndr Relat Disord. 2018; https://doi.org/10.1089/met.2018.0003.

Kristiansson K, Perola M, Tikkanen E, Kettunen J, Surakka I, Havulinna AS, et al. Genome-wide screen for metabolic syndrome susceptibility Loci reveals strong lipid gene contribution but no evidence for common genetic basis for clustering of metabolic syndrome traits. Circ Cardiovasc Genet. 2012;5(2):242–9. https://doi.org/10.1161/CIRCGENETICS.111.961482.

Lamster IB, Pagan M. Periodontal disease and the metabolic syndrome. Int Dent J. 2017;67(2):67–77. https://doi.org/10.1111/idj.12264.

Li X-H, Lin H-Y, Wang S-H, Guan L-Y, Wang Y-B. Association of microalbuminuria with metabolic syndrome among aged population. Biomed Res Int. 2016;2016:9241278. https://doi.org/10.1155/2016/9241278.

Lucero D, Miksztowicz V, Gualano G, Longo C, Landeira G, Álvarez E, et al. Nonalcoholic fatty liver disease associated with metabolic syndrome: influence of liver fibrosis stages on characteristics of very low-density lipoproteins. Clin Chim Acta. 2017;473:1–8. https://doi.org/10.1016/j.cca.2017.08.006.

Marchetti E, Monaco A, Procaccini L, Mummolo S, Gatto R, Tetè S, et al. Periodontal disease: the influence of metabolic syndrome. Nutr Metab (Lond). 2012;9(1):88. https://doi.org/10.1186/1743-7075-9-88.

Marsland AL, McCaffery JM, Muldoon MF, Manuck SB. Systemic inflammation and the metabolic syndrome among middle-aged community volunteers. Metab Clin Exp. 2010;59(12):1801–8. https://doi.org/10.1016/j.metabol.2010.05.015.

Matsunaga T, Muramatsu M-A. Knowledge-based computational search for genes associated with the metabolic syndrome. Bioinformatics. 2005;21(14):3146–54. https://doi.org/10.1093/bioinformatics/bti484.

Mazidi M, Rezaie P, Kengne AP, Mobarhan MG, Ferns GA. Gut microbiome and metabolic syndrome. Diabetes Metab Syndr Clin Res Rev. 2016;10(2):S150–7. https://doi.org/10.1016/J.DSX.2016.01.024.

Mealey BL. Periodontal disease and diabetes. A two-way street. J Am Dent Assoc. 2006;137(Suppl):26S–31S. 137/suppl_2/26S [pii]

Missouri. Metabolic syndrome screening and monitoring tool. 2018.

Molavi B, Rasouli N, Kern PA. The prevention and treatment of metabolic syndrome and high-risk obesity. Curr Opin Cardiol. 2006;21(5):479–85. https://doi.org/10.1097/01.hco.0000240586.76344.f5.

Monteiro R, Azevedo I. Chronic inflammation in obesity and the metabolic syndrome. Mediators Inflamm. 2010;2010 https://doi.org/10.1155/2010/289645.

Moore JX, Chaudhary N, Akinyemiju T. Metabolic syndrome prevalence by race/ethnicity and sex in the United States, National Health and Nutrition Examination Survey, 1988–2012. Prev Chronic Dis. 2017;14:160287. https://doi.org/10.5888/pcd14.160287.

Morita T, Yamazaki Y, Mita A, Takada K, Seto M, Nishinoue N, et al. A cohort study on the association between periodontal disease and the development of metabolic syndrome. J Periodontol. 2010;81(4):512–9. https://doi.org/10.1902/jop.2010.090594.

Motamed N, Rabiee B, Roozafzai F, Zamani F, Faraji AH, Maadi M, et al. Metabolic syndrome and cardiovascular risk assessment tools' estimations of 10-year cardiovascular risk: a population-based study. Acta Cardiol. 2017:1–8. https://doi.org/10.1080/00015385.2017.1410335.

Mulè G, Calcaterra I, Nardi E, Cerasola G, Cottone S. Metabolic syndrome in hypertensive patients: an unholy alliance. World J Cardiol. 2014;6(9):890–907. https://doi.org/10.4330/wjc.v6.i9.890.

Musskopf ML, Daudt LD, Weidlich P, Gerchman F, Gross JL, Oppermann RV. Metabolic syndrome as a risk indicator for periodontal disease and tooth loss. Clin Oral Investig. 2017;21(2):675–83. https://doi.org/10.1007/s00784-016-1935-8.

den Engelsen C, Koekkoek PS, Gorter KJ, van den Donk M, Salome PL, Rutten GE. High-sensitivity C-reactive protein to detect metabolic syndrome in a centrally obese population: a cross-sectional analysis. Cardiovasc Diabetol. 2012;11(1):25. https://doi.org/10.1186/1475-2840-11-25.

National Cholesterol Education Program (NCEP) Expert Panel on Detection, Evaluation, and Treatment of High Blood Cholesterol in Adults (Adult Treatment Panel III), Grundy SM, Cleeman JI, Daniels SR, Donato KA, Eckel RH, Franklin BA, et al. Third Report of the National Cholesterol Education Program (NCEP) Expert Panel on Detection, Evaluation, and Treatment of High Blood Cholesterol in Adults (Adult Treatment Panel III) final report. Circulation. 2002;106(25):3143–421. https://doi.org/10.1161/circulationaha.105.169404.

Nesbitt MJ, Reynolds MA, Shiau H, Choe K, Simonsick EM, Ferrucci L. Association of periodontitis and metabolic syndrome in the Baltimore Longitudinal Study of Aging. Aging Clin Exp Res. 2010;22(3):238–42. Retrieved from http://www.ncbi.nlm.nih.gov/pubmed/20634647

NHLBI. Metabolic syndrome | National Heart, Lung, and Blood Institute (NHLBI). 2018. https://www.nhlbi.nih.gov/health-topics/metabolic-syndrome. Retrieved 30 June 2018.

Nibali L, Tatarakis N, Needleman I, Tu Y-K, D'Aiuto F, Rizzo M, Donos N. Association between metabolic syndrome and periodontitis: a systematic review and meta-analysis. J Clin Endocrinol Metabol. 2013;98(3):913–20. https://doi.org/10.1210/jc.2012-3552.

Nojiri S, Daida H. Atherosclerotic cardiovascular risk in Japan. Jpn Clin Med. 2017;8:117906601771271. https://doi.org/10.1177/1179066017712713.

Nolan PB, Carrick-Ranson G, Stinear JW, Reading SA, Dalleck LC. Prevalence of metabolic syndrome and metabolic syndrome components in young adults: a pooled analysis. Prev Med Rep. 2017;7:211–5. https://doi.org/10.1016/j.pmedr.2017.07.004.

Ofori SN, Odia OJ. Risk assessment in the prevention of cardiovascular disease in low-resource settings. Indian Heart J. 2016;68(3):391–8. https://doi.org/10.1016/j.ihj.2015.07.004.

Palomo IG, Gutiérrez CL, Alarcón ML, Jaramillo JC, Segovia FM, Leiva EM, et al. Increased concentration of plasminogen activator inhibitor-1 and fibrinogen in individuals with metabolic syndrome. Mol Med Rep. 2009;2(2):253–7. https://doi.org/10.3892/mmr_00000092.

Patel P, Abate N. Body fat distribution and insulin resistance. Nutrients. 2013;5(6):2019–27. https://doi.org/10.3390/nu5062019.

Pencina MJ, D'Agostino RB, Larson MG, Massaro JM, Vasan RS. Predicting the 30-year risk of cardiovascular disease: the Framingham heart study. Circulation. 2009;119(24):3078–84. https://doi.org/10.1161/CIRCULATIONAHA.108.816694.

Peyrol J, Riva C, Amiot M. Hydroxytyrosol in the prevention of the metabolic syndrome and related disorders. Nutrients. 2017;9(3):306. https://doi.org/10.3390/nu9030306.

Phelan M, Kerins DM. The role of plasminogen activator Inhibitor-1 in the metabolic syndrome and its regulation. J Food Res. 2014;3(6):36–53. https://doi.org/10.5539/jfr.v3n6p36.

Ridker PM, Buring JE, Cook NR, Rifai N. C-reactive protein, the metabolic syndrome, and risk of incident cardiovascular events: an 8-year follow-up of 14 719 initially healthy American women. Circulation. 2003;107(3):391–7. Retrieved from http://www.ncbi.nlm.nih.gov/pubmed/12551861

Ridker PM, Wilson PWF, Grundy SM. Should C-reactive protein be added to metabolic syndrome and to assessment of global cardiovascular risk? Circulation. 2004;109(23):2818–25.

Roberts CK, Hevener AL, Barnard RJ. Metabolic syndrome and insulin resistance: underlying causes and modification by exercise training. In: Comprehensive physiology, vol. 3. Hoboken, NJ, USA: John Wiley & Sons, Inc.; 2013. p. 1–58. https://doi.org/10.1002/cphy.c110062.

Saad MF, Lillioja S, Nyomba BL, Castillo C, Ferraro R, De Gregorio M, et al. Racial differences in the relation between blood pressure and insulin resistance. N Engl J Med. 1991;324(11):733–9. https://doi.org/10.1056/NEJM199103143241105.

Sah SK, Khatiwada S, Pandey S, Kc R, Das BKL, Baral N, Lamsal M. Association of high-sensitivity C-reactive protein and uric acid with the metabolic syndrome components. SpringerPlus. 2016;5:269. https://doi.org/10.1186/s40064-016-1933-y.

Saito M, Shimazaki Y, Nonoyama T, Tadokoro Y. Number of teeth, oral self-care, eating speed, and metabolic syndrome in an aged Japanese population. J Epidemiol. 2018; https://doi.org/10.2188/jea.JE20170210.

Saklayen MG. The global epidemic of the metabolic syndrome. Curr Hypertens Rep. 2018;20(2):12. https://doi.org/10.1007/s11906-018-0812-z.

Sanz Y, Olivares M, Moya-Pérez Á, Agostoni C. Understanding the role of gut microbiome in metabolic disease risk. Pediatr Res. 2015;77(1):236–44. https://doi.org/10.1038/pr.2014.170.

Sárközy M, Zvara A, Gyémánt N, Fekete V, Kocsis GF, Pipis J, et al. Metabolic syndrome influences cardiac gene expression pattern at the transcript level in male ZDF rats. Cardiovasc Diabetol. 2013;12:16. https://doi.org/10.1186/1475-2840-12-16.

Sherling DH, Perumareddi P, Hennekens CH. Metabolic syndrome. J Cardiovasc Pharmacol Ther. 2017;22(4):365–7. https://doi.org/10.1177/1074248416686187.

Shillinglaw B, Viera AJ, Edwards T, Simpson R, Sheridan SL. Use of global coronary heart disease risk assessment in practice: a cross-sectional survey of a sample of U.S. physicians. BMC Health Serv Res. 2012;12:20. https://doi.org/10.1186/1472-6963-12-20.

Similä T, Auvinen J, Puukka K, Keinänen-Kiukaanniemi S, Virtanen JI. Impaired glucose metabolism is associated with tooth loss in middle-aged adults: The Northern Finland Birth Cohort Study 1966. Diabetes Res Clin Pract. 2018;142:110–9. https://doi.org/10.1016/J.DIABRES.2018.05.035.

Singh O, Gupta M, Khajuria V. Lipid profile and its relationship with blood glucose levels in metabolic syndrome. Natl J Physiol Pharm Pharmacol. 2015;5(2):134–7. https://doi.org/10.5455/njppp.2015.5.051120141.

Srikanthan K, Feyh A, Visweshwar H, Shapiro JI, Sodhi K. Systematic review of metabolic syndrome biomarkers: a panel for early detection, management, and risk stratification in the west Virginian population. Int J Med Sci. 2016;13(1):25–38. https://doi.org/10.7150/ijms.13800.

Tanaka A, Takeuchi K, Furuta M, Takeshita T, Suma S, Shinagawa T, et al. Relationship of toothbrushing to metabolic syndrome in middle-aged adults. J Clin Periodontol. 2018;45(5):538–47. https://doi.org/10.1111/jcpe.12876.

Taylor JY, Kraja AT, de Las Fuentes L, Stanfill AG, Clark A, Cashion A. An overview of the genomics of metabolic syndrome. J Nurs Scholarsh. 2013;45(1):52–9. https://doi.org/10.1111/j.1547-5069.2012.01484.x.

Teixeira FC, Pereira FEF, Pereira AF, Ribeiro BG. Metabolic syndrome's risk factors and its association with nutritional status in schoolchildren. Prev Med Rep. 2017;6:27–32. https://doi.org/10.1016/J.PMEDR.2017.02.002.

Terfve C, Sabidó E, Wu Y, Gonçalves E, Choi M, Vaga S, et al. System-wide quantitative proteomics of the metabolic syndrome in mice: genotypic and dietary effects. J Proteome Res. 2017;16(2):831–41. https://doi.org/10.1021/acs.jproteome.6b00815.

Tomiyama H, Higashi Y, Takase B, Node K, Sata M, Inoue T, et al. Relationships among hyperuricemia, metabolic syndrome, and endothelial function. Am J Hypertens. 2011;24(7):770–4. https://doi.org/10.1038/ajh.2011.55.

Toolkit. Metabolic monitoring. 2018, 2–3.

de Toro-Martín J, Arsenault B, Després J-P, Vohl M-C. Precision nutrition: a review of personalized nutritional approaches for the prevention and management of metabolic syndrome. Nutrients. 2017;9(8):913. https://doi.org/10.3390/nu9080913.

VanWormer JJ, Boucher JL, Sidebottom AC, Sillah A, Knickelbine T. Lifestyle changes and prevention of metabolic syndrome in the Heart of New Ulm Project. Prev Med Rep. 2017;6:242–5. https://doi.org/10.1016/J.PMEDR.2017.03.018.

Villareal DT, Aguirre L, Gurney AB, Waters DL, Sinacore DR, Colombo E, et al. Aerobic or resistance exercise, or both, in dieting obese older adults. N Engl J Med. 2017;376(20):1943–55. https://doi.org/10.1056/NEJMoa1616338.

Watz H, Waschki B, Kirsten A, Müller K-C, Kretschmar G, Meyer T, et al. The metabolic syndrome in patients with chronic bronchitis and COPD: frequency and associated consequences for systemic inflammation and physical inactivity. Chest. 2009;136(4):1039–46. https://doi.org/10.1378/CHEST.09-0393.

WHO. Obesity and overweight. 2018. http://www.who.int/news-room/fact-sheets/detail/obesity-and-overweight. Retrieved 30 June 2018.

Willers J, Hahn A. Risk assessment using two different diagnostic tools: metabolic syndrome and cardiovascular risk SCORE (SCORE)—data from a weight reduction intervention study. Food Nutr Sci. 2013;4:1028–36. https://doi.org/10.4236/fns.2013.410134.

Wittcopp C, Conroy R. Metabolic syndrome in children and adolescents. Pediatr Rev. 2017; https://doi.org/10.1007/s11936-006-0045-3.

Chapter 11
Health Information Technology Considerations of Medical and Dental Data Integration

Miguel H. Torres-Urquidy, Valerie Powell, Shin-Mey Rose Yin Geist, Sushma Mishra, Monica Chaudhari, and Mureen Allen

11.1 Achieving Interoperability of Medical and Dental Records

In this chapter, we explore and consider several of the technical, knowledge, and data issues that impact electronic health records. These issues include security of applications and data, privacy of information, the ability to accurately identify uniquely a participant across all healthcare domains, usability and context-based information retrieval, and clinical decision support. These generally applicable informatics issues are then examined with a specific goal of integrating medical and dental health information. The reader will notice that we are not including content related to controlled terminologies, standardization, ontologies, and vocabularies. Given their importance, we separated and dedicated a whole chapter to these important topics. Still, the reader needs to keep in mind that the aspects of integration are many and ideally, integration will be more easily achieved when using a comprehensive strategy.

M. H. Torres-Urquidy (✉)
Centers for Disease Control and Prevention, Atlanta, GA, USA
e-mail: miguel@forwardthinkingconcepts.org

V. Powell · S. Mishra
Robert Morris University, Pittsburgh, PA, USA
e-mail: powell@rmu.edu; mishra@rmu.edu

S.-M. R. Y. Geist
University of Detroit Mercy, Detroit, MI, USA
e-mail: geistsh@udmercy.edu

M. Chaudhari
Cancer Research and Biostatisticians, Seattle, WA, USA
e-mail: monicach@crab.org

M. Allen
United Health Group, New York City, NY, USA

A. Acharya et al. (eds.), *Integration of Medical and Dental Care and Patient Data*, Health Informatics, https://doi.org/10.1007/978-3-319-98298-4_11

11.2 Physicians' Dental Data Needs and Oral Healthcare Providers' Medical Data Needs: The Clinical Rationale

11.2.1 Physicians' Needs for Dental Records

Physicians require dental records:

- For diagnosing and assessing systemic diseases and health status of their patients
- For coordination and collaboration of healthcare
- For research purposes
- For forensic purposes

More than 200 systemic diseases can present oral symptoms and/or signs. Dental records prepared by an alert dentist provide invaluable information for early diagnosis and monitoring the progress of these diseases. Conditions most common or highly relevant to oral health with respect to systemic disease are presented in this section. Please also see Contact Points in the book for pertinent literature on individual categories of diseases and conditions where medical-dental collaboration is valuable for patient care or research.

11.2.2 Oral Healthcare Providers' Medical Data Needs

With advances in medical and dental sciences and technology, many dental patients present with multiple medical conditions that may require modifications in dental management. It is essential to have patients' relevant medical information accurately stated and updated in the record so a risk and benefit assessment can be done for every dental treatment, and that certain precautions be taken, to deliver dental care safely and efficiently. A patient's self-reported health history is not always reliable (Pakhomov et al. 2008; Leikauf et al. 2009). For example, a patient may not report the status of COPD, which precludes supine positioning during long periodontal procedures. A patient may not report clearly and precisely about his or her cancer status and cancer treatment plan to permit the dentist to decide which dental treatment procedure takes priority. In general, a patient's medical record should be included in his or her dental record because dental care is delivered to a whole person. However, for practical purposes, information with high relevancy needs to be sought. This includes medical data needed for assessing the risk of:

- Office emergencies
- Post-surgery bleeding
- Post-treatment infection
- Certain other conditions

In addition to the above, when coordinating the preparation of patients for HCT, BMT, or other organ transplant, for chemotherapy and/or radiation therapy, and for implantation of various devices, relevant medical data is also needed.

11.3 Standardized/Structured Messages Facilitate Efficient Information Sharing and Benefit Patient Care

Due to the medical advances and evolution of medical subspecialties, large portions of the population, especially those with chronic medical conditions, often receive healthcare from multiple specialists. Care coordination by sharing patients' health information among different specialists becomes essential for quality of care to maximize the resources of the healthcare system. The key to care coordination is communication, which takes the form of consultation or referral.

Consultation or referral is a process involving three steps:

- *Initiation of the process*: confirming relevant patient information, providing reasons for the consultation or referral, and requesting specific information.
- *Responding*: The response to this consultation provides direct answers to the request.
- *Interpretation*: The final step of this process is interpretation of the response and making clinical decisions. When these three steps are carried out adequately and in a timely manner, the process can be efficient, benefiting patients and reducing costs for the healthcare system. Each step has its own challenges of knowledge, time, manpower, and sometimes, financial demand.

It has been widely recognized that communication among healthcare providers regarding consultation/referral can be time consuming, labor intensive, and many times, futile. It is a major source of inefficiency and a quality issue in the healthcare system (Geist and Geist 2008a, b; O'Malley and Reschovsky 2011a, b).

This section will focus on the knowledge part of the consultation-referral, address the importance of standardized-structured communications and indicate how these can greatly streamline the consultation/referral process.

Knowing what information to request or answer in the consultation/referral is the key to efficient communication. The information should be relevant and current, meaning problem-focused information and the current understanding of the disease and paradigm of management. This relevant information can be organized into a concise standardized/structured communication message (Geist and Geist 2008a, b).

Resources for standardized/structured communication messages are derived from standards of care and clinical practice guidelines in prevention, detection, evaluation, and treatment of various diseases.

Many health organizations either regularly update their clinical practice guidelines or develop new guidelines for managing patients with various diseases. The Institute of Medicine defines guidelines as "systematically developed statements to assist practitioner and patient decisions about appropriate health care for specific clinical circumstances" (Field and Lohr 1990). Health care organizations also develop and update scientific statements, scientific advisories, and position statements. These publications serve as tools to increase healthcare professionals' knowledge and awareness of effective, state-of-the art science related to the causes, prevention, detection, or management of specific diseases, or to provide rapid, clear and consistent statements of the organization's position on scientific issues.

Published periodically every 5–6 years, depending on the scientific evidence that has emerged, these publications reflect major paradigm shifts in the understanding of disease behavior and management.

The American Diabetes Association (ADA) publishes their clinical practice guidelines as clinical practice recommendations, which consist of position statements on various topics related to diabetes. These statements are reviewed annually and updated as needed. *Standards of Medical Care in Diabetes* is one of these position statements and is published every January (American Diabetes Association 2011). The American Heart Association publishes guidelines on various topics on cardiovascular diseases such as prevention of endocarditis (Wilson et al. 2007a, b), myocardial infarction management (ACC/AHA 2008) and many others.

These clinical practice guidelines or scientific statements, being current, evidence-based, widely recognized, and deeply influential, not only provide assistance in clinical decision making. They also establish the parameters of interdisciplinary conversation and have a major impact on consultation concerns and consultant responses. In essence, they provide the common ground for communication and the structure of the consultation questions.

By compliance with standards of care or clinical practice guidelines, many interdisciplinary communications can be brief and to the point to avoid redundancy and confusion.

An example would be the primary care provider (in this case a dentist) requesting a specialist (in this case a cardiologist) to provide a pre-surgical cardiovascular risk assessment for a patient who reported a history of heart attack 3 months ago. Communication can be standardized and structured by following the current ACC/AHA 2007 Guidelines on Perioperative Cardiovascular Evaluation and Care for Non-cardiac Surgery (Fleisher et al. 2007a, b). These current guidelines provide an algorithm to direct the clinician to reach a clinical decision. The dentist needs to request verification of the date of the heart attack, the extent of the infarct as well as residual LV function, and the severity of coronary artery disease. Once this information is obtained from the cardiologist, the dentist should be able to reach a clinical decision on when and how to provide dental care by using the algorithm (see Fig. 11.1).

Routinely requesting a formal pre-surgical cardiovascular risk assessment, however, can cause unnecessary delay and increase costs.

11.3.1 Other Examples of Clinical Practice Guidelines That Influence Interdisciplinary Consultations

11.3.1.1 Hypertension

Hypertension is one of the most ancient diseases and is a major global health issue. The history of hypertension has shown that in the 1930s (Moser 2006), high blood pressure was considered a natural process and should be left alone. In the 1940s,

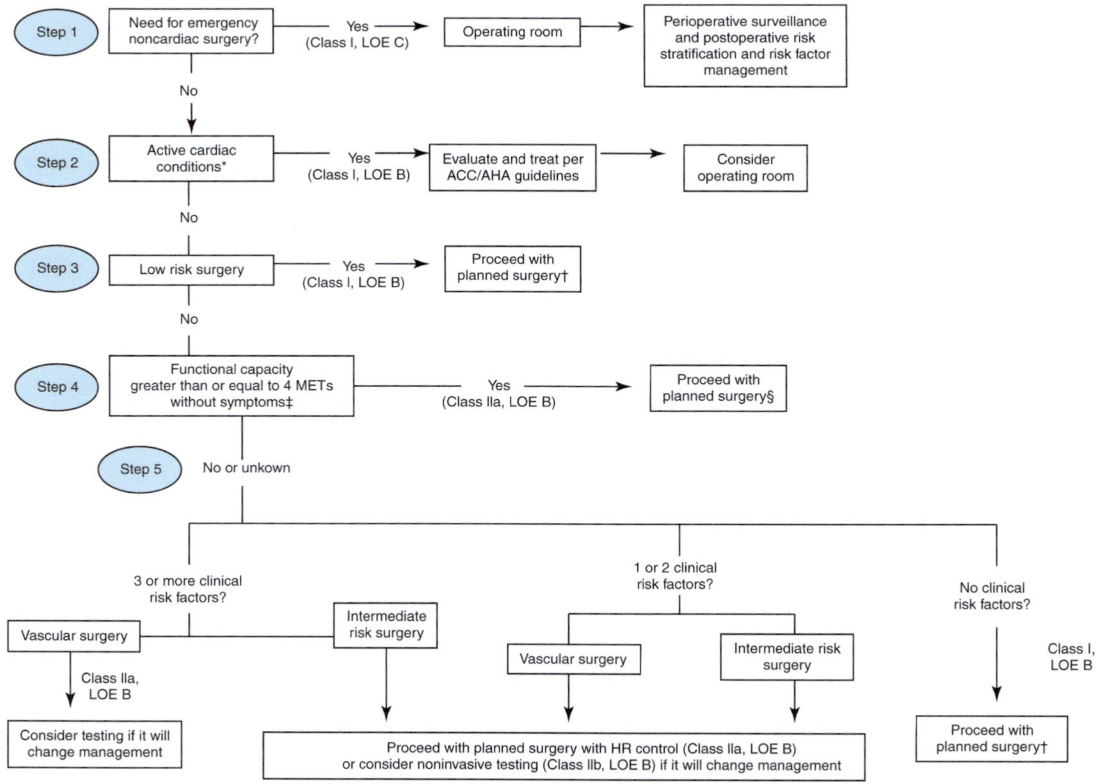

Fig. 11.1 Cardiac evaluation and care algorithm for non-cardiac surgery based on active clinical conditions, known cardiovascular disease or cardiac risk factors for patients 50 years of age or greater (Fleisher et al. 2007a, b). (Reprinted with permission Circulation. 2007;116:e418–e500 ©2007 American Heart Association, Inc.)

hypertension was diagnosed only when blood pressure was greater than 180/110. Until the 1950s, elevated blood pressure was still considered necessary for the adequate perfusion of vital organs. Over the next half-century, the definition, prevention, diagnosis and treatment of hypertension have gone through tremendous changes. The changes in concepts and management are well reflected in the national guidelines: the Joint National Committee on Prevention, Detection, Evaluation, and Treatment of High Blood Pressure (JNC) Reports. These reports are published as clinical practice guidelines by a committee that is sponsored by the National Heart, Lung, and Blood Institute (NHLBI), a branch of the National Institutes of Health of the US Department of Health and Human Services. From the first JNC report in 1976 to the seventh, and final, JNC report published in 2003 (Lenfant et al. 2003), committees have been formed every 4–6 years to issue new sets of guidelines. They update the management of hypertensive patients based on the scientific understanding of the physiology, epidemiology, pathology, and availability of pharmaceutical therapeutic agents. The guidelines guide physicians, other health care providers, patients and the public on new definitions, classifications, treatment rationales, and options in the management of hypertension and its complications. In the first JNC report, no specific action was recommended unless the diastolic pressure was ≥105 mmHg. There were no recommendations for the staging of hypertension based on systolic pressure. There were fewer than 30 drugs available to treat hypertension at that time. In the seventh JNC report (Lenfant et al. 2003), normal blood pressure for adults 18 years and older was defined as <120/80 mmHg. Prehypertension was defined for individuals whose blood pressure fell between 120/80 and 140/90 mmHg. Individuals with prehypertension who also have diabetes or kidney disease should be considered candidates for appropriate drug therapy if a trial of lifestyle modification fails to reduce their BP to 130/80 mmHg or less. JNC seven suggests that all people with hypertension (BP ≥140/90 mmHg) be treated. The treatment goal for individuals with hypertension and no other compelling conditions is <140/90 mmHg. Based on recent evidence, the seventh JNC emphasizes the importance of systolic blood pressure as a major risk factor for CVDs. There were more than 100 antihypertension drugs available at the time of publication of the seventh report of JNC.

All these changes have had a major impact on interdisciplinary communication. Dentists know when to refer patients for hypertension evaluation and treatment. Dentists also know how to manage dental patients with hypertension without sending unwarranted consultations to request permission from physicians to treat dental patients who have hypertension.

11.3.1.2 Heart Murmurs and Antibiotic Prophylaxis for Prevention of Infective Endocarditis

Heart murmurs are abnormal sounds either heard during the heart cycle, by stethoscope, or detected on an echocardiogram. A heart murmur may have no pathological significance or may be an important clue to the presence of valvular or other structural heart abnormalities. A murmur that has no pathological significance is often referred to as an innocent, functional, or physiologic murmur. Innocent murmurs are common in children and are quite harmless. Other causes of innocent heart murmur are pregnancy, fever, thyrotoxicosis (a condition resulting from an overactive thyroid gland), or anaemia.

11.3.1.3 Pathologic Heart Murmurs (Organic Heart Murmurs) That Are Caused by a Variety of Valvular Defects

Prior to the current American Heart Association (AHA) guidelines regarding the prevention of infective endocarditis (IE), an organic heart murmur had great clinical significance. This was because previous AHA guidelines on antibiotic prophylaxis (AP) for IE prevention recommended AP for many heart conditions; the list was long and complex. An organic heart murmur was often used as a surrogate marker to identify conditions for which AP was recommended because almost all heart conditions recommended previously for AP were associated with an organic (pathologic) heart murmur. An organic heart murmur thus had great clinical significance (Dajani et al. 1997; Bonow et al. 2006). When a patient reported a heart murmur without further information regarding its nature (organic or innocent), its clinical significance was somewhat ambiguous. Clarification of the nature of the heart murmur was a major reason for medical consultations and contributed to inefficiencies in health care (Geist and Geist 2008a, b; Lessard et al. 2005).

The AHA 2007 guidelines on AP for IE prevention (Wilson et al. 2007a, b) excluded many of the conditions associated with organic heart murmur from the list of conditions that are reasonable for AP, such as aortic stenosis and mitral valve prolapse (MVP) with regurgitation and about a dozen other heart conditions. The new guidelines defined a clear and short list of heart conditions for which AP is reasonable, thus making the pursuit of the nature of a heart murmur an insignificant clinical issue in this respect (Fig. 11.2).

- Prosthetic cardiac valve or prosthetic material used for cardiac valve repair;
- Previous IE;
- Congenital heart disease (CHD)[1]
  - Unrepaired cyanotic CHD, including palliative shunts and conduits;
  - Completely repaired congenital heart defect with prosthetic material or device, whether placed by surgery or by catheter intervention, during the first 6 months after the procedure[2];
  - Repaired CHD with residual defects at the site or adjacent to the site of a prosthetic patch or prosthetic device (which inhibit endothelialization).
- Cardiac transplantation recipients who develop cardiac valvulopathy.

[1] Except for the conditions listed above, antibiotic prophylaxis is no longer recommended for any other form of CHD.

[2] Prophylaxis is reasonable because endothelialization of prosthetic material occurs within 6 months after the procedure.

Fig. 11.2 Cardiac conditions associated with the highest risk of adverse outcome from endocarditis for which antibiotic prophylaxis for dental procedures is reasonable (Wilson et al. 2007a, b)

Prosthetic cardiac valve or prosthetic material used for cardiac valve repair
Previous IE
Congenital heart disease (CHD)*
Unrepaired cyanotic CHD, including palliative shunts and conduits
Completely repaired congenital heart defect with prosthetic material or device, whether placed by surgery or by catheter intervention, during the first 6 months after the procedure†
Repaired CHD with residual defects at the site or adjacent to the site of a Prosthetic patch or prosthetic device (which inhibit endothelialization)
Cardiac transplantation recipients who develop cardiac valvulopathy

* Except for the conditions listed above, antibiotic prophylaxis is no longer recommended for any other from of CHD.

†Prophylaxis is reasonable because endothelialization of prosthetic material occurs within 6 months after the procedure.

With these changes, the reasons for and requested information in consultations have drastically reduced and the increased clarity has improved the efficiency in communication. Dentists simply need to confirm with cardiologists if their patients have any of the heart conditions associated with the highest risk of adverse outcome from endocarditis for which antibiotic prophylaxis for dental procedures is reasonable. (See Appendix A for a standard/structured consultation form.)

11.3.1.4 Diabetes

The American Diabetes Association (ADA) publishes standards of medical care in *Diabetes* every January. The standards contain current treatment and possible complications, and therefore serve as tools for risk and benefit assessment for all health care providers who manage patients with diabetes (American Diabetes Association 2011).

The ADA's clinical recommendations are closely linked to other major diabetes care organizations such as the World Health Organization (WHO) and the International Diabetes Federation (IDF). These recommendations provide a standardized message, such as patient's target A1c level and risk for hypoglycemia, microvascular and macrovascular complications risk and management, insulin-resistance-risk-control, and many other diabetes issues. When an oral healthcare provider consults with a physician regarding dental care for a patient who has diabetes, questions of current A1c level and A1c target should be routinely asked.

11.3.1.5 Coronary Artery Stent

Coronary angioplasty, also called percutaneous coronary intervention (PCI), is a procedure designed to open clogged coronary arteries. More than 70% of the PCI include the placement of stent(s) in the artery to prop it open. In 2006, there were 652,000 PCI procedures with stents, of which approximately 76% were drug-eluting stents and 24% bare-metal stents. Individuals with coronary stent(s) are recommended to take dual antiplatelet therapy: thienopyridines (clopidogrel or ticlopidine) in combination with aspirin to reduce the incidence of major adverse cardiac events and stent thrombosis.

In 2007, the American Heart Association, American College of Cardiology, Society for Cardiovascular Angiography and Interventions, American College of Surgeons, and American Dental Association jointly published a Science Advisory: Prevention of Premature Discontinuation of Dual Antiplatelet Therapy in Patients with Coronary Artery Stents (Grines et al. 2007). It is recommended that individuals with bare-metal stents should stay on the dual antiplatelet therapy for 3 months, individuals with drug-eluting stents for 12 months. There should be coordination of care between the patient's cardiologist and other healthcare providers who perform invasive or surgical procedures and are concerned about perioperative and postoperative bleeding. These healthcare providers must be made aware of the potentially catastrophic risk of premature discontinuation of thienopyridine therapy. Dental practitioners are strongly discouraged from manipulating patients' antiplatelet therapy. The advisory stated that there is little or no indication for interruption of antiplatelet drugs for dental procedures. When concerned about prolonged bleeding during or after invasive dental procedures, dental practitioners should either postpone the procedure or consider using local hemostasis measures. The same issue was also addressed in the American College of Chest Physicians practice guidelines on the perioperative management of antithrombotic therapy (Douketis et al. 2008).

These advisory and current guidelines provide relevant information for dental practitioners before even initiating the consultation to ask about discontinuance or alteration of the antiplatelet regimen.

11.3.1.6 Chronic Kidney Disease

Prior to 2002, different terms were used to describe chronic kidney disease: diminished renal reserve, renal insufficiency, renal failure, and end-stage renal disease (ESRD). Severity of kidney malfunction was measured with abstract criteria such as percentage of nephrons' function loss. These non-specific terms and vague disease stage criteria made interdisciplinary and even intradisciplinary communication difficult, with negative consequences to patients' care.

In 2002 The National Kidney Foundation's (NKF-USA) Kidney Disease Outcomes Quality Initiative (KDOQI) published a guideline on chronic kidney disease (CKD), in which a new definition of chronic kidney malfunction and criteria for staging the severity of the malfunction were introduced (Kidney Disease Outcome Quality Initiative 2002). The term chronic kidney disease (CKD) was proposed for a spectrum of function loss based on the level of glomerular filtration rate (GFR). In 2005, KDIGO (Kidney Disease: Improving Global Outcomes), an independent non-profit organization under the administration of NKF, endorsed this definition and staging system (Levey et al. 2005). From that point on, global communication regarding chronic kidney disease was improved. Nevertheless, the definition and staging system are not perfect; while they have attained global acceptance, there are also controversies. The main concern was the over- and misdiagnosis of CKD and possible overuse of specialty resources. The position of KDOQI and KDIGO is that current definition/staging of CKD is simple and easy to apply (Eckardt et al. 2009). It raises awareness of CKD and improves the prognosis, in the long run benefiting patients and reducing the costs of the healthcare system. In response to these controversies, KDIGO has convened a workgroup to develop global clinical practice guidelines for the definition, classification/staging, and prognosis of CKD. The consensus has been reached to keep the current definition for CKD with the addition of clinical diagnosis and albuminuria staging to modify the classification system (Levey et al. 2011). The future guidelines will facilitate improved interdisciplinary communication even more.

11.3.1.7 Renal Dialysis

Individuals undergoing long-term renal dialysis (hemodialysis (HD)) have a dialysis access which can be an arteriovenous (AV) fistula or a synthetic graft. Patients undergoing peritoneal renal dialysis (PD) have a PD catheter dialysis access. Hemodialysis access serves as a lifeline to the patient because it provides access for blood going through the dialysis machine and returning to the body. Infection of the access can be a serious complication; emergent access must be made and new long-term access has to be made. Due to the invalid focal infection theory, patients with hemodialysis access had been given antibiotic prophylaxis for any invasive medical or dental procedure causing transient bacteremia to prevent access infection. New evidence indicates that the majority of hemodialysis access infections are most often caused by staphylococci, gram-negative bacteria, or other microorganisms in association with surgery when the access was placed, or resulting from wound or other active infections. There is no convincing evidence that microorganisms associated with transient bacteremia from dental procedures cause infection of these accesses. In 2003, the AHA published a scientific statement on nonvalvular cardiovascular device-related infections. The statement does not recommend antibiotic prophylaxis after HD access placement for patients who undergo routine dental, respiratory, gastrointestinal, or genitourologic procedures causing transient bacteremia. Prophylaxis is only recommended for patients when they undergo incision and drainage of infection at other sites or replacement of a hemodialysis access (Baddour Larry et al. 2003).

11.3.2 Permanent Pacemaker and Implantable Cardioverter-Defibrillator (Cardiovascular Implantable Electronic Device)

Because of the focal infection theory, patients with pacemakers and implanted defibrillators had been given antibiotic prophylaxis for any invasive medical or dental procedure causing transient bacteremia to prevent infection of the devices.

According to the AHA's 2003 statement on nonvalvular cardiovascular device-related infections, individuals with pacemakers and defibrillators only need antibiotic prophylaxis when undergoing incision and drainage of an abscess or replacement of a pacemaker or defibrillator (Baddour Larry et al. 2003). Based on new evidence, in 2010 the American Heart Association published a scientific statement to update guidelines on permanent pacemaker (PPM) and implantable cardioverter-defibrillator (ICD) infections and their management. The statement does not recommend antibiotic prophylaxis for dental or other invasive procedures not directly related to device manipulation to prevent cardiovascular implantable electronic device (CIED) infection (Baddour Larry et al. 2010).

11.3.3 Patients Who Are Taking Oral Anticoagulants

Warfarin is a synthetic vitamin K antagonist. It has been used as an oral anticoagulant since the 1950s for the primary and secondary prevention of venous thromboembolism, for the prevention of systemic embolism in patients with prosthetic heart valves or atrial fibrillation, for the primary prevention of acute myocardial infarction in high-risk individuals, for the prevention of stroke, recurrent infarction, or death in patients with acute myocardial infarction. Although warfarin is effective, this medication is both challenging to clinicians and patients. The anticoagulation status of the patient must be closely monitored by a laboratory test—the international normalized ratio (INR)—to keep the patient in a narrow therapeutic range without causing a bleeding problem. Many kinds of food are rich in vitamin K; consumption of too much vitamin K-rich food will cancel the anticoagulant effect of warfarin. Patients on warfarin must follow dietary instructions. Many medications also interact with warfarin. Many clinicians, including dentists who provide surgical procedures to patients taking this medication, often face the dilemma of continuing or discontinuing warfarin therapy or adjusting the dosage for fear of prolonged bleeding after surgery. These issues were addressed in the American College of Chest Physicians' Evidence-Based Clinical Practice Guidelines (eighth edition) in the Perioperative Management of Antithrombotic Therapy section (Douketis et al. 2008). The guideline developers recommend continuance of warfarin therapy around the time of dental procedures and co-administration of an oral prohemostatic agent to control local bleeding.

Dabigatran is an alternative to warfarin. It provides an anticoagulant effect similar to warfarin but does not need INR monitoring. Dabigatran is a direct thrombin inhibitor and is not a vitamin K antagonist. Dabigatran has been approved for use in Europe, Britain, and Canada since 2008 to prevent blot coagulation. In October 2010, the drug was approved by the U.S. Food and Drug Administration for prevention of stroke in patients with non-valvular atrial fibrillation. Its use is recommended by the American College of Cardiology Foundation/American Heart Association as a Class I recommendation (Wann et al. 2011).

11.3.4 Patients Who Are Taking Antiplatelets

Consultation requests to physicians asking if a patient's antiplatelet regimen should be altered for dental surgery is one of the unwarranted reasons for consultation (Geist and Geist 2008a, b), and are often done because of fear of post-operative bleeding. However, stopping a patient's antiplatelet therapy can carry a risk for fatal thrombosis. This issue was addressed in the section on coronary artery stents.

11.3.5 Bleeding Time (BT) and Platelet Function Assay-100 (PFA-100)

In assessing perioperative excessive bleeding, clinicians often request BT or PFA-100. The College of American Pathologists (CAP) and the American Society of Clinical Pathologists (ASCP) published a position statement in 1998 stating that BT cannot reliably identify individuals who have recently ingested aspirin or who have a drug-induced platelet defect. It concluded, "in the absence of a bleeding history, BT does not predict the risk of bleeding associated with surgery" (Peterson et al. 1998). Currently, no laboratory tests are predictive of surgical bleeding in patients taking antiplatelets.

PFA-100 is a sensitive test for drug effects; however, its value in prediction of surgical bleeding is not established. Patient history is the most cost-effective screening tool in predicting surgical bleeding.

The current American College of Chest Physicians Evidence-Based Clinical Practice Guidelines on the Perioperative Management of Antithrombotic Therapy recommend against the routine use of platelet function assays to monitor the antithrombotic effect of aspirin or clopidogrel in patients who are receiving antiplatelet drugs (Douketis et al. 2008).

In summary, the evidence-based clinical practice guidelines, scientific statements, advisory statements, and position statements from various specialty organizations provide parameters for interdisciplinary communication.

11.3.6 Cancer Patient Management

The National Cancer Institute of the U.S. Institutes of Health has developed and maintains a comprehensive online database of the most current, credible, and accurate information regarding cancer patient management. This database is also called Physician Data Query (PDQ). The PDQ contains peer-reviewed summaries on cancer treatment, screening, prevention, genetics, complementary and alternative medicine, and supportive care. It also includes a registry of cancer clinical trials from around the world, and directories of physicians, professionals who provide genetics services, and organizations that provide cancer care. The PDQ is provided in professional and patient versions to facilitate communication among healthcare providers and between patients and their care providers (National Cancer Institute 2010).

Oral complications of chemotherapy and head/neck radiation can be quite significant. The PDQ contains the current standard information for head and neck radiation therapy, including dosage, delivery methods, prevention and management of oral mucositis, infections, taste alterations, salivary dysfunction, dental decay, truisms, and risk levels of osteoradionecrosis. It also addresses prevention and management of the oral complications of various cancers and hematopoietic stem cell transplantation (National Cancer Institute 2011).

These information resources will serve as a risk/benefit assessment tool and will provide common language for communication.

11.3.7 Limitations of Structured Communication

Today, it is every healthcare provider's responsibility to update his/her knowledge in practice guidelines in order to practice team-based care. Communication is a dynamic process, and the content of the communication varies as the disease pattern changes and treatment advances. The strength of standard/structured communication can sometimes become a limitation to a clinician who is not abreast of current knowledge. A standard/structured consultation form may need to be updated often and may restrict free information flow.

However, limitations always can be overcome by continuing education that is designed to bring all parties of healthcare providers up to date. Various medical healthcare specialist organizations and oral healthcare organizations should work together to share each other's expertise and advocacy so patients will benefit from integrated and coordinated health services. The health system will benefit from cost reduction with collaboration in care and reduction of unwarranted consultations and laboratory tests.

Adaptation of an electronic health record system will reduce the administrative burden of time and the tasks of generating new consultation forms and transmitting consultation requests and responses.

11.4 Designing and Implementing Efficient Structured Communication Among a Patient's Medical and Dental Providers

For efficiency of information sharing, confidentiality of patient information, record keeping, and legal purposes, interdisciplinary communication takes the form of consultation and referral so that it can be well documented and easy to retrieve. The process of consultation/referral involves request, response, and interpretation to reach a clinical decision. Each step of the process has its challenges. The biggest one is the content of the request and response. Once the content of the consultation/referral form is standardized by applying knowledge of current clinical practice guidelines and/or scientific statements, the requests and responses can be organized into a concise and structured communication message to improve the quality of the consultation/referral and consequently the efficiency of patient care (Geist and Geist 2008a, b).

Principles of designing efficient structured communication among a patient's medical and dental providers consist of:

- *Request Forms*: Designing a straightforward request form with standard questions based on current standards of care or clinical practice guidelines, and
- *Answer Lists*: Providing a standard answer list in the response for the consultant to check.

For example, a primary care provider (in this case a dentist) requests a specialist (in this case a cardiologist) to provide information for cardiovascular risk assessment for a patient with a reported history of myocardial infarction (MI) who needs two teeth extracted under local anesthesia. Instead of asking the cardiologist about the patient's risk from dental treatment, the oral healthcare provider should ask specific questions regarding the date, extent, and treatment for the MI, and outcome of that treatment; in other words, the patient's current cardiac status. Once the information is received, the oral healthcare provider will plug the information into the algorithm provided in the ACC/AHA 2007 guidelines on perioperative cardiovascular evaluation, care for noncardiac surgery (Fleisher et al. 2007a, b), and take necessary precautions for indicated treatment.

For a dental patient who is reported to have diabetes mellitus, oral healthcare providers should issue a standardized/structured consultation requesting the most recent HbA1c level and glycemic control target (see the consultation form Appendix A).

When an oral healthcare provider considers giving a dental patient antibiotic prophylaxis (AP) to prevent infective endocarditis (IE), he or she should provide the cardiologist with a list of heart conditions for which AP is reasonable. This should take the form of a checklist which should be clear, concise and efficient. The list of conditions is based on the American Heart Association's 2007 evidence-based practice guidelines on IE prevention (Wilson et al. 2007a, b) and is well recognized as common ground for communication. See the consultation form Appendix B.

When a consultation is to be sent to a cancer patient's oncologist, it can be designed as follows (Fig. 11.3):

On the other hand, when an oncologist refers a cancer patient to an oral healthcare provider to prepare the oral cavity for radiation therapy or chemotherapy, the same strategy can be used to design the referral as follows (Fig. 11.4):

When a hemophilia patient or patients with other bleeding disorders need dental care, the hematologist can refer the patient to an oral healthcare provider by offering preparation of the patient to coordinate the dental care, or the oral healthcare

Fig. 11.3 Oncology consult form for a cancer patient regarding part or future bisphosphonate therapy

Referral:

Mr./Ms. ______________ will need
chemotherapy / radiation therapy for ______________ cancer.
Please assess his / her dental needs and prepare his / her oral cavity for the therapy to minimize the discomfort and the risk for oral infection and other complications during and after the therapy.

Chemotherapy / radiation therapy will be initiated on
________ , 20 _______
Chemotherapy agent(s) include:

____

The areas of the radiation will be

____

The total radiation dosage will be

____

The radiation delivery mechanism will be

____

Request:	*from Dental Provider:*	*Date:*

Mr./Ms. ______________ reports a history of ______________ cancer. Comprehensive oral examination reveals that he/she has a dental diagnosis of ______________ and needs __________________ treatment. Please provide the following information to facilitate the dental treatment of Mr./Ms. ______________

Response:	*from Medical Provider:*	*Date:*

Current cancer status of Mr./Ms. ______________
Was Mr./Ms. ______________ given IV bisphosphonates? YES ____ NO _____
Is Mr./Ms. ______________ currently taking IV bisphosphonate? YES ____ NO _____
Is IV bisphosphonate therapy planned for the future? YES ____ NO _____

Fig. 11.4 Oral health referral form for a cancer patient needing chemotherapy or radiation therapy

provider can request the hematologist to prepare the patient for the dental care. This is an example of mutual respect of each other's expertise and collaboration to improve the efficiency of patient care.

When there are no clear clinical practice guidelines to follow, and there is a conflict of opinion regarding treatment, a clear statement should be made either in the request or in the response. For example, currently there are controversies regarding antibiotic prophylaxis (AP) for dental treatment of patients with artificial joints. The purpose of the consultation in this case is to inform the orthopedic surgeon that since there is no clear evidence indicating a benefit from this practice the oral healthcare provider would leave the decision regarding AP to the orthopedic surgeon. If the surgeon believes that it would be beneficial to the patient then he or she should prescribe the antibiotics of choice and take the responsibility for administering the medication. See the Appendix A for an example consultation.

11.4.1 Transmission Methods

How to transmit and receive standardized/structured consultation or referral in a timely fashion is another challenge. In designing an efficient way to meet this challenge one must examine the pitfalls of the traditional consultation and referral transmission mechanism.

11.4.2 Illegibility

Traditional consultation letters are written on blank forms, with the dentist's or physician's often illegible writing. This can be a major barrier to communication among healthcare workers. This problem would be prevented by electronic communications.

11.4.3 Demands on Time and Manpower

The traditional paper-based handwritten consultation is a time consuming and labor intense process. The patient usually carries it to the physician and brings it back to the oral healthcare provider. Sometimes it is mailed to the patient or the physician and returned by mail. These paper forms may be lost during the process. In recent years, many hospitals and clinics have adopted electronic health record systems (EHR). Consultation requests are transmitted to the consultants through facsimile then scanned and stored in the EHR, and the returned responses are received and stored in the same manner. This has shortened the transmission time and improved record keeping, but it demands extra manpower to track the facsimile and do the scanning. A recent study has shown that nurse care managers or non-physician staff members contribute positively to the process of communication (O'Malley and Reschovsky 2011a, b). However, there are times when the consultation requests can only be answered by physicians, such as when comments on laboratory results or treatment decisions are required. In such cases, the nurse care manager or non-physician staff must track down the physician for the response, which is not always easy to accomplish in a timely manner.

11.4.4 Implementation Through Health Information Technology (HIT)

Today, electronic health records (EHRs) are common in medical and dental practice. Although not all systems are compatible with each other by default or by choice to protect patient's confidentiality, each system has the capacity to electronically generate, transmit and store the standardized/structured consultation/referral.

Some major healthcare corporations have already yielded positive results in electronic consultation/referral because their systems are used by large numbers of primary care providers and specialists (Chen and Yee 2011; Stoves et al. 2010). This may not be feasible for small, individual practices. One easy solution: an electronically generated consultation request can be sent through email to a consultant, who can directly answer and return the request form electronically. The consultation can then be stored in the patient's electronic health record. This direct communication between the primary care health care provider and specialist eliminates the need to involve additional personnel who can delay a response and leads to the possible breach of confidentiality.

In conclusion, although the time has not yet arrived for all healthcare providers to have universal access to their patients' medical and dental electronic records, HIT can definitely improve the efficiency of the consultation/referral process and consequently patient care.

11.5 Towards an Integrated Electronic Health (EHR) System: Compliance, Security, and Privacy Concerns

11.5.1 Introduction

An electronic health record (EHR) is a collection of medical information about individual patients stored in an electronic manner. It contains personally identifiable information about a patient such as social security number or medical record number, home address, and health related details. An individual's personal medical information could have sensitive information about emotional problems, sexually transmitted disease, substance abuse, genetic predisposition to diseases, or sexual minority status, information potentially adversely affecting major employment opportunities or to which social stigma is attached (Cannoy and Salam 2010). Considering that an individual's personal health information is declared "privileged" by the government, it is surprising to find that as many as 400 people may have access to one's personal medical information throughout the typical care process (Cannoy and Salam 2010). It is important to reassure the patients that their information is kept confidential. Such reassurance encourages patients to share all their health information, to the best of their knowledge, with care providers.

The terms electronic health record (EHR) and electronic medical record (EMR) have been used synonymously in the literature; however, in 2008 the National Alliance for Health Information Technology suggested that the term EMR be used for electronic record systems that are not interoperable and that EHR be used when health information is shared electronically among multiple entities. On the other hand, the personal health record (PHR) is the electronic version of an individual's health record that the person has access to via the web. Several organizations are providing the patients access to their private records or to portions of them, such as laboratory test results. In this chapter, EMR signifies separate systems used by various organizations to record health information electronically whereas EHR refers to an integrated database of electronic health records that provides access for several entities who are sharing it. Integrating all the medical information of a person electronically for regional or nationwide use, something that is proposed in the EHR concept, has significant implications. Having a single point of access to the entire medical history of a patient bears certain challenges. Among the major widespread concerns are; where will this data reside, what would the access mechanism be and who owns the responsibility of maintaining the security and privacy standards of such records and who owns the information? Lack of interoperability is a common concern as a barrier to successful health information exchanges in an integrated health information environment.

There have been several initiatives by the government in the United States in the form of regulations, guidelines, and monetary incentives to expedite the process of integrating health information from disparate sources. The Health Insurance Portability and Accountability Act (HIPAA) of 1996 is a major step towards digitization of health records with a clear focus on security and privacy of patients' personal health information. The American Recovery and Reinvestment Act of 2009 (ARRA) provides monetary incentives to medical providers for using EHR systems rather than paper counterparts (Austin et al. 2010). Considerable effort is required to standardize the electronic systems so that interoperability issues can be dealt with effectively. The Certification Commission for Health Information Technology (CCHIT) is currently modifying its criteria to conform to the ARRA-defined requirements and is working closely with the Department of Health and Human Services (HSS), the Health Information Technology (HIT) Policy Committee and the Office of the National Coordinator for Health Information Technology (ONC) to influence national EHR certification policy. On February 17, 2009, U.S. President Barack Obama signed into law HR 1, the American Recovery and Reinvestment Act, which allocates $19.2 billion dollars in funding to support the adoption and use of health information technology also known as a the "Health Information Technology for Economic and Clinical Health Act" or the "HITECH Act" (U.S. Department of Health and Human Services 2011). Impetus from federal and state governments towards digitization of patient health records is aimed at avoiding errors in medical judgment from health care providers, reducing cost of healthcare delivery, and improving overall care for the patient (Jha et al. 2009). Increasing popularity and adoption of EHRs is geared towards improving the, quality of healthcare provided in the nation. The objective is better patient-provider communication, better communication among providers delivering care to the same patient, integration of records from different health care disciplines and subspecialties and accessibility and aggregation of records among different health care delivery sites to provide a holistic health profile for a patient. Such benefits are not without associated risk of exposure of personally identifiable information and compromise in digital health data resulting in patient anguish and possible damage to career and provider embarrassment and possible liability. It is crucial that providers utilizing EMRs address the challenges to security and privacy issues of EHR technology. Anecdotal evidence and media reports about medical security breaches suggest a rather weak preparedness on the part of the health service providers in assuring security of health data. Several security, privacy, and compliance issues must be addressed within the context of creating a universal electronic health record system that provides a single point of access to patient health information.

This section explores the security, privacy, and compliance challenges in EHRs and outlines some solutions to these issues. The next section explores the regulatory requirements for security and privacy of health care records primarily from HIPAA. It also discusses the guidelines for PHI for ensuring security and privacy of health records. The third section lists the common challenges that we are facing in securing the information in an integrated environment. The fourth section outlines broad steps in dealing with the security and privacy concerns of EHRs. The final section presents the conclusion for this chapter.

11.5.2 Regulations and Guidelines

The Health Insurance Portability and Accountability Act (HIPAA) of 1996 protects the privacy of medical records of patients by preventing unauthorized disclosure and improper use of patients' protected health information (PHI). There have been federal support and impetus for migrating to electronic medical records over the years. With considerable emphasis and monetary investment in the 1990s on the computerization of health services operations, the possibility of data manipulation and non-consensual secondary use of personally identifiable records has tremendously increased (Baumer et al. 2000). HIPAA declares PHI "privileged," protecting individuals from losses resulting from the fabrication of their personal data. Businesses affected by HIPAA are directed to protect the integrity, confidentiality, and availability of the electronic PHI they collect, maintain, use, and transmit.

Three major components of HIPAA for the security and privacy of electronic records are:

11.5.2.1 The Security Rule

The security rule of HIPAA is concerned about the personal health information in electronic form. The law states that private information of individuals must be kept safe from damage of any kind. The purpose of this clause is to protect electronic patient information from alteration, destruction, loss, and accidental or intentional disclosure to unauthorized persons. HIPAA establishes behavioral standards and requires covered entities to develop practices that adhere to these behavioral standards.

The security rule requires compliance actions in the following categories:

- *Administrative safeguards*: this requires formal practices to manage security and personnel from the side of the healthcare service provider. Ensuring correct administrative safeguards entails a correct approach to governing the information security of the organization, putting correct controls in place and frequently monitoring and upgrading such controls.

- *Physical safeguards*: An important piece of the security solution of an organization lies with physical protection of the data, computers, and the physical premises where it resides. This would entail creating correct physical security controls in the form of authorization controls for physical access to the computers and premises. Another important source of critical data is disposal of paper versions of the protected data or of digital media on which protected data are stored. Adequate mechanisms need to be created to deal with physical threats to data security.
- *Technical safeguards*: This category of safeguard requires creating detailed access control mechanisms to declare and monitor information access. It is also important to make sure that data in transit (moving from one point to another in the healthcare domain) is secure.
- *Organizational requirement*: This requirement assures that employees understand the serious implications for maintaining the integrity and security of data that they deal with on a daily basis. The employee should have explicit business associate contract provisions so that they can affirm agreement regarding the role that is required for them.
- *Policies, procedures and documentation*: These requirements stipulate that correct security policies and procedures are in place to protect the data.

Meeting the security rule requirements entails coming up with a comprehensive security plan that has detailed procedures for addressing risks at several levels in the organization and that proactively addresses those risks. Examples of the planning steps include establishing security certification processes for employees and contractors, keeping employee records constantly updated to indicate the level of security appropriate to each job position, termination of role or employment, assessing the compliance of the Management Information Systems (MIS) department with the Security Rule standards and explicitly stating consequences for noncompliance with new security rules (Choi et al. 2006).

11.5.2.2 The Privacy Rule

The privacy rule of HIPAA applies to PHI in all forms, including oral, written, and electronic forms. The purpose of the privacy rule is to "meet the pressing need for national standards to control the sensitive health information and to establish real penalties for the misuse or improper disclosure of this information" (Choi et al. 2006). The rules established within the privacy dimension of HIPAA, apply to all aspects of use of personal health records including medical records, claims and payment information, and almost all additional information related to a patient's health care. The privacy rule protects the individual's right of dictating how and when the personal information of the patient can be released. It is meant to empower an individual to play an important role in managing one's own health records. It allows patients to have a participatory approach to data management by giving them the specific right to access their medical records and request amendments, to allow or not allow access to their information in certain circumstances, and be aware of their privacy rights in this domain.

Transactions among various participants in the healthcare industries must communicate effectively and electronically patient information. Successfully meeting this requirement necessitates that the privacy and security covenants also be met.

This regulation has forced companies to revisit and reorganize their business processes. Compliance with HIPAA is not just a matter of technical products ensuring safe and secure data collection, transaction, and storage; rather, compliance is an issue of "organizational change management" (Mishra and Chin 2008). It requires instituting new structures and patterns for health care organizations to coordinate care efficiently, trust other's intentions, and responsibly maintain and protect sensitive data (Huston 2001). HIPAA influences healthcare organizations at the basic infrastructure level, thus demanding re-evaluation at all levels, including the creation and implementation of technical solutions. Employing and adapting to technical solutions requires not only proper planning but also an overhaul in organizational processes (Mishra and Chin 2008). Even though more than one-third of the rules in HIPAA address administrative security requirements, many organizations focused disproportionately on technology rather than on administrative safeguards. The different types of security required by the HIPAA security rule were also not well understood by participating organizations. It is critical to establish a consistent method for linking patients with the electronic records to assure exchanging health information about the correct patient.

In the United States, the American Recovery and Reinvestment Act of 2009 (ARRA) provides monetary incentives to medical providers for using EHR systems rather than paper counterparts (Austin et al. 2010). In October 2009, CCHIT augmented its certification criteria with additional security criteria and provided corresponding black-box test scripts. The security criteria provide specific requirements intended to establish a minimum level of security of an EHR system. The purpose of CCHIT certification is to confirm that certified EHR systems maintain a minimum level of accuracy, reliability, security, and interoperability. These characteristics are known as software quality factors (Austin et al. 2010). Regional or state-level efforts to exchange health information also will have to reconcile the differences among participants in how security policies are implemented. Organizations in ten states are working to develop and test a set of model policy requirements to bridge policy gaps for authentication and audit across these organizations.

In the case of personal health records (PHRs), which are becoming popular, security and privacy concerns have led to guidelines proposed by the government. The Office of the National Coordinator for Health Information Technology (ONC) issued a "Nationwide Privacy and Security Framework for Electronic Exchange of Individually Identified Health Information" in 2008. This framework suggests eight principles for establishing a consistent approach that meets privacy and security challenges of online PHRs and electronic health information exchange. An organization operating a PHR or Health Information Exchange (HIE) service has to follow the guidelines regardless of whether it is explicitly covered by HIPAA. These principles are expected to guide the actions of all health care-related persons and entities that participate in a network for the purpose of electronic exchange of individually identifiable health information. These principles are not intended to apply to individuals with respect to their own individually identifiable health information.

The proposed eight principles are:

- *Individual access*: Personal health information should be accessible to individuals to manage their health care. HIPAA covered entities generally make it difficult for individuals to access their personal healthcare records online (Brown 2009). This principle favors easy access to individuals for their health records.
- *Correction*: In case of a mistake in an individual's personal healthcare records, the individual should be able to correct that mistake. There should be a clear process to allow changes by the individual and to record the changes for documentation. In case of disagreement, there should be a process for documenting the disagreement as well. The HIPAA privacy rule recognizes that individuals should play an important role in ensuring accuracy of their health record. Individuals have the right to have a covered entity under HIPAA amend their PHI in a designated record set. In case a correction is made, the covered entity is entitled to inform its business associates and others who are known to have their PHI that the record was amended.
- *Openness and Transparency*: Healthcare providers should aim for complete openness and transparency to the individuals about policies, procedures, and technologies employed to collect and disseminate individually identifiable information. The information should be provided in easily understandable format to the individual, providing details about who accesses the information, how is it transmitted, how is it used, and what control the individual has of it.
- *System Complexity*: With the health information technologies evolving into increasingly complex systems, with better access to health information, larger storage capacity, and interoperability across networks, it is important that the individuals whose information is stored in these systems trust the technologies and the care providers to keep their information safe. Openness and transparency is thus essential in establishing this trust through adequate information provided to the individuals about how the system is being used. Health information organizations (HIOs) and entities that participate in HIOs should provide clear notice of their policies and procedures regarding how they use and disclose individuals' identifiable health information and how they will protect the privacy of this information.
- *Individual Choice*: Individuals should have the control over deciding what specific part of the personally identifiable information should be disclosed and to whom. The individual choice principle of the Privacy and Security Framework emphasizes that the opportunity and ability of an individual to make choices with respect to the electronic exchange of their individually identifiable health information is an important aspect of building trust (U.S. Department of Health and Human Services 2011). The Privacy and Security Framework (PSF) also recommends that the options available for choices should depend on the nature

of information being exchanged and the purpose of the exchange. The privacy rule empowers the individuals to participate actively in managing their own information.

- *Collection, Use and Disclosure Limitations*: Health information about individuals should be collected, used, and disclosed as required by the policies and procedures. The privacy rule generally requires covered entities to take reasonable steps to limit the use or disclosure of PHI to the minimum necessary to accomplish the intended purpose. This principle also suggests that for routine or recurring requests and disclosures, covered entities must implement reasonable policies and procedures (which may be standard protocols) to limit information disclosures or requests. It also suggests that a covered entity should limit the business associate's uses and disclosures of PHI to be consistent with its own policies and procedures. The business associate may not have the similar stringent policies about the use of PHI, hence the restriction.
- *Data Quality and Integrity*: There should be reasonable care taken to ensure that data being collected and transmitted is complete, accurate, and timely. It is also important to ensure that it has not been altered or destroyed in an unauthorized manner.
- *Safeguards Principle*: there should be reasonable assurance that administrative, technical, and physical safeguards are provided to ensure confidentiality, integrity, and availability of data. It is important to protect the personally identifiable data from inappropriate access, use, or disclosure. The Safeguards Principle in the Privacy and Security Framework emphasizes that trust in electronic health information exchange can only be achieved if reasonable administrative, technical, and physical safeguards are in place.
- *Privacy Rule*: the HIPAA privacy rule supports the Safeguards Principle by requiring covered entities to implement appropriate administrative, technical, and physical safeguards to protect the privacy of protected health information (U.S. Department of Health and Human Services 2009).

11.5.2.3 Accountability

All the guidelines should be followed and implementation should be verified through auditing, monitoring, and other procedural and technical processes.

The Accountability Principle in the Privacy and Security Framework emphasizes that guidelines should be followed and all the activities and mechanisms in accordance with HIPAA compliance should be reported. This principle is important to build trust in the electronic exchange of individually identifiable information. The privacy rule in HIPAA provides the foundation for accountability within an electronic health-information-exchange environment. It requires covered entities to comply with administrative requirements and extend such obligations to business associates. This rule also establishes mechanisms for addressing non-compliance with privacy standards through a covered entity's voluntary compliance, a resolution agreement, and corrective action plan or imposing civil penalties (U.S. Department of Health and Human Services 2009).

The Certification Commission for Healthcare Information Technology (CCHIT) is an independent, voluntary, private-sector initiative that has been designated by the Department of Health and Human Services (HHS) as a recognized certification body for electronic health records (EHRs) and their networks (Brown 2009). CCHIT has modified its criteria to certify PHRs. It is likely that CCHIT certification will become the commonly accepted requirement for PHRs as well (Brown 2009).

11.5.3 Challenges with Integrated Electronic Health Records

The U.S. health care system faces multiple challenges such as increasing cost and inconsistent quality. It is perceived that the electronic health records have the potential to improve the efficiency and effectiveness of health care providers. The American Recovery and Reinvestment Act of 2009 makes national, integrated health information systems a priority. Even though there is a broad consensus on benefits of such an integrated system, health care providers were initially slow to adopt it. A study by Jha et al. (2009) reported that, at that time, only 17% of U.S. physicians used either a minimally functional or comprehensive electronic-records system. As of 2015, however, 87% of office based physicians had adopted any EHR, and 78% had adopted a certified EHR (Office of the National Coordinator for Health Information Technology, Health IT Dashboard 2018). Integration efforts pose serious challenges to organizations in terms of technical preparedness as well as organizational willingness. Employing and adapting to technical solutions requires not only proper planning but also an overhaul in organizational processes. Some of the areas identified as major challenges for integration of electronic medical records are:

11.5.3.1 Getting Patient Consent

There is confusion about the "correct" way of obtaining patient permission to disclose personal health information. There are several reasons to determine prevalent practice (Dimitropoulos and Rizk 2009):

- A lack of understanding about HIPAA requirements to get patient permission for certain disclosures. Organizations have interpreted and executed this requirement differently.
- A set of different state laws that lack clear guidance on when to seek permission and when not to seek permission.
- Ethical and moral obligations to get the permission before sharing any information.
- Organizational policies require getting permission as an added security layer to their security practices.

There is also confusion about the terms used for obtaining patients' permission. This is due to use of different terms in the HIPAA privacy rule for different purposes (Dimitropoulos and Rizk 2009). Adding to the confusion is the variance in state laws of terms such as *consent*, *authorization*, and *release*, to describe a patient's written permission to disclose health information.

11.5.3.2 Ensuring Privacy and Security of Patient Information

HIPAA requires a certain level of preparedness from organizations implementing the security and privacy rules of this legislation. Various organizations' interpretations of HIPAA requirements to secure information and protect privacy vary significantly adding to the confusion about how integrated health information should be treated. There is a general lack of understanding about privacy rule implications to allow disclosure of health information for treatment, payment, and health care operations. Also, the state laws add to the confusion with reference to when the rule is being applied or how it is it being applied.

The primary causes of variation identified in security policies were attributable to a general misunderstanding about appropriate security practices, including what is technically available and what provisions can be applied more broadly (Dimitropoulos and Rizk 2009). Some organizations get concerned when they do not find the participating organization to be dealing with security requirements effectively. The security rule addresses administrative, physical, and technical security. Even though more than one-third of the rule addresses administrative security requirements, many organizations focused disproportionately on technology rather than on administrative safeguards (Dimitropoulos and Rizk 2009). An overemphasis on technical safeguards is unable to protect the organization from insider threats to security which is significantly more common compared to vulnerabilities originating outside an organization.

11.5.3.3 Data Access Mechanisms and Authorization Techniques

There is a need to develop standard authentication and authorization protocols to be implemented with electronic systems holding health data. Organizations require a fair amount of trust on other participating members to share their records with a reasonable assurance that the other party is keeping the information secure. In an integrated environment, data should flow seamlessly from one system to another resulting in several access points across the systems. Considering the critical nature of the data in such systems, our existing access control models must be used innovatively.

11.5.3.4 Linking Data to a Unique Person

If organizations intend to share data across databases to realize the vision of one record per patient, there have to be predefined agreed upon ways of linking the databases such that records are accurately identified. If the correct record for a patient is not identified, that might lead to serious clinical and privacy threats. It is important because different organizations involved in providing care to a patient use locally assigned patient identifiers which lose meaning outside the organizational boundaries. Correctly identifying patients and providers not only is critical in the delivery of high quality care and for electronic HIE, but also is a fundamental issue in other information security domains, such as authentication and authorization (Dimitropoulos and Rizk 2009).

Even though we have seen a lot of progress in adoption of EHRs in recent years, a lot needs to be achieved. Most of the providers are not realizing the full benefits from an EHR since they shy away from using all its capabilities. The use of EHR technology improves efficiency and safety but the way it is being used currently restricts it to the data that is fed in the system or data in the linked systems. The information has to be entered manually and there is no easy access to the historical records of a specific patient.

11.5.3.5 Data Storage and Handling

HIPAA requires healthcare providers to be more stringent with storing and handling of patient data, within the system as well as during transmission of the information to other systems. Transmission of information from one system to another requires use of encryption techniques. Benaloh et al. (2009) argue for using encryption control measures for patient health records. The approach calls for patient enabled encryption keys such that the patient participates in their own security management of the data.

11.5.3.6 Disaster Recovery Preparation

Disasters, natural or man-made, could prove catastrophic to the information held in systems. With a greater emphasis on storing the patient information electronically, comes an increased responsibility to plan for disaster recovery techniques for such systems. The systems also require enhanced interoperability to deal with data from various sources.

The challenges in complying with regulatory requirements lie in the ever changing nature of technology and the associated security vulnerabilities. It is important to continuously assess, evaluate, and address these challenges proactively. As the EHR is implemented in provider practices, a full-risk assessment of the administrative, technical and physical safeguards must be addressed. Each HIPAA security rule specification should be addressed and procedures should be put in place to minimize risk.

11.5.4 Addressing These Challenges

Security violations in electronic health records, such as unauthorized access or unauthorized alteration of individual information could lead to potential problems for all the involved parties. Though the concept of EHR is appealing to improve the effectiveness of processing health care data, caution is needed while designing and deploying the system. The amount of damage resulting from a compromised EHR would be significantly greater, than that in a paper-based system (Goldschmidt 2005). To encourage healthcare service consumers and providers to use electronic health records it is crucial to instill confidence that the electronic health information is well protected and that consumers' privacy is assured (Liu et al. 2007). The traceability of data in a computer system also has to be considered an asset in controlling information or containing damage from an unauthorized access. This does not happen with paper records; unauthorized information access is not tracked *or* monitored. This does not mean there should not be concern about attempts to gain access to electronic medical records for unauthorized or criminal purposes. Some of the common solutions to the integration of electronic health records are provided below:

11.5.4.1 Common Agreement on Patient Consent for Disclosure

The development of a common approach to obtaining and managing patient consent for disclosure is critical. There are several state laws that have more stringent standards for security and privacy than HIPAA, which does not preclude state laws being enforced. Due to differing expectations statewide, organizations cannot come up with a standard privacy requirement that can satisfy all the security needs for participating organization in HIEs. Several options are being considered by state and federal bodies to come up with satisfactory solutions for interstate sharing of information.

11.5.4.2 Harmonizing State Privacy Laws

It is important to harmonize state privacy laws to enable a nationally integrated HIE. This has to be a coordinated effort among states to help prevent the codification of policies that could make nationwide electronic HIE impossible. There are several ongoing initiatives in this direction.

11.5.4.3 Standard Access Control and Authorization Policies

More work is required to establish how security and privacy policies will be implemented among participants. There has to be an agreement by the involved parties not only on the content of such policies but also a consensus on implementation and adoption approaches as well. The access control models should be based on a "need to know" basis (Kurtz 2003). It's better to provide access based on the role of the participant in the organization than a blanket access power to persons or organizations. The care providers should access only the records of patients for whom they are providing care.

11.5.4.4 Inter-Organizational Agreements (IOAs)

There have to be clearly defined inter-organizational agreements between organizations sharing the data in electronic health record systems. These agreements provide the basis of trust in the relationship between participating organizations. There is an ongoing effort to get consensus from the partners on creating a legal agreement in case of any breach of trust. The IOA Collaborative has developed a core set of privacy and security provisions and plans to pilot-test two model agreements for interstate electronic HIEs—one agreement for a public health setting and the other for exchange among private entities (Dimitropoulos and Rizk 2009).

11.5.4.5 Educating the Consumer and the Provider

Electronic HIEs can be a new concept to consumers nationwide and thus require a widespread effort to educate the consumer about the pros and cons of such a collaborative effort. Such an effort will engage consumers in the discussion about security of the records and will make them informed participants in this ongoing effort. One of the key findings in the assessment of variation was that many health care providers misunderstand the capabilities and benefits of electronic HIEs and have concerns about the security of electronic health record (EHR) systems (Dimitropoulos and Rizk 2009). The efforts are directed towards disseminating consistent educational information to providers about the benefits of EHRs and electronic HIE, with a focus on privacy and security, to help encourage their participation in electronic HIE.

11.5.4.6 Standardization and Interoperability

In order to make patient information shareable across several healthcare providers, it is important to standardize the system and EMR specifications. The aim of this sharing of information should be a single record for a patient that provides the complete medical history compiling information from all the primary care physicians, surgeons, dentists, pharmacies, or any other healthcare provider the patient has visited. This concept of total integration leads to development of the electronic healthcare record (EHR). As challenging as it might be, EHR truly is far behind in its implementation, except in certain environments, such as the Department of Veterans Affairs.

11.5.4.7 Audit Controls and Monitoring

Continuous audit control and monitoring should be provided to ensure the integrity of data. Auditing system logs provides insights into data access on a "need to know" basis and developing such audit trails would be beneficial in the long run. Random and directed review of the audit trail should be accomplished regularly to test compliance with confidentiality policies. It is crucial to review the feeder systems for audit trail capabilities, as these could be vulnerable without proper information security and auditing capabilities.

11.5.4.8 Clear Policies, Procedures and Controls

Policies, controls, and procedures for accessing data should be clearly defined. These policies should be communicated very well to the users through regular training and education. Regular backup of the database must be established to include the capability to reload the database in case of disaster.

11.5.4.9 Disaster Recovery Plan

Design of the disaster recovery plan should be carried out to assure minimum risk of systems downtime and data loss in case of a calamity. Disaster recovery plans are crucial for the data recovery process especially in the health care domain. Eventually, all of the records of the patients will be in electronic form and loss of access to this data could jeopardize patient care. Care should be taken to provide the correct services for the risk involved. Backup copies of data with fail-over capabilities are important to maintain. There should be stringent mechanisms in place to ensure continued operation and data integrity in case of a disaster (Kurtz 2003).

11.5.4.10 Physical Security of the Information

Physical protection of important information in the form of printers, disposal of copies in paper or digital form, and computers on which the data resides should be ensured.

11.5.4.11 Integrating Dental Records with EHR

There has been little effort in integrating the dental records into the EHR, with the primary exception of certain U.S. Federal EHR technologies. According to Groen and Powell (2010), "While patient interaction with PHR systems is still very limited, the National Dental EDI Council (NDEDIC) has recognized their importance and begun to focus on ensuring the participation of dental insurance stakeholders in the development of PHR systems." Further, according to Groen and Powell, "UHIN (the Utah Health Information Network) is an example of a state health information network that supports the dental community and is focused on helping to reduce costs for dental practices. Dental claims, payments, reports and X-rays can be transferred electronically through UHIN."

11.5.5 Conclusion

The Health Insurance Portability and Accountability Act (HIPAA) of 1996 mandates the privacy, security, and electronic transaction standards for maintaining the patient information for all healthcare providers. HIPAA targets two goals (Choi et al. 2006): insurance flexibility (electronic records that can be easily accessed and transferred thus preventing refusal of coverage due to change of jobs) and administrative ease (reducing healthcare cost due to standardizing the transactions). Hence, electronic data interchange is an important element in assisting the organizations to meet with high patient load and enhance business partner relationships in healthcare organizations. HIPAA seeks to validate and assist with the inevitability of electronic data transactions, while also addressing privacy and security issues that may stem from converting to the use of potentially vulnerable electronic transactions. The main challenge ahead is to continue work toward a common set of privacy and security policies and practices that respect local preferences in each state yet facilitate nationwide electronic HIE. For the success of integrated electronic health record technology, it is crucial to create a broad base of support from various stakeholders and develop consensus-based polices that could be broadly adopted and shared. This section explores various issues and concerns in creating EHR and discusses several possible ways of meeting such challenges.

11.6 Matching Patients to Achieve Unique Patient Identification

The medical and dental insurances and care systems that have evolved separately with little integration are now exploring a joint outcomes assessment approach to confirm and quantify the link between systemic and oral health by measuring the two-way impact on clinical, economic, and humanistic outcomes, such as patient health-related quality of life.

One such joint outcomes research was conducted using the linked data from both Washington Dental Service (WDS) and Group Health Cooperative (GH). WDS is a founding member of the Delta Dental Plans Association delivering dental care to more than two million people through employer-sponsored programs. GH is a nonprofit health care system that coordinates care and coverage for more than half a million residents of Washington state and Idaho. Secondary enrollment data from WDS and GH, clinical (laboratory, pharmacy and diagnosis) data from GH, and claims data from WDS were used on enrollees continuously and dually insured between 2002 and 2006.

The inception of this research project pivoted on a strategy devised to identify the same subjects between WDS and GH, i.e. to uniquely identify individuals. This strategy has been discussed at length by Theis et al. (2010). The ability to successfully match individuals' records in non-related databases entailed identifying a number of overlapping variables with personal information, their information richness, and the accuracy with which they are recorded in individual databases. Generally, the challenge in uniquely matching a patient across different databases is that across healthcare entities data standards may differ, personal identifiers may be coded differently, and data update and retention rules may be applied differently. Incorrectly specified information from keying-in-errors may add to these challenges resulting in higher non-match rates with larger datasets. On the other hand, too few overlapping variables may increase the likelihood of duplicate matches resulting in misclassification bias. (Blakely and Salmond 2002).

To optimize matching, two approaches, deterministic and probabilistic, are usually used for record linkage based on the reliability of the overlapping identifiers. While deterministic linkage requires an exact match on one or more identifiers used iteratively to link and verify the linkage, probabilistic matching uses information from many variables and allows for disagreement by assigning weights to all possible record pairs. When reliable identifiers are available, deterministic approaches are usually preferred because they achieve acceptable results, are less cumbersome, and require less development time than probabilistic matching. (Liu 1999; Gill et al. 1993; Roos and Wajda 1991) Because of the enormity of data with half a million subscribers to be matched, we conducted an initial test to assess the performance of the deterministic linkage approach in a sub-sample.

We first explored the linkage utility of personal identifiers within respective databases by examining them for missing or invalid values and their consistency over time. The GH database was inspected for the time period 2004–2005. The variables in GH database with the greatest number of unique values, and thus potentially the most discriminating, were social security number (SSN), telephone number, last name, first name, and date of birth. However, significant year-to-year variability in telephone number, city, and zip code made these variables less suitable for deterministic linkage.

The SSN, while collected, was not used as the principal personal identifier in either of the databases and was found missing for nearly 100% of dependents of the WDS subscribers. Unlike GH that retained a unique patient identifier for each individual across all enrolment-disenrollment cycles, a new unique identifier was assigned at WDS when an enrolee changed employer groups. This caused duplication of records with multiple identifiers for the same individual, also termed as 'weak warm body mapping'. This term is coined due to the implications it bears on tying (mapping) the histories of an individual (a warm body) that are captured by the system under different identifiers over different periods.

Figure 11.5 illustrates the differences between the GH and WDS approaches to coded patient identifiers within their respective systems.

To avoid problems emanating from weak warm body mapping and the frequent absence of dependents' SSN, we inspected WDS records for subscribers and dependents separately for the entire study period 2002–2006. The issue of weak warm body mapping was resolved by ensuring existence of a unique identifier within the WDS database for both dependants and subscribers on a combination of personal identifiers like subscribers' member-id (most of the time it was the subscribers' SSN also shared by their dependents), last name, first name, and birth date.

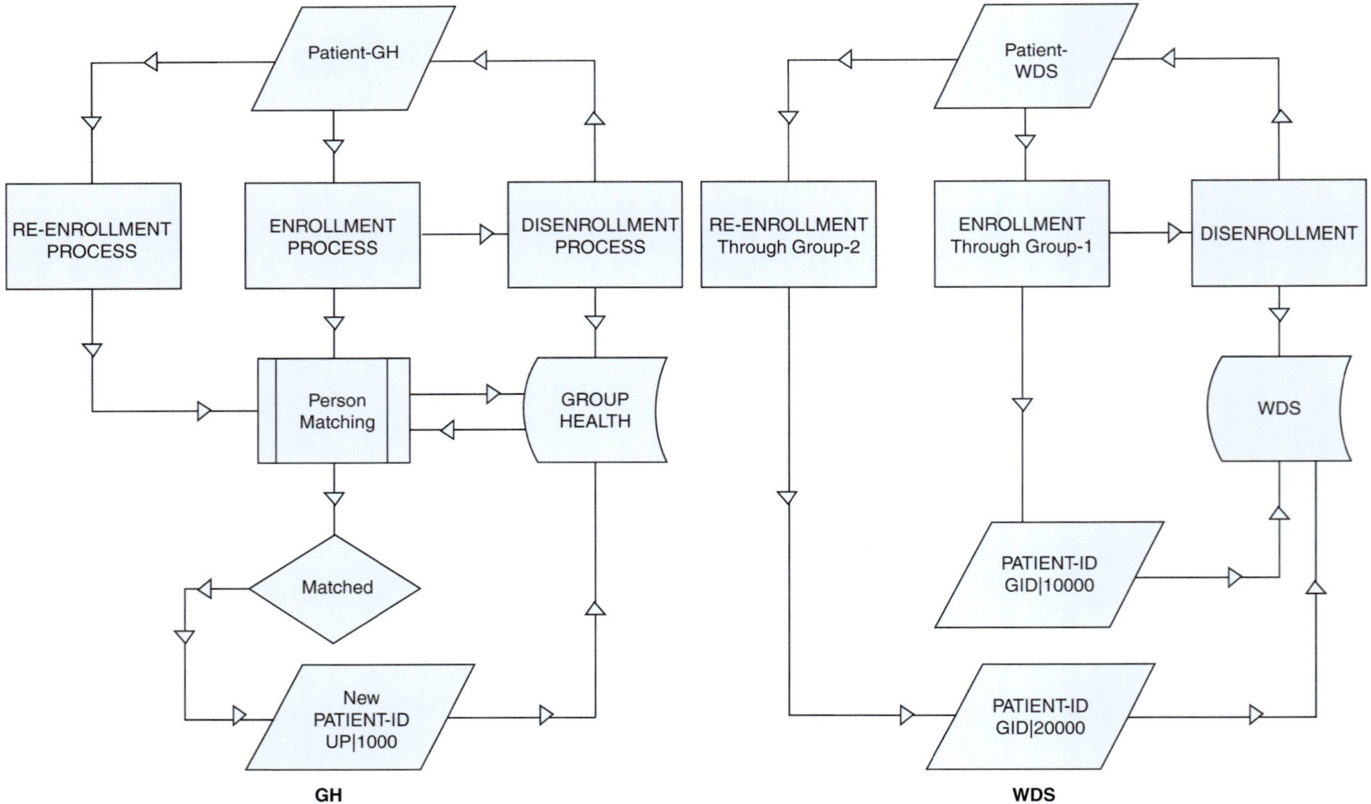

Fig. 11.5 GH and WDS approaches to coded patient identifiers. The figure is intended to reflect broadly the difference between the two systems and is not representative of the true processes

All subscribers had unique SSNs but there were a few who had more than one SSN on the unique combination of last name, first name, and birth date if it was not missing or on the combination of last name and first name if birth date was missing. Such subscribers were not included in the study. We also made sure that all the subscribers included in the study had a single unique identifier in the database on the above combination. The dependents of only the selected subscribers who had a single unique identifier in the database for the combination of their first name, last name, and subscriber's member-id were included in the study. This ensured reliable traceability of their dental history and benefits within the WDS database. See Fig. 11.6 for the decision flow used to manage the weak warm body mapping.

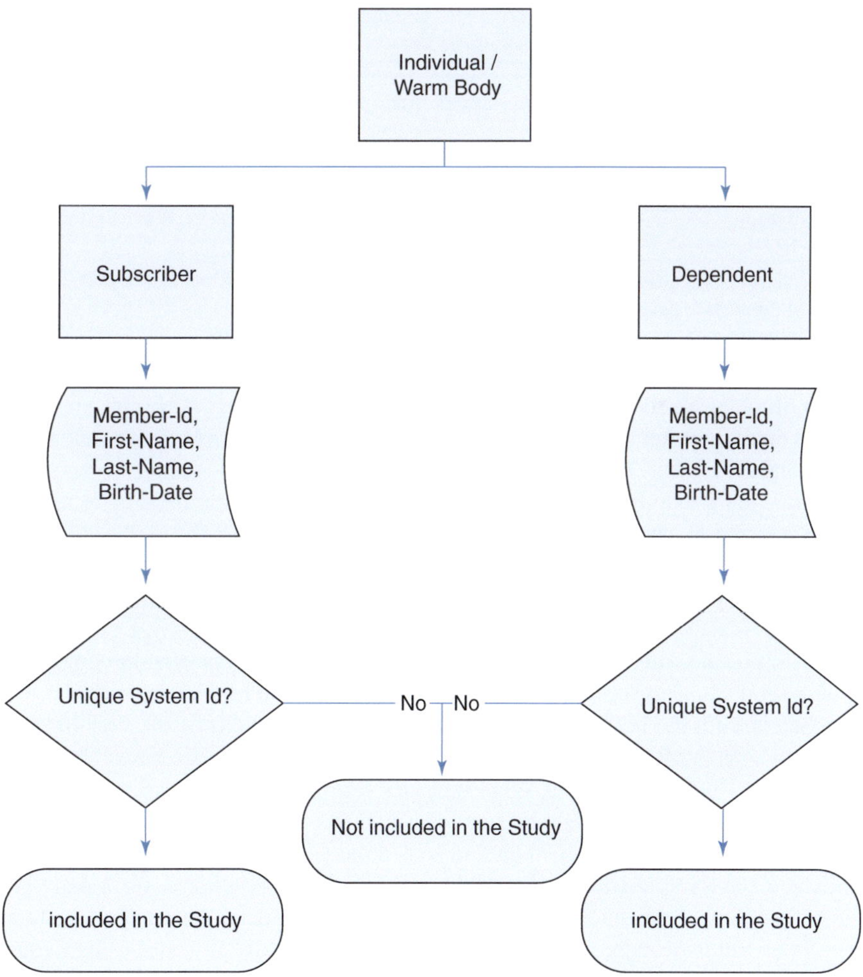

Fig. 11.6 Weak warm body decision flow

Table 11.1 Test match-merges of WDS data to four GH plans with known WDS dental coverage

Data elements examined	Number of unique matches (% agreement with WDS)
Social security number[a]	97.7
Social security number + last name[a]	96.9
Social security number + birth date[a]	97.3
Last name + first name + birth date[a]	96.0

[a]Duplicates on each of the four combinations were deleted from both datasets

Table 11.2 Linkage results of WDS data to GH data among persons aged 40–74 with 5-year continuous enrollment*

Exact merge	% of individuals linked in agreement with GH
SSN	41
SSN + last name + first name + birth date	36
n − 1 deterministic merge	
SSN + last name + first name	37
Last name + first name + birth date	51
SSN + first name + birth date	37
SSN + last name + birth date	38
Total of the n − 1 Deterministic merge*	**55**

*Duplicate social security numbers, last names, first names or birth dates were deleted from each merge group in both datasets

To test our confidence in the four linkage variables, SSN, last name, first name, and birth date, we then performed four deterministic linkages with four employer groups dually insured by GH and WDS, restricted to adults born between January 1, 1932, and December 31, 1961 and enrolled in 2004 or 2006. To improve matching precision, the Group Health and WDS datasets were then standardized by removing duplicates and names were cleaned (e.g. removing prefixes, suffices, punctuation). Subsequently, as shown in Table 11.1, the linkage showed 96% or higher exact matches of the minimum of the total unique identifiers from WDS and GH respectively with matches on just SSN, SSN + last name, SSN + birth date, last name + first name + birth date. This also suggested that insurance data are homogeneous; employer groups send identical administrative data to both dental and health care insurers.

Content with the high degree of matching on combinations of the four linkage variables, we finally developed the entire linked dataset for our research study, including all individuals from WDS and GH who met the study criteria. Only a subset of the population would be successfully linked. An $n - 1$ deterministic linkage strategy was then performed on four sets of merges with three of the four merge variables: (1) SSN, last name, first name; (2) last name, first name, birth date; (3) SSN, first name, birth date; and (4) SSN, last name, birth date. We grouped the four $n - 1$ deterministic merges into one dataset and removed all duplicates using Group Health's unique identifier to obtain our final linked population (n = 78,230). Using this approach, we showed (Table 11.2) that a relatively simple deterministic approach, within a narrow time frame and with demographic variables commonly collected by dental and medical insurance carriers, results in high-quality record linkage.

In order to protect confidentiality, all personal identifiers were stored on a computer file that only the GH analyst could access. WDS sent SSNs separately from names and birth dates through a Web-based application (Secure File Transfer). Once the linkage was complete, personal identifiers (excluding the unique system identifier which is usually a cryptic number for each enrollee) were destroyed and replaced by study identifiers. To protect confidentiality and privacy, the study identifiers were used to combine medical and dental information on the same individuals.

Now that we had a validated method to identify uniquely the same individual across the GH and WDS databases, we were able to examine the actual joint outcomes research question, i.e. what is the nature and degree of association between periodontal disease and diabetes.

11.7 Improved Electronic Healthcare Technologies (EHT) Through the Harmonization of Application Design and Clinician Needs

11.7.1 Introduction

There is general excitement as the healthcare industry lumbers slowly but surely to full electronic integration of healthcare systems. In 2004, President Bush decreed that every American should have an electronic health record by 2014; since then the clock has been ticking. Many public-private collaborations since 2004 have been formed to accelerate the adoption and use of electronic health records. Until the funded mandate of the American Recovery and Reinvestment Act (ARRA) to adopt and use electronic health records the momentum of adoption by healthcare providers had been relatively slow.

The electronic health record (EHR) is only one component of what is essential for electronic integration. There are many other components essential for a fully integrated healthcare system including, but not limited to, laboratory information systems (LISs), medication management systems, registry systems, patient health records (PHRs), and biometric devices, etc., which collectively represent electronic health technologies (EHTs). It is imperative that attention be paid to these technologies to increase their acceptance and use by healthcare providers.

For many years the adoption of electronic health technologies, especially EHRs, has been woefully lacking. There are a number of factors that will drive the adoption and successful use of these technologies including, (1) whether they seamlessly integrate with the clinical workflow to support context-specific delivery of care, (2) their relative ease of use and (3) the completeness of the data. If EHTs support all three of these criteria then resistance to their adoption will decline precipitously.

11.7.2 Context-Specific Delivery of Information to Improve Care

At this point, you might be wondering why should the developers of EHTs pay attention to the clinical workflow or much less try to integrate seamlessly into the workflow. The answer is unmet information needs. There are a number of studies (Covell et al. 1985) indicating that during healthcare encounters, providers often have information needs that go unmet. These needs exist even when healthcare providers interact with EHTs (Allen et al. 2003) Healthcare providers typically rely on the information at hand (memory, reference textbooks, journals, and colleagues) to help make decisions about a specific aspect of a patient's care. The difficulty with relying on these is that memory can be faulty or limited, reference textbooks often do not contain the latest treatment protocols, journals are too numerous and too detailed, and colleagues are often unreliable. Clearly, a better method is needed. This is where EHTs can play an important role. EHTs are capable of providing the knowledge to support the provider in the decision-making process. EHTs should seamlessly supplement the information requirements of the health care provider in a timely, context-specific manner. In addition, EHTs should be capable of reusing data entered in the health record to drive context-specific care. To facilitate this capability EHTs need to take into account the clinical workflow, the ability to capture structured and codified data from all aspects of documentation, and the ability to collate and reuse data once they are stored in the electronic record.

Information captured through structured, codified data facilitates the ability to deliver context-specific information at the point of care, including links to guidelines or protocols, clinical decision support, performance measurement, the measurement of individual patient, and population management.

The factors essential for context-specific information retrieval are discussed below and an example of each is provided. For each of the examples the context is indicated by **bold** text and the resultant information and action based on the context is indicated by <u>underlined</u> text:

(a) **Who requires the information**? EHTs should understand that information needs of users might vary. Within the clinical context the EHT should anticipate the needs of a medical student, resident, or specialist.

Example 1

Dr. Jones, an **oncologist**, is reviewing Mrs. Black's electronic medical record. Mrs. Black, a **40 year old female with leukemia, has failed standard treatment**. As he prepares to update the treatment section of her record, he sees <u>an alert entitled "Treatment Options"</u>. As he opens the alert, he sees <u>a list of treatment studies, a list of published references about failed leukemia treatment, and finally a number of experimental treatment protocols that are available</u> for Mrs. Black, including <u>a clinical trial</u> for patients who have already received and failed standard therapy.

Dr. Jones reviews the various recommended treatment options and determines the best options for Mrs. Black. On Mrs. Black's arrival, Dr. Jones reviews the treatment options with her.

In this example, the doctor has access to a clinical decision support tool that tracts treatment protocols.

(b) **What does the user want**? Context-specific information needs will vary from one user to the next. A medical student might need information to help him learn a topic whereas a specialist might need cutting edge information to help manage a difficult patient. A nurse's needs might be different from those of a physician.

Example 2

Mr. Smith is a **50 year old diabetic**, who was just **admitted to the hospital** for **treatment of a leg ulcer**. Nurse White starts to review Mr. Smith's record, including the treatment sections, where she sees the <u>clinical protocol for diabetic leg ulcers</u>. There are a number of <u>standing orders</u> relevant to Mr. Smith's care including <u>wound cultures, blood tests, etc</u>.

In this example, the nurse has access to an electronic clinical protocol, which will guide how she cares for the patient.

(c) **Who does the user need information about**? Health needs about individuals vary. The context-specific information needs about a 50 year old woman is different from that of a 20 year old woman. Specifically, context-specific needs will vary based on the socio-economic status, ethnicity, age, or gender of the patient.

Example 3

Dr. Jackson, **a dentist**, is meeting with **a new patient** Mr. Brown who **has diabetes, and hypertension**, both of which are **apparently well-controlled**. As Dr. Jackson reviews Mr. Brown's electronic record, she notices the clinical data available from his previous providers. She notices, based on his record, that Mr. Brown is overdue for a routine dental prophylaxis. In addition, Dr. Jackson notices that recently Mr. Brown's **blood glucose readings** on his home monitor are **higher than usual**. Dr. Jackson suspects, based on Mr. Brown's signs and symptoms that he <u>has gingivitis</u>, which she <u>confirms on examination</u>.

In this example, the user has all the relevant information to make critical decisions relevant to the patient's condition.

(d) **Where is the user when he has the information needed**? The needs of the user in the emergency room will differ from the user in the ambulatory center.

Example 4

Mrs. Anderson is in the **emergency room** complaining of **shortness of breath and mild indigestion. She is 45**, and **slightly overweight. The emergency room physician** taking care of her pulls up her ambulatory healthcare record. He notes that apart from **mild heartburn and smoking** Mrs. Anderson has no other history. The ER physician enters his clinical findings into Mrs. Anderson's record and as he begins to enter her diagnosis, he reviews a list of potential diagnoses. As he reviews this list, he notices that one of the potential diagnoses is a heart attack. He quickly orders a blood test that confirms that Mrs. Anderson is having a heart problem and she is admitted. Afterwards, he reviews the recommendation and learns that women with a cardiac problem usually present with atypical symptoms when compared to men.

In this example, the system takes into context the user and the location and determines the appropriate potential diagnoses.

To date, current systems are not capable of using context-specific information to drive workflow. However, developers and researchers are beginning to add intelligent electronic health technology incrementally.

11.7.3 Usability

The usability of an interface is of critical importance for the accurate use of any application. Healthcare technologies have their own specific set of usability issues. A good user interface (UI) enhances the users' experience. It is well known that user satisfaction with an application is often driven by the friendliness and intuitiveness of the UI. Measurable benefits that stem from a good UI include workflow efficiency and data accuracy. Logically, the effects of a bad UI are the opposite of the good UI, namely, user dissatisfaction, workflow inefficiency, and data inaccuracies. Users typically will not interact with applications with non-intuitive interfaces.

A bad UI may even be dangerous. Poor usability has the potential to introduce a set of errors that affect the patient's health. Issues include selecting incorrect medications from a pick list, ordering the incorrect dose of a medication, etc. (Horsky et al. 2005; Koppel et al. 2005). Because of the possibility of a disastrous error caused by the UI, there is a need to study formally the user interface of EHTs to determine how they affect the clinical workflow and more importantly how they influence care. Ultimately, there is a need to develop standardized user interfaces that have been proven to mitigate the risk for errors attributable to the UI (Armijo et al. 2009).

Example 5

Dr. Bailey is a busy dentist. He pulls up his patient's electronic medical record, and notices that that his patient, James, is a 5 year old male, weighing 50 lbs. who is complaining of a toothache. After his examination Dr. Bailey concludes that James has an early dental infection and using his electronic prescribing system decides to prescribe Augmentin. As he enters the order, Dr. Bailey scrolls through the drop-down menu of all antibiotics including many variants of Augmentin. There is no context associated with the list of Augmentin so Dr. Bailey selects the first antibiotic on the list and sends the prescription electronically to the pharmacy. At the pharmacy, when James' mother goes to pick up the prescription the pharmacist is concerned. The pharmacist confirms that the prescription is for a child and calls the doctor's office. It seems that in his haste, Dr. Bailey selected the incorrect medication strength.

In this example, the design of the user interface results in an error on the part of the user.

With EHTs, it is now possible to present a large volume of information all at the same time. This places an additional cognitive burden on the user to determine what is relevant, or worse to ignore information that is irrelevant and potentially harmful. If EHTs are to be successful, they need to present information to the user in such a manner as to minimize the cognitive burden on the user.

Example 6

Dr. Hendricks examines Mrs. Boxer and diagnoses a dental abscess. Dr. Hendricks determines that the best course of action is to incision and drain the abscess. Prior to the procedure, he reviews Mrs. Boxer's electronic record and notes her list of active medical conditions and her history of mitral valve prolapse. He reviews the list of past medical conditions and determines that he can proceed with the procedure. Just prior to the incision and drainage, the patient, seeing the scalpel in Dr. Hendricks' hand tells the doctor that she developed a heart infection after a previous surgery. Dr. Hendricks stops and reviews every part of Mrs. Boxer's electronic record. After some time, Dr. Hendricks finds the relevant information in the medical summaries. The medical summary in question was in a folder buried in the electronic record with 20 other summaries and the contents were not indexed for search.

In this example, the user is forced to review the entire document in the medical record to find the relevant information. There is not a simple method available to facilitate retrieval of all the relevant information.

The design of an EHT can contribute to user error. All information stored in an EHT should be indexed, catalogued, and searchable. EHTs that require the user to search consistently and proactively all components of the EHT to find all relevant information will lead to potentially life-threatening errors. Obscure data buried within an EHT can lead to the user not having all the relevant information readily available. However, giving the user a simple method of searching all the content in the EHT ensures that he finds the relevant information.

Ultimately, usability is a critical component of EHTs. It is not sufficient for healthcare providers to have technologies in their offices for documentation, it is imperative that these technologies take into consideration how healthcare providers process information and how they look for information. In addition, these technologies should have failsafe mechanisms to prevent errors of omission and commission.

To encourage the development of safe EHTs there needs to be a better understanding of the technologies, how these can lead to user errors and how such errors can be mitigated. There is a need for studies to identify the best practices with respect to the development of the user interface of EHTs. The results of these studies should be codified as recommendations and guidelines that all EHT are required to adhere to in order to minimize the likelihood of errors.

11.7.4 The Totality of the Data

The success or failure of EHTs will depend on the totality of the data available to the healthcare provider. Clinical decisions are driven by the availability of data at the point of care. Data are generated each time a patient interacts with the healthcare system and even today, as we transition to EHTs, the data are still siloed and often not accessible across the healthcare system. For the healthcare system to be effective, data available electronically in one system should be available to other systems. The test result for a patient should be available to all of the treating healthcare providers (with the appropriate authority and consent) and not just the ordering physician. Essentially all available data should be accessible to the healthcare provider at the time of decision-making.

The aggregation of a patient's data from multiple disparate sources is crucial. Whether forming a centralized database or using a record locator system to find the patient records on distributed systems, it is critical that at the time the healthcare provider needs to make a decision about a patient, he can view all the data available for that patient.

Example 7
Mr. Brown pays a visit to Dr. Smith for the first time. He has a Personal Health Record which supports codified data. Before he arrived at the office, Mr. Brown was able to download a copy of his records and send a structured copy to the doctor's office so that the data can be imported into the Dr. Smith's medical record. In the office, Dr. Smith reviews and accepts the data from Mr. Brown's PHR. Based on this new information Dr. Smith receives an alert that shows deficits in Mr. Brown's care including persistent hypertension and elevated blood glucose. In addition, Dr. Brown sees a list of best practices for Mr. Smith many with which have been complied. For those measures and alerts that have not been complied with Dr. Smith has the ability to order the necessary tests and/or medications.

In this example, the completeness of the data from the PHR enabled Dr. Smith to provide very personalized care.

Example 8
Mrs. Jones is in the dentist's office for a toothache. As Dr. Roberts asks her about her medical history, Mrs. Jones knows that she has a low blood count but she cannot remember how low. Fortunately, Dr. Roberts has an electronic dental record, which is connected to a health information network that receives data from other healthcare providers, laboratories, and pharmacies. As he does a quick check of her laboratory records, he realizes that she has a very low platelet count that could potentially lead to life-threatening bleeding if he attempts an invasive procedure in the office.

In this example, the critical piece of data was available only because the dentist had access to the medical lab tests from another provider.

11.8 Electronic Decision Support in Medicine and Dentistry

11.8.1 Medicine and Dentistry: Differences in Electronic Decision Support

One of the constant themes throughout this book is the idea that systemic health and oral health are connected and that despite the historical separation of medicine and dentistry, both professions can benefit from increased use of health IT and informatics. In some cases, the designs and developments that influence medicine are equally applicable to dentistry, like an enterprise master patient index. Unfortunately, electronic clinical decision support (CDS) has developed differently for medicine and dentistry. In this chapter, we examine how this occurred, review some of the differences, speculate on why CDS is less robust in dentistry, and explore ways to improve CDS in dentistry.

11.8.2 Historical Drivers of CDS Divergence

In the early days of health IT, computer technology was limited only to large medical institutions that could afford computer technology. The cost of the hardware, software, maintenance and support were distributed across a large number of providers, administrators, etc. In contrast, dentists usually worked in small solo or group practice and in isolation from other dentists. The same cost for health IT was born by a much smaller number of people. Thus, it is not surprising the dentists were unable to incorporate computer technology early. The one dental institution that could afford health IT was a dental school. However, these entities saw little or no benefit in acquiring computer technology, nor did they have the manpower to develop such systems.

11.8.3 Clinical Drivers of CDS Divergence

CDS systems in medicine, especially in hospitals, thrive on the integration with the electronic patient record. The CDS process takes into consideration all the patient data already in the system and produces warnings, alerts, and other automatic analysis.

Some of the early seminal works on medical CDS include:

- Musen et al. (Shortliffe 2001) described several classic examples of CDS systems in medicine. Musen mentioned that although early prototypes were developed in the sixties, full fledged applications did not start appearing until a decade later.
- The Leeds Abdominal Pain System developed by F.T. deDombal, using Bayes theorem, was developed to help in the identification of acute abdominal pain including appendicitis, diverticulitis, perforated ulcer, etc. The Leeds system (Shortliffe 2001), used sensitivity, specificity, and disease prevalence data of signs and symptoms to calculate the probability of the possible explanations.
- In 1976, Shortliffe and colleagues developed MYCIN which focused on the management of patients with infection through the prescription of antibiotics. MYCIN used as knowledge a set of production rules commonly used in the field of artificial intelligence.
- Years later, in 1985, a system devoted to the identification of possible diagnoses was developed by Randy Miller and colleagues at the University of Pittsburgh.

They developed the Quick Medical Reference (QMR) (Bankowitz et al. 1989). QMR represented medical knowledge by using "disease profiles," which in turn were a synthesis of information collected "from review of the published literature and expert opinion. Disease profiles consisted of a list of all history, physical, and laboratory data reported to occur in the given disease." As well, each finding would have a sensitivity level and a positive predictive value.

Although these and other systems were not fully adopted, they provided the foundation under which current expert systems work in hospitals.

In dentistry, White (1996) and more recently Mendonca (2004) conducted a review of the state of CDS in dentistry which, like medical CDS, has been available for several years (Walker 1967). These systems can be found in subspecialties such as dental emergencies, orofacial pain, oral medicine, oral radiology, orthodontics, pulpal diagnosis, and removable prosthodontics. Examples include:

- The Diagnostic Aid Resource Tool (DART) for oral medicine. This software contains a diagnostic module which through a "statistical data-base manager" retrieves diseases matching the possible patient diagnoses.
- ORAD (White 1989) provides decision support in the interpretation of radiographic lesions. ORAD requests information through 16 questions which then are analyzed using Bayesian methods. ORAD is capable of diagnosing up to 140 possible diseases and is currently available on the Internet.
- Invisalign provides decision support with orthodontic cephalometric analyses and treatment planning procedures (Melkos 2005). Currently it is possibly the most commonly used decision support system in dentistry.
- OralCDx (Sciubba 1999) assists in the identification of precancerous lesions using oral brush biopsies. OralCDx utilizes a neural network-based image processing system to detect oral epithelium cancerous or precancerous cells.
- Both Invisalign and OralCDx, provide decision support over the distance and operate more like a lab test than the traditional decision support.

In medicine, the driving force behind CDS has been the challenge of dealing with uncertainty when diagnosing disease and delivering treatment. The diagnostic space in medicine requires physicians to consider a large number of possibilities. Further, in medicine, diagnosis is a very important and distinct process. A diagnostic session includes the selection of diagnostic procedures followed by an interpretation of the results. Thus, the medical profession has invested more resources in creating tools that would assist in reducing uncertainty. Decision support includes finding diagnoses, reminders for prevention, disease management, and drug dosing and prescribing (Garg et al. 2005) among many others such as adherence to guidelines (Mickan et al. 2014).

In dentistry decision-making is intrinsically linked to the definition of a diagnosis-treatment complex. Uncertainty is not as strong a component of the diagnostic reasoning as in medicine. For example, the diagnosis of common dental problems (caries, missing teeth, periodontal problems) is a simple determination of present or not. Most of the diagnostic information usually is obtained at initial examination through direct observation or using immediate, at hand, methodologies. Emphasis on treatment instead of diagnosis is enforced by the fact that dentists are not reimbursed for diagnoses. They are paid for treatment. Further, in order to obtain third party payments, a diagnosis is not a necessary element of the paperwork, only the treatment. Hence dentists are trained to focus more on treatment planning than on diagnosis in dental school.

11.8.4 Why Electronic Decision Support Is Less Common in Dentistry than in Medicine?

There are several reasons why this seems to be the case. In this section, we focus in three possible explanations of why CDS is less common in dentistry.

11.8.5 Our Level of Understanding of the Way We Diagnose Patients

Since the 1950s, there have been several efforts in medicine to define and formalize the underlying cognitive processes occurring when humans search and identify diagnosis. Ledley and Lusted (1959) dissected how physicians use "complex reasoning" and provided systematization to the intangible processes that occur in the physician's mind. Ledley et al. introduced the mathematical concepts of symbolic logic; probability and value theory which have helped us operationalize diagnostic reasoning. Subsequent efforts in medicine built on this key paper and created a large array of decision support tools from as early as the sixties (Warner et al. 1964). Thus, the amount of effort invested by the medical profession in understanding these processes is far larger than in dentistry. There are divisions in medical schools, professional associations, and dedicated journals in the area medical decision-making that contrast with the lack of the same in dentistry.

In dentistry, several efforts have been made to understand the way dentists reach diagnoses especially for caries (Crespo et al. 2004; Bader and Shugars 1997a). However, our understanding is limited since diagnostic information is not routinely recorded in dental records (Bader and Shugars 1997b). Both groups identified that dentists use cognitive structures called "illness scripts" and that "these scripts develop from continuous exposure to patients." Bader points out; dentists follow a pattern recognition process that is inextricably linked to treatment decisions instead of a pure diagnostic approach.

11.8.6 Application Areas

Physicians have to deal with significant uncertainty and sometimes pursue treatment without a clear diagnosis (Sox 1988). Physicians define a preliminary diagnosis and initiate treatment expecting a specific response in order to define subsequent actions, while taking into consideration incoming additional diagnostic information. Physicians also have to decide between a large array of diagnostic tests that vary in terms of availability and cost but also risk and specificity. Thus, medicine can greatly benefit from the use of decision support tools that ameliorate uncertainty at the diagnostic level.

On the other hand, Abbey observes, "the dentist is often more challenged by deriving the treatment plan than by deciphering the diagnosis" (Weed 1991). Abbey continues by saying that in medicine the varieties in clinical presentation of systemic diseases with "superimposed signs and symptoms" require physicians to select a different array of diagnostic aids that subsequently help in reaching a diagnosis. In dentistry, the possible signs and symptoms are confined to the head and neck region. Additionally, dentists routinely use a limited number of diagnostic aids compared to medicine (although new dental diagnostic aids have appeared in recent years). "Dental radiography is mostly morphological rather than quantitative," Abbey continues. Also, dentists rely heavily on personal capabilities including his/her senses and information obtained directly from patients. Use of laboratory data is limited.

11.8.7 The Way Knowledge Is Represented and the Inference Mechanisms

According to both White and Mendonça, several knowledge representation mechanisms include algorithmic systems that use "logical classification methods." One advantage of these systems is that they do not require large datasets. However, they lack flexibility and if a change needs to be made these systems would struggle to meet this requirement. Usually well-understood diagnostic processes would fit this category well; in the case of dentistry, we have examples of decision support systems that use this principle in oral pathology (Rudin 1994). In the case of statistical systems, ORAD is a classical example where, using a Bayesian method, it analyses the responses from 16 questions and provides a diagnosis from 140 possible lesions. In the area of rule-based systems in dentistry, we found a system called RHINOS which provides differential diagnoses for headache and facial pain. Finally, there is a dental system that uses neural networks for the prediction of the location and relationships between past and present dental conditions (Okuda et al. 1997).

As we have shown, the application of different inference mechanisms is common in dentistry. However, most of these systems usually appear as prototypes in academic units and are not present in dental offices. The inability to migrate CDS to the dental office is for one or more of the following reasons:

- Traditional dental practice, on a day to day basis, does not require CDS (the clinician is good enough to make satisfactory decisions);
- There are no external factors that would increase the need for better decision making, for example evaluation of treatment quality or the necessity of always present treatment alternatives;
- The status quo of computer technology prevents the implementation of CDS and
- A combination of some or all of these.

11.8.8 What Needs To Be Done in Order to Increase the Adoption of Electronic Decision Support in Dentistry?

Current dental software lacks the proper human interface that could facilitate an easy integration in regular dental practice. This problem needs to be solved before any subsequent steps can be taken into incorporating other functionality such as CDS into dental practice. As mentioned before, current successful decision support systems are not necessarily integrated within the software in use in offices. Preliminary studies point toward that direction (Thyvalikakath, personal communication). Additionally other areas needing further study are:

11.8.9 Health and the Use of Diagnostic Information

The profession needs to step toward an "oral physician" model, moving away from being "denturists" (a focus on diagnosis and science rather than dental procedures) and being more involved in the systemic aspects of patient health. Population age is projected to increase and thus the longevity of our patients. As a direct consequence of an aging population, chronic diseases are going to be more common, thus, dental practitioners should be able to proactively deal with patients with complex medical histories. For example, a dentist as an oral physician can increase their role as early detectors of patients' systemic problems and intervening in modifying health related habits.

11.8.10 Education

Dental education programs should incorporate the concept of using informatics tools to facilitate the diagnosis and treatment planning. Currently, dental education does not consider the use of information technology to facilitate these steps in clinical practice.

11.8.11 Justification

Developers should correctly identify the needs of dentists and justify the implementation of CDS. We should avoid the approach of having a hammer looking for a nail as has been common amongst our medical counterparts. As described before, there are intrinsic differences between medicine and dentistry, thus developers need to identify where decision support would maximize the effectiveness of the practicing dental professional. Proponents of higher accountability, guidelines, and evidence based practice would agree that decision support could foster these areas in dentistry; however, it is important to identify what are the specific areas in which dentistry would really benefit from the tool. Furthermore, we need to also formally provide evidence of their effectiveness (Oosterkamp et al. 2016).

11.8.12 Workflow

A key element in decision support is the ability of systems to provide the information when it is needed and that it does not interrupt other critical or more important activities. It is necessary to understand the dental office as a healthcare delivery system and not as a "one-size fits all" customer when developing software applications.

11.8.13 Mobility and Flexibility

With the advent of mobile computing (tablets, smartphones, watches, and other mobile delivery technologies) we are seeing an uptake in the implementation of direct and indirect decision support. Taking a phone out of one's pocket and looking up a medication is a tangible and valid way to improve the clinician's decision making. Formal analyses demonstrate that such flexibility will be a great differentiator in CDS adoption (Mickan et al. 2013, 2014).

11.8.14 Professional Environment and Interactions with the Rest of the Health Care Delivery System

The complexity of certain medical treatments will increase in the middle term because of advancements in other areas, such as genetics. This will require dentists to interact in new ways with fellow healthcare professionals thus creating a need to join a multidisciplinary health delivery system. The dentist will have to coordinate his/her actions at new levels of complexity. Additionally, evidence-based dentistry, quality, pay per performance, and other elements that are common in the other areas of health care will start influencing the way we interact with patients, thus will be necessary the implementation of decision support tools.

Regardless, both dentists and physicians will continue to see the emergence of decision support tools. Fortunately, increasingly we will be able to assess the outcomes resulting from the use of CDS (Garg et al. 2005). As evidence of their beneficial effects and best practices implementation becomes widespread (Varghese et al. 2018), we then must plan clinical environments were CDS will be the norm and not the exception.

Disclaimer The views presented in this chapter are solely of the authors and do not necessarily represent the views of the US Government, Department of Health and Human Services and/or the Centers for Disease Control and Prevention.

References

Physicians' Dental Data Needs and Oral Healthcare Providers' Medical Data Needs: The Clinical Rationale

Leikauf J, Federman AD. Comparisons of self-reported and chart-identified chronic diseases in inner-city seniors. J Am Geriatr Soc. 2009;57(7):1219–25. Epub 2009 May 21

Pakhomov SV, Jacobsen SJ, Chute CG, Roger VL. Agreement between patient-reported symptoms and their documentation in the medical record. Am J Manag Care. 2008;14(8):530–9.

Standardized/Structured Messages Facilitate Efficient Information Sharing and Benefit Patient Care

ACC/AHA. Performance measures for adults with ST-elevation and non-ST-elevation myocardial infarction. A report of the American College of Cardiology/American Heart Association task force on performance measures (writing committee to develop performance measures for ST-elevation and non-ST-elevation myocardial infarction). Circulation. 2008;118:2596–648.

American Diabetes Association. Standards of medical care in diabetes – 2011. Diabetes Care. 2011;34(Suppl 1):S11–61.

Baddour Larry M, Bettmann Michael A, Bolger Ann F, et al. Nonvalvular cardiovascular device-related infections AHA scientific statement—2003. Circulation. 2003;108:2015.

Baddour Larry M, Epstein Andrew E, Erickson Christopher C, et al. Update on cardiovascular implantable electronic device infections and their management a scientific statement from the American Heart Association 2010, endorsed by the Heart Rhythm Society. Circulation. 2010;121:458–77.

Bonow RO, Carabello BA, Kanu C, et al. ACC/AHA 2006 guidelines for the management of patients with valvular heart disease: a report of the American College of Cardiology/American Heart Association task force on practice guidelines (writing committee to revise the 1998 guidelines for the management of patients with valvular heart disease): developed in collaboration with the society of cardiovascular anesthesiologists: endorsed by the society for cardiovascular angiography and interventions and the society of thoracic surgeons. Circulation. 2006;114(5):e84–231.

Dajani AS, Taubert KA, Wilson W, et al. Prevention of bacterial endocarditis. Recommendations by the American Heart Association. Circulation. 1997;96(1):358–66.

Douketis JD, Berger PB, Dunn AS, et al. The perioperative management of antithrombotic therapy: American college of chest physicians evidence-based clinical practice guidelines (8th edition). Chest. 2008;133(6 Suppl):299S–339.

Eckardt KU, Berns JS, Rocco MV, Kasiske BL. Definition and classification of CKD: the debate should be about patient prognosis—a position statement from KDOQI and KDIGO. Am J Kidney Dis. 2009;53(6):915–20.

Field MJ, Lohr KN, editors. Clinical practice guidelines: directions for a new program, institute of medicine. Washington, DC: National Academy Press; 1990. p. 38.

Fleisher LA, Beckman JA, Brown KA, et al. ACC/AHA 2007 guidelines on perioperative cardiovascular evaluation and care for noncardiac surgery: a report of the American College of

Cardiology/American Heart Association task force on practice guidelines (writing committee to revise the 2002 guidelines on perioperative cardiovascular evaluation for noncardiac surgery) developed in collaboration with the American society of echocardiography, American Society of Nuclear Cardiology, Heart Rhythm Society, Society of Cardiovascular Anesthesiologists, Society for Cardiovascular Angiography and Interventions, Society for Vascular Medicine and Biology, and Society for Vascular Surgery. J Am Coll Cardiol. 2007a;50(17):e159–241.

Geist SM, Geist JR. Improvement in medical consultation responses with a structured request form. J Dent Educ. 2008a;72(5):553–61.

Grines CL, Bonow RO, Casey DE Jr, et al. Prevention of premature discontinuation of dual antiplatelet therapy in patients with coronary artery stents: a science advisory from the American Heart Association, American College of Cardiology, Society for cardiovascular angiography and interventions, American College of Surgeons, and American Dental Association, with representation from the American College of Physicians. Circulation. 2007;115(6):813–8.

Kidney Disease Outcome Quality Initiative. K/DOQI clinical practice guidelines for chronic kidney disease: evaluation, classification, and stratification. Am J Kidney Dis. 2002;39:S1–246.

Lenfant C, Chobanian AV, Jones DW, et al. Seventh report of the joint national committee on the prevention, detection, evaluation, and treatment of high blood pressure (JNC 7): resetting the hypertension sails. Hypertension. 2003;41(6):1178–9.

Lessard E, Glick M, Ahmed S, Saric M. The patient with a heart murmur: evaluation, assessment and dental considerations. J Am Dent Assoc. 2005;136:347–56.

Levey AS, Eckardt KU, Tsukamoto Y, et al. Definition and classification of chronic kidney disease: a position statement from kidney disease: improving global outcomes (KDIGO). Kidney Int. 2005;67:2089–100.

Levey AS, de Jong PE, Coresh J, et al. The definition, classification and prognosis of chronic kidney disease: a KDIGO controversies conference report. Kidney Int. 2011;80(1):17–28.

Moser M. Historical perspectives on the management of hypertension. J Clin Hypertens. 2006;8(8 Suppl 2):15–20.

National Cancer Institute. Oral complications of chemotherapy and head/neck radiation PDQ. Bethesda: National Institutes of Health; 2010. Available at: http://www.cancer.gov/cancertopics/pdq/supportivecare/oralcomplications/HealthProfessional. Accessed 10 June 2018

National Cancer Institute. PDQ® oral complications of chemotherapy and head/neck radiation. Bethesda: National Cancer Institute; 2011. http://cancer.gov/cancertopics/pdq/supportivecare/oralcomplications/HealthProfessional. Accessed 8 May 2011

O'Malley AS, Reschovsky JD. Referral and consultation communication between primary care and specialist physicians. Arch Intern Med. 2011a;171(1):56–65.

Peterson P, Hayes TE, Arkin CF, et al. The preoperative bleeding time test lacks clinical benefit: College of American Pathologists' and American Society of Clinical Pathologists' position article. Arch Surg. 1998;133(2):134–9.

Wann LS, Curtis AB, Ellenbogen KA, et al. ACCF/AHA/HRS focused update on the management of patients with atrial fibrillation (update on dabigatran): a report of the American College of Cardiology Foundation/American Heart Association task force on practice guidelines. J Am Coll Cardiol. 2011;57(11):1330–7. Epub 2011 Feb 14

Wilson W, Taubert KA, Gewitz M, et al. Prevention of infective endocarditis: guidelines from the American Heart Association. Circulation. 2007a;116(15):1736–54.

Designing and Implementing Efficient Structured Communication Among a Patient's Medical and Dental Providers

Chen AH, Yee HF Jr. Improving primary care-specialty care communication: lessons from San Francisco's safety net: comment on "referral and consultation communication between primary care and specialist physicians". Arch Intern Med. 2011;171(1):65–7.

Fleisher LA, Beckman JA, Brown KA, et al. ACC/AHA 2007 guidelines on perioperative cardiovascular evaluation and care for noncardiac surgery: a report of the American College of Cardiology/American Heart Association task force on practice guidelines (writing committee to revise the 2002 guidelines on perioperative cardiovascular evaluation for noncardiac surgery) developed in collaboration with the American society of echocardiography, American Society of Nuclear Cardiology, Heart Rhythm Society, Society of Cardiovascular Anesthesiologists, Society for Cardiovascular Angiography and Interventions, Society for Vascular Medicine and Biology, and Society for Vascular Surgery. J Am Coll Cardiol. 2007b;50(17):e159–241.

Geist SM, Geist JR. Improvement in medical consultation responses with a structured request form. J Dent Educ. 2008b;72(5):553–61.

O'Malley AS, Reschovsky JD. Referral and consultation communication between primary care and specialist physicians. Arch Intern Med. 2011b;171(1):56–65.

Stoves J, Connolly J, Cheung CK, et al. Electronic consultation as an alternative to hospital referral for patients with chronic kidney disease: a novel application for networked electronic health records to improve the accessibility and efficiency of healthcare. Qual Saf Health Care. 2010;19(5):e54.

Wilson W, Taubert KA, Gewitz M, et al. Prevention of infective endocarditis: guidelines from the American Heart Association. Circulation. 2007b;116(15):1736–54.

Towards an Integrated Electronic Health (EHR) System: Compliance, Security and Privacy Concerns

Austin A, Smith B, Williams L. Towards improved security criteria for certification of electronic health record systems. In Proceedings of SEHC'10, Cape Town; 3–4 May 2010.

Baumer DL, Earp JB, Payton FC. Privacy of medical records: IT implications of HIPAA. ACM Comput Soc. 2000;30(4):40–7.

Benaloh J, Chase M, Horvitz E, Lauter K. Patient controlled encryption: ensuring privacy of electronic medical records. CCSW'09. Chicago, 13 Nov 2009.

Brown B. Improving the privacy and security of personal health records. J Health Care Compliance. 2009;11(2):39–40. 68

Cannoy S, Salam A. A framework for healthcare information assurance policy and compliance. Commun ACM. 2010;53(3):126–31.

Choi Y, Caption K, Krause J, Streeper M. Challenges associated with privacy in health care industry: implementation of HIPAA and the security rules. J Med Syst. 2006;30(1):57–64.

Dimitropoulos L, Rizk S. A state-based approach to privacy and security for interoperable health information exchange. Health Aff (Millwood). 2009;28(2):428–34.

Goldschmidt PG. HIT and MIS: implications of health information technology and medical information systems. Commun ACM. 2005;48(10):69–74.

Groen P, Powell VJH. Electronic dental records (EDR): 'open source' and commercial-off-the shelf (COTS) solutions. Virtual Medical Worlds. 2010. http://www.hoise.com/vmw/10/articles/vmw/LV-VM-08-10-5.html. 23 Aug 2010.

Huston T. Security issues for implementation of e-medical records. Commun ACM. 2001;44(9) https://doi.org/10.1145/383694.383712.

Jha AK, DesRoches CM, Campbell EG, et al. Use of electronic health records in U.S. hospitals. N Engl J Med. 2009;360:1628–38.

Kurtz G. EMR confidentiality and information security. J Health Inf Manag. 2003;17(3):41–8.

Liu V, May L, Caelli W, Croll P. A sustainable approach to security and privacy in health information systems. In Proceedings of 18th Australasian conference on information systems security & privacy in health IS, Toowoomba, 5–7 Dec 2007.

Mishra S, Chin AG. Assessing the impact of governmental regulations on the IT industry: a neo-institutional theory perspective. In Subramanian R, editor. Computer security privacy politics. 2008:36–53.

Office of the National Coordinator for Health Information Technology. Health IT dashboard. 2018. https://dashboard.healthit.gov/quickstats/quickstats.php. Accessed 16 June 2018.
U.S. Department of Health and Human Services. Nationwide privacy and security framework for electronic exchange of individually identified health information 2008. 2011. www.hhs.gov/healthit/documents/NationwidePS_Framework.pdf. Accessed 23 Feb 2011.
U.S. Department of Health and Human Services. HITECH Act enforcement interim final rule. 2009. http://www.hhs.gov/ocr/privacy/hipaa/administrative/enforcementrule/hitechenforcementifr.html. Accessed 23 Feb 2011.

Matching Patients to Achieve Unique Patient Identification

Blakely T, Salmond C. Probabilistic record linkage and a method to calculate the positive predictive value. Int J Epidemiol. 2002;31(6):1246–52.
Gill L, Goldacre M, Simmons H, et al. Computerised linking of medical records: methodological guidelines. J Epidemiol Community Health. 1993;47(4):316–9.
Liu S. Development of record linkage of hospital discharge data for the study of neonatal readmission. Chronic Dis Can. 1999;20(2):77–81.
Roos LL, Wajda A. Record linkage strategies. Part I: Estimating information and evaluating approaches. Methods Inf Med. 1991;30(2):117–23.
Theis MK, et al. Case study of linking dental and medical healthcare records. Am J Manag Care. 2010;16(2):e51–6.

Improved Electronic Healthcare Technologies (EHT) Through the Harmonization of Application Design and Clinician Needs

Allen M, Currie LM, Graham M, et al. The classification of clinicians' information needs while using a clinical information system. AMIA Annu Symp Proc. 2003;2003:26–30.
Armijo D, McDonnell C, Werner K (2009) Electronic health record usability: interface design considerations. AHRQ Publication No. 09(10)-0091-2-EF. Rockville: Agency for Healthcare Research and Quality.
Covell DG, Uman GC, Manning PR. Information needs in office practice: are they being met? Ann Intern Med. 1985;103(4):596–9.
Horsky J, Kuperman GJ, Patel VL (2005) Comprehensive analysis of a medication dosing error related to CPOE. J Am Med Inform Assoc; 12(4):377–382.
Koppel R, Metlay JP, Cohen A, et al. Role of computerized physician order entry systems in facilitating medication errors. JAMA. 2005;293(10):1197–203.

Electronic Decision Support in Medicine and Dentistry

Bader JD, Shugars DA. What do we know about how dentists make caries-related treatment decisions? Community Dent Oral Epidemiol. 1997a;25(1):97–103.
Bader JD, Shugars DA. A case for diagnoses. J Am Coll Dent. 1997b;64(3):44–6.
Bankowitz RA, et al. A computer-assisted medical diagnostic consultation service. Implementation and prospective evaluation of a prototype. Ann Intern Med. 1989;110(10):824–32.
Crespo KE, Torres JE, Recio ME. Reasoning process characteristics in the diagnostic skills of beginner, competent, and expert dentists. J Dent Educ. 2004;68(12):1235–44.

Garg AX, Adhikari NKJ, McDonald H, et al. Effects of computerized clinical decision support systems on practitioner performance and patient outcomes. A systematic review. JAMA. 2005;293(10):1223–38.

Ledley RS, Lusted LB. Reasoning foundations of medical diagnosis; symbolic logic, probability, and value theory aid our understanding of how physicians reason. Science. 1959;130(3366):9–21.

Melkos AB. Advances in digital technology and orthodontics: a reference to the invisalign method. Med Sci Monit. 2005;11(5):PI39–42.

Mendonca EA. Clinical decision support systems: perspectives in dentistry. J Dent Educ. 2004;68(6):589–97.

Mickan S, Atherton H, Roberts NW, et al. Use of handheld computers in clinical practice: a systematic review. BMC Med Inform Decis Mak. 2014;14:56. https://doi.org/10.1186/1472-6947-14-56.

Mickan S, Tilson JK, Atherton H, et al. Evidence of effectiveness of health care professionals using handheld computers: a scoping review of systematic reviews. Med Internet Res. 2013;15(10):e212. https://doi.org/10.2196/jmir.2530.

Okuda T, Yoshida T, Hotta M (1997) A dental condition prediction system with artificial neural networks and fuzzy inference systems. Orlando: IEEE.

Oosterkamp BC, Wafae A, Schols JG, et al. Effectiveness of a clinical guideline to improve dental health among orthodontically treated patients: study protocol for a cluster randomized controlled trial. Trials. 2016;17(1):201. https://doi.org/10.1186/s13063-016-1325-1.

Rudin JL. DART (diagnostic Aid and resource tool): a computerized clinical decision support system for oral pathology. Compendium. 1994;15(11):1316. 1318, 1320 passim

Sciubba JJ. Improving detection of precancerous and cancerous oral lesions. Computer-assisted analysis of the oral brush biopsy. U.S. Collaborative OralCDx Study Group. J Am Dent Assoc. 1999;130(10):1445–57.

Shortliffe EH. Medical informatics: computer applications in health care and biomedicine. 2nd ed. New York: Springer; 2001. p. xxvii, p. 854

Sox HC. Medical decision making. Boston: Butterworths; 1988. p. 406.

Varghese J, Kleine M, Gessner SI, et al. Effects of computerized decision support system implementations on patient outcomes in inpatient care: a systematic review. J Am Med Inform Assoc. 2018;25(5):593–602. https://doi.org/10.1093/jamia/ocx100.

Walker GF. Cephalometrics and the computer. J Dent Res. 1967;46(6):1211.

Warner HR, Toronto AF, Veasy LG. Experience with Baye's theorem for computer diagnosis of congenital heart disease. Ann N Y Acad Sci. 1964;115:558–67.

Weed LL. Knowledge coupling: new premises and new tools for medical care and education. New York: Springer; 1991. p. xxv, p. 362

White SC. Computer-aided differential diagnosis of oral radiographic lesions. Dentomaxillofac Radiol. 1989;18(2):53–9.

White SC. Decision-support systems in dentistry. J Dent Educ. 1996;60(1):47–63.

Chapter 12
Biosurveillance and Dentistry

Miguel H. Torres-Urquidy

12.1 Dentistry and Modern Public Health Surveillance

The public health environment (like the rest of healthcare) is changing and incorporating digital strategies at the forefront of their responses to public health events and routine public health interventions. The H1N1 pandemic, SARS, Ebola epidemic, and Zika pandemic are recent global events of public health concern (Fineberg 2014; Dixon et al. 2014; Fauci and Morens 2016). In addition, other local crises such as the US opioid epidemic (US Department of Health and Human Services 2017), have reinforced the need to establish bidirectional communications between clinical practices and public health authorities. As a result, organized healthcare has established and adopted protocols to rapidly handle patients and related risks adequately. It is now common in clinical practices to hear the question "have you travelled abroad recently?" or "have you been to places experiencing a public health emergency?" Furthermore, guidance from public health authorities can be seen posted throughout halls or clinical spaces in practices. These messages and warnings are now also part of electronic health records and patients are questioned and treated accordingly. Public health authorities (federal, state, and local) continue to develop strategies to reach both clinicians and the general public and having the capacity to handle electronic health record data is a high priority for all of them.

In the case of surveillance, there are a myriad of mechanisms to collect, distribute, and aggregate information (Groseclose and Buckeridge 2017). In addition, in the US, the public health surveillance effort is highly distributed where, depending on the type of condition, funding stream, and/or regulation, the authority and scope of responsibility of the different public health agencies is spread across geographical boundaries. Furthermore, local, state, and/or federal priorities can modify the way surveillance gets conducted. Whether responding to public health emergencies,

M. H. Torres-Urquidy
Centers for Disease Control and Prevention, Atlanta, GA, USA
e-mail: miguel@forwardthinkingconcepts.org

A. Acharya et al. (eds.), *Integration of Medical and Dental Care and Patient Data*, Health Informatics, https://doi.org/10.1007/978-3-319-98298-4_12

adjusting to local geographic conditions or events (e.g. hurricanes) or new evidence, requires public health surveillance efforts to remain flexible.

Another trend that is important to recognize is how evidence is gathered, synthesized, and made available. Big Data, cloud, and edge (mobile) computing are enabling more organizations to develop their own public health insights (Griebel et al. 2015). Large hospital systems, data consortiums, and public health partnerships are empowering the academic community, health insurance companies, and employers to design and implement their own public health interventions. In summary, population health (Kindig and Stoddart 2003) is steadily solidifying and expanding the number of those who are part of the public health system.

In this chapter, we focus on the response efforts to bioterrorism and, although such a term is less in vogue nowadays, it is a constant element of worry among public health planners. It is also important given that systems and mechanisms put in place to identify, prevent, and respond to such bioterrorism events are likely to be used in many other public health situations. This is not to take away from other traditional public health surveillance approaches and very successful interventions (such as national surveys and water fluoridation), yet in the case of dentistry and biosurveillance, there is plenty of room to grow and integrate.

12.2 Dentistry and Bioterrorism

During March 27 and 28 of 2003, the American Dental Association and the US Public Health Service sponsored the conference "Dentistry's Role in Responding to Bioterrorism and Other Catastrophic Events" (Palmer 2003; National Institute of Dental and Craniofacial Research, 2004). This meeting reviewed several aspects of bioterrorism and the dental profession: the nature of biological pathogens and its oral manifestations, what needed to be communicated, how dentists should participate, etc. Dr. Michael C. Alfano described the difficulties that biological pathogens create for clinicians because "they are so insidious." While discussing the anthrax mailings after September 11th he pointed out that: "… early symptoms appeared so they resembled the aches, fever, and malaise of flu so those affected delayed seeking treatment, a delay that has proven fatal in some cases". Lieutenant Colonel Ross H. Pastel of the US Army Medical Research Institute of Infectious Disease (USAMRIID) listed the "Category A" pathogens as defined by the Centers for Disease Control and Prevention, and those are: smallpox, anthrax, plague, botulinum toxin, tularemia, and viral hemorrhagic fever. He also described an outbreak of smallpox in Yugoslavia in 1972 and the measures that had to be taken to control it. Dr. Michael Glick described the oral manifestations of smallpox showing "signs 24 h before skin rash. These oral signs include tongue swelling, multiple mucosa vesicles, ulceration, and mucosal hemorrhaging. Oral signs are also evident in inhalation and gastro-intestinal anthrax. In oropharyngeal anthrax the mucosa appears edematous and congested; there may be neck swelling, fever, and sore throat".

Dr. Ed Thompson, at the time Deputy Director of the Centers for Disease Control and Prevention, mentioned that "None of the new counter-bioterrorism measures can be effective unless local health practitioners are vigilant in observing and reporting a possible disease outbreak. Such surveillance—knowing what to look for and whom to report to—is critical and applies not only to suspected bioterrorist agents, but to a list of reportable diseases which has grown to include such entities as West Nile virus and Severe Acute Respiratory Syndrome (SARS)." Dr. Sigurs O. Krolls presented the response at the local level and he "stressed the importance of communication and the need for redundant systems", "to keep all the parties informed". He also posed the question "Can dentists recognize signs and systems of contagious diseases?", and emphasized that education is essential. Dr. Louis DePaola made several recommendations that can be key in the scope of this paper by saying "dentists can contribute to bioterrorism surveillance by being alert to clues that might indicate a bioterrorism attack. Such surveillance would note if there is an influx of people seeking medical attention with non-traumatic conditions and flu-like or possibly neurological or paralytic symptoms… or even specific signs of a bioterrorist agent. Patterns of school or work absence, appointment cancellations or failures to appear, could also be indicators." Dr. DePaola made clear that in cases of limited release of bioterrorist agents, dentists "have little to offer" but "a widespread attack can certainly tap into dental professional skills in recognition, isolation and management". In addition, Dr. Guay (Guay 2002) lists all the possible roles in which dentists can participate including "education, risk communication, diagnosis, surveillance and notification, treatment, distribution of medications, decontamination, sample collection and forensic dentistry."

These recommendations provide initial knowledge that can drive the development of integrated health records. It is also important to understand that integration needs to occur within existing technologies such as electronic dental records (EDR), previously called the computer-based oral health record and respective electronic health standards. The final recommendation from the meeting stated that to play an important role in biodefense a serious amount of coordination and preparation will be required, not only from dentists but from other groups, most likely requiring medical and dental data integration.

12.3 The Computer-Based Oral Health Record (COHR) and Computer Ownership

The COHR, as described by Rhodes (1996), "can provide a structure for documentation that goes beyond the concept of a blank form on a page, it includes a glossary of dental terminology for the entire content of the form as well as knowledge bases and expert systems that can enhance the practitioner's diagnostic and treatment planning decisions". He also acknowledges that one of the advantages of this type of documentation is that it "is much more transportable". He also recognizes the need for standardized methods for collecting information from dentists. Schleyer and Eisner (1997) defined several scenarios where the COHR is used in a "shared" environment where several healthcare providers interact and information is seamlessly communicated, improving the decisions made by clinicians. Delrose and Steinberg (2000) discuss how the "Digital Patient Record" enhances clinical practice by providing "better quality information" to the clinician. Although all of these benefits sound promising and encouraging some still express concern about the lack of standards among different information systems, which translates into communication breakdowns (Schleyer 2003). On the other hand, Heid et al. (2002) list all the steps that are currently being taken by different organizations such as the ADA in order to produce a standardized COHR. Other examples of standardization can be found in a paper presented by Narcisi (1996) where ADA's participation as a voting member in the American National Standards Institute has allowed EDI or the COHR to be discussed and improved at a national level, now much commonly known as the Electronic Dental Record or EDR.

Additional influences in the standardization of the EDR are the security regulations mandated by HIPAA, the Health Insurance Portability and Accountability Act of 1996. Dentists are required to "adopt practices necessary for compliance" (Sfikas 2003; Chasteen et al. 2003). These and other regulations (Szekely et al. 1996) will encourage homogeny among different system vendors. Computer ownership, on the other hand, has increased steadily during the last 25 years. According to Schleyer et al. (2003) in 1976 only 1% of dental professionals used computers in their practices compared to 85% in 2000. Additionally, similar trends in Internet connectivity where described. Acharya et al. (2017) reported that chairside Internet utilization increased to 72% in 2017.

12.4 Dentists, Source of Information for Detecting Biosurveillance Events

Given the previous background (levels of adoption/utilization) it is plausible to consider using EDRs as a monitoring source for public health events. Next, we present a blueprint for developing a biosurveillance system.

12.5 Proposed Approach

The purpose of developing an electronic health surveillance system is to gather information from patients directly (Wagner et al. 2006) by detecting signs and/or symptoms, or indirectly by obtaining other types of information such as over-the-counter medication sales, patients' no-shows, usage of Internet search engines, keywords, etc. In this particular case, the proximity of contact between the dentist and the patient is equivalent to a medical inspection in terms of immediacy and/or closeness. Such signs and symptoms can be easily detected if the dentist is properly prompted to search for them. This is just one example of how a system could provide assistance in the detection of a bioterrorism incident.

But, before describing our proposed approach, it would be important to describe the principles behind biosurveillance systems including those such as syndromic surveillance as well as the technical aspects behind them (Tsui et al. 2003). As an example, we describe the Realtime Outbreak Disease Surveillance Laboratory (RODS Lab). RODS Lab uses data obtained directly from chief complaints in the emergency departments of hospitals to construct time series and other forms of aggregated data, to characterize the health status of a specific population. These aggregated data are then assessed by detection algorithms, which can issue alerts in case patterns in the data suggest the emergence of a bioterrorism event.

When implementing such systems, it is important to take into consideration the scale and number of possible contributors. Traditional biosurveillance systems use information collected from hospitals and/or health systems. In the case of large implementations, with dissimilar technologies, careful consideration needs to occur to manage and integrate different kinds of data sources, in our example, EDRs. With this in mind, we proposed a set of elements for creating a biosurveillance system based on EDR data.

The proposed approach should work at multiple levels:

- Communications: The system would have to provide a mechanism to alert the dentist if there is suspicion that a bioterrorist attack may be happening. The mechanism would increase the dentist's awareness in case of finding suspicious signs or symptoms in a patient. This can be triggered by the patient's characteristics such as geographic location of residence, etc.
- Surveillance: Automated collection of information from the patient's EDR. The system would report to a central database, signs or symptoms of interest. The aggregation of this data could generate information that would eventually detect the presence of patterns that may lead to the early detection of such events.
- Reuse of data: Collection of additional information, which combined with other sources, can be useful in terms of detecting or tracing some incident. Patient "no-shows" is the primary example, that, if combined with others such as work or school absenteeism can provide a relevant pattern for public health officials.

12.6 Use Case Example

Dr. X, who practices in a community 20 min away from Capitol City, installed a new clinical management system 2 months ago. Among the features that were included in this new clinical management system (CMS), a bioterrorism detection module was added. She felt curious because of recent news she read in the newspaper about possible attacks against the US and decided to install the feature. She read about how the module would work in combination with the CMS she just bought. The educational information provided with the software instructed Dr. X, that in case a patient victim of a bioterrorism attack happens to be seen in her practice, the software would collect information and would send it to public health officials. When installing the software, Dr. X was asked if she agreed to share such information with public health authorities and she approved.

During the week, a patient walked into Dr. X's dental office. The patient presented some signs that indicated the presence of a disease of unclear origin. An epidemiologic study later would show that the patient was present at a football stadium when an infectious agent was released (Fig. 12.1). Although, at that time his medical history showed no indication of a systemic disease, the presence of multiple *oral vesicles* prompted the dentist to make an annotation into the COHR. The system, by using a natural language processing engine, detected the sign and sent this information to a central database. The patient was discharged and instructed to take some support medication to treat the oral ulcers. The next day, the central database pinpointed the presence of an out of the ordinary increase in the number of cases with the same signs and symptoms around that region. When the presence of this peak was detected, the central server sent a request to the dentist's computer for additional information. One of the requested elements was if there was any use of medication for treating oral ulcers. Fortunately, this information was available. The central database crossed this with the information of other surveillance systems together with the information from other patients that happened to have similar clinical signs and/or symptoms. Dr. X received an email from a public health official asking her to communicate to the local health department to discuss information about one her patients.

The case depicted above simulates the release of smallpox during a football game. In the case of smallpox, oral symptoms include tongue swelling, multiple oral mucosal vesicles, ulceration, and mucosal hemorrhaging (National Institute of

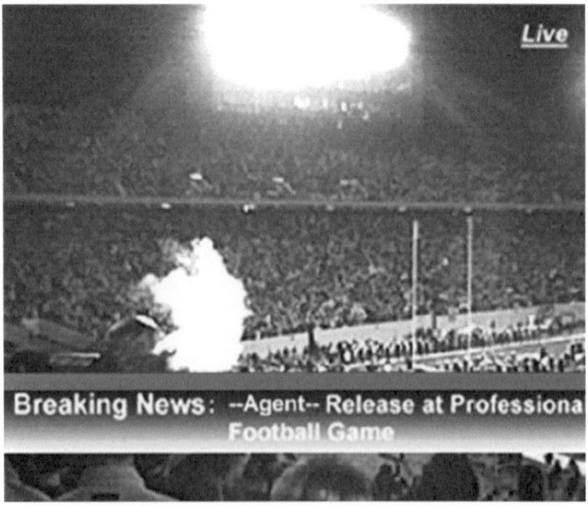

Fig. 12.1 Biosurveillance systems should be cognizant of different kinds of events since this can be linked to issues of public health concern

Dental and Craniofacial Research 2004). Dentists could be alerted by an electronic system to search for such signs or they can be detected automatically. In case of a high incidence within a group of patients, in a confined area, public health officials get to be notified.

In our hypothetical case there are issues that need to be addressed in order to make such a detection system feasible:

12.7 System Design

As described by Schleyer et al. (2006) and Acharya et al. (2017), 85% of dentists in the US use a computer in their practices. Given the current number of dentists in the US, this figure would generate an estimate of 166,000 computers in dental practices, all possibly eligible to be public health surveillance data sources.

Ideally, a biosurveillance system would rely on existing EDRs already implemented by practices. Currently there are many clinical management software packages in the dental market (Toth 2015). It is possible to create modular software that would interact with the practice management system, and allow for "querying" for specific clinical data. Additionally, a natural language processing engine could be embedded into the application in order to detect variations of data input in the EDR. Nevertheless, it is necessary to obtain a detailed list of the oral manifestations of diseases that are likely to be found in patients. Successful implementations of similar systems have been shown to work successfully (Chapman et al. 2001; Ivanov et al. 2002), and using the same approach for our system seems technically feasible.

This collected information later would be sent to a central server in order to be analyzed and interpreted.

12.8 Software Architecture

The components of our system would be as follows (Fig. 12.2):

- Thin client: a software application distributed for data collection. It would be conformed of a "querying" mechanism, combined with a natural language processing engine and a communication module. This software client should be as thin as possible to reduce the workload on the dentist's equipment and should be embedded as a plug-in for current clinical management systems. Vendors should be contacted to ask for their collaboration in the development of such an application to ensure maximum compatibility and integrity of data collection. In case the dentist uses a cloud based EDR, the "client" would collect information from the cloud service and would then resubmit the information to the central server.
- Central servers: server software in charge of integrating all the data collected from dental offices. It has to be capable of handling simultaneous requests from multiple users. This server would integrate all the data and would perform an

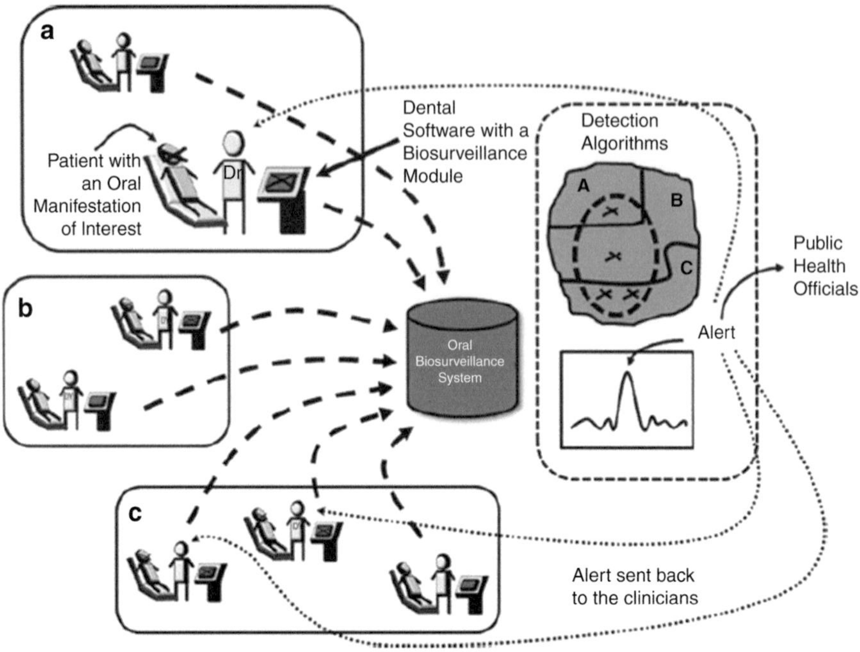

Fig. 12.2 System architecture of a biosurveillance system using information from dental practices

analysis with the intention of detecting anomalies. It would be recommended that redundant servers should be located in different data centers with mirroring capabilities to guarantee their survivability in case of technical difficulties.

- Communication network: the transmission of information should be done using the Internet. This, of course, would essentially depend on the practitioner's current connectivity. If that is not available, backup connection to the central servers should be established.

12.9 Standards

Dentistry uses several standards for transmission of health related information. Clinical management systems use standard-based technology to transmit information (Narcisi 1996; Chasteen et al. 2003; Szekely et al. 1996). As we describe elsewhere in this book, the development, implementation, and use of electronic standards among dentists is on the rise and this can expedite the implementation of a biosurveillance system. The use of standards can also open the opportunity to link EDR systems with other, already existing, public health surveillance systems.

12.10 Security and Redundancy

Information security remains a constant challenge given the constant unveiling of software and hardware vulnerabilities. As a result of this, a maintenance process should be in place to make sure that the components of the surveillance system remain secure and up-to-date. On the server side, redundancy should be provided so downtime is reduced. The system should be developed so mirrored servers are always up and running. Data integrity mechanisms should also be considered as well as other industry best practices.

12.11 Privacy and Confidentiality

Privacy and Confidentiality are important issues that need to be incorporated as part of a robust biosurveillance system and distinct regulations such as HIPAA require protecting patient information (Frist 2002; Chasteen et al. 2003; Bayer and Colgrove 2002; Etzioni 2002; Ivanov et al. 2002). In our use case we described the use of several sources of information for detecting a bioterrorist attack. We described how syndromic information, which initially should be de-identified, is transmitted to a central database. Later, after the suspicion of a bioterrorist attack, more information is requested (medications) and more inferences are made. This, although technically possible, would require allowing for sharing clinical information with public health authorities. This leads to the discussion about "individual rights" vs. "common good". Although HIPAA addresses public health (Gesteland et al. 2003; Lumpkin 2001), some other implications may arise and the health professionals including dentists, physicians, and public health officials, and patients should discuss and address such issues.

Careful consideration has to be given to which information is required to detect a bioterrorist attack, while also keeping in mind that it is always important to reduce, as much as possible, the collection and transmission of patients' information over the Internet or any other network.

12.12 Detection Algorithms and Evaluation

A detection algorithm has to be created or adapted in order to determine the presence of a bioterrorist attack. Some algorithms have proven their effectiveness (Wong et al. 2003) and it is likely that, from these, a new analysis should be done in order to select or create one that addresses the particular needs of our system.

A study was conducted to assess the feasibility of using oral manifestations in order to detect disease outbreaks (Torres-Urquidy et al. 2009). Torres-Urquidy and colleagues found it is feasible to use oral signs and symptoms to create biosurveillance signals. In their study, the most promising signals were those for botulism and smallpox. For data extraction, the investigators used natural language processing followed by the use of statistical methods such as moving average (MA) to serve as part of a detection algorithm.

The system should also be thoroughly evaluated, before and after implementation. Evaluation prior to implementation can be performed using simulated data. Simulation and modeling techniques (Reshetin and Regens 2003) have been used to estimate the effects of a bioterrorist attack. The same techniques can be used to evaluate our system. In the study by Torres-Urquidy et al. (2009), the investigators utilized synthetic outbreaks to test the performance of different signals. From their evaluation process, they learned, for instance, how many cases would be necessary to occur for the system to reach certain detection thresholds.

12.13 Dissemination and Collaboration

Several dental organizations have shown publicly their support of measures to prepare in case of bioterrorism events. The American Dental Association and local dental societies play an important role in disseminating information about the system in coordination with local, state, and federal public health agencies.

12.14 Conclusion

On March 2018, the Journal of the American Dental Association reported on an outbreak of bacterial endocarditis associated with infection control practices at an oral surgery practice (Ross et al. 2018). Their investigation occurred as a result of a clever infectious disease physician noticing the occurrence of two patients with no known risk factors being diagnosed with E. faecalis endocarditis.

Per the investigation conducted by the New Jersey Department of Health (NJDOH), in coordination with the NJ Board of Dentistry, further cases were identified. The NJDOH utilized their NJ Discharge Data Collection System (NJDDCS) to identify the other cases using ICD-9 billing diagnostic codes. This lead to the identification of 15 cases linked to the practice. Due to the time that had passed since the original cases occurred, there was no chance to use molecular sequencing or matching. As a result of the infection, 12 patients underwent surgery and one died. This is an example, where, in the future, biosurveillance systems could play a significant role in identifying real time or near real time increases of cases (or in an expanded geographical area) that compel further investigation. Again, biosurveillance systems could be of benefit, not only in extreme circumstances (like catastrophic man made public health events), but also as part of ongoing public health activities.

As mentioned by Dr. DePaola (National Institute of Dental and Craniofacial Research 2004) dentists may "have little to offer" in specific biosurveillance scenarios, yet the integration of different technologies can change this perception. Goldenberg et al. (2002) described over-the-counter medication sales as a technique for discovering disease outbreaks and stated that their approach may be "more timely" than traditional medical or public health approaches. Medical cases that result from bioterrorism attacks do not produce symptoms until they have fully developed, so it is likely that different patterns can be detected before the patients start reaching the Emergency Department. In the case of dentistry, Torres-Urquidy et al. (2009) established that using oral manifestations may allow for detecting a bioterrorism event up to 24 h prior to other signals using other forms of surveillance.

Public health events, at least at their inception, are intrinsically local events. Dr. Krolls (National Institute of Dental and Craniofacial Research 2004; Munson and Vujicic 2016) in his final remarks during his presentation at the Dentistry's Role Conference Against Bioterrorism, said, "dentists may pick up tell-tale information about what is happening in the community. After all, dentists spend more time with their patients than any other health specialty."

Disclaimer The views presented in this chapter are solely of the authors and do not necessarily represent the views of the US Government, Department of Health and Human Services and/or the Centers for Disease Control and Prevention.

References

Acharya A, Schroeder D, Schwei K, Chyou PH. Update on electronic dental record and clinical computing adoption among dental practices in the United States. Clin Med Res. 2017;15(3-4):59–74. https://doi.org/10.3121/cmr.2017.1380. Epub 11 Dec 2017

Bayer R, Colgrove J. Bioterrorism, public health and the law. Health Aff (Millwood). 2002;21(6):98–101.

Chapman WW, Bridewell W, Hanbury P, et al. Evaluation of negation phrases in narrative clinical reports. Proc AMIA Symp. 2001:105–9.

Chasteen JE, Murphy G, Forrey A, Heid D. The health insurance and portability and accountability act: practice of dentistry in the United States: privacy and confidentiality. J Contemp Dent Pract. 2003;1(4):59–70.

Delrose DC, Steinberg RW. The clinical significance of the digital patient record. J Am Dent Assoc. 2000;131(Suppl):57S–60S.

Dixon MG, Schafer IJ, Centers for Disease Control and Prevention (CDC). Ebola viral disease outbreak—West Africa, 2014. MMWR Morb Mortal Wkly Rep. 2014;63(25):548–51.

Etzioni A. Public health Law: a communitarian perspective. Health Aff. 2002;21(6):102–4.

Fauci AS, Morens DM. Zika virus in the Americas—yet another arbovirus threat. N Engl J Med. 2016;374:601–4.

Fineberg HV. Pandemic preparedness and response—lessons from the H1N1 influenza of 2009. N Engl J Med. 2014;370(14):1335–42. https://doi.org/10.1056/NEJMra1208802.

Frist B. Public health and national security: the critical role of increased federal support. Health Aff. 2002;21(6):117–30.

Gesteland PH, Gardner RM, Tsui FC, et al. Automated syndromic surveillance for the 2002 Winter Olympics. J Am Med Inform Assoc. 2003;10(6):547–54. Epub 4 Aug 2003
Goldenberg A, Shmueli G, Caruana RA, Fienberg SE. Early statistical detection of anthrax outbreaks by tracking over-the-counter medication sales. Proc Natl Acad Sci U S A. 2002;99(8):5237–40.
Griebel L, Prokosch HU, Köpcke F, et al. A scoping review of cloud computing in healthcare. BMC Med Inform Decis Mak. 2015;15:17. https://doi.org/10.1186/s12911-015-0145-7.
Groseclose SL, Buckeridge DL. Public health surveillance systems: recent advances in their use and evaluation. Annu Rev Public Health. 2017;38:57–79. https://doi.org/10.1146/annurev-publhealth-031816-044348.
Guay AH. Dentistry's response to bioterrorism: a report of a consensus workshop. J Am Dent Assoc. 2002;133:1181–7.
Heid DW, Chasteen J, Forrey AW. The electronic oral health record. J Contemp Dent Pract. 2002;1(3):043–54.
Ivanov O, Wagner MM, Chapman WW, Olszewski RT. Accuracy of three classifiers of acute gastrointestinal syndrome for syndromic surveillance. Proc AMIA Symp. 2002:345–9.
Kindig D, Stoddart G. What is population health? Am J Public Health. 2003;*93*(3):380–3.
Lumpkin JR. Air, water, places, and data—public health in the information age. J Public Health Manag Pract. 2001;7(6):22–30.
Munson B, Vujicic M. Number of practicing dentists per capita in the United States will grow steadily. Health Policy Institute. American Dental Association. 2016. http://www.ada.org/~/media/ADA/Science%20and%20Research/HPI/Files/HPIBrief_0616_1.pdf. Accessed 17 June 2018.
Narcisi JP. The American dental association's commitment to electronic data interchange. J Dent Educ. 1996;60(1):28–32.
National Institute of Dental and Craniofacial Research. Dentistry's role in responding to bioterrorism and other catastrophic events. 2004. https://web.archive.org/web/20180104212106/https://www.nidcr.nih.gov/careersandtraining/DentistryCatastrophicEvents.htm. Accessed 17 June 2018.
Palmer C. Dental leaders review roles in bioterrorism response. ADA NEWS. 2003. https://web.archive.org/web/20060219190632/http://www.ada.org/prof/resources/pubs/adanews/adanewsarticle.asp?articleid=390. Accessed 17 June 2018.
Reshetin VP, Regens JL. Simulation modeling of anthrax spore dispersion in a bioterrorism incident. Risk Anal. 2003;23(6):1135–45.
Rhodes PR. The computer-based oral health record. J Dent Educ. 1996;60(1):14–8.
Ross KM, Mehr JS, Greeley RD, et al. Outbreak of bacterial endocarditis associated with an oral surgery practice: New Jersey public health surveillance, 2013 to 2014. J Am Dent Assoc. 2018;149(3):191–201. https://doi.org/10.1016/j.adaj.2017.10.002. Epub 2 Feb 2018
Schleyer TK. Integrating dental office technology—the next frontier. Dent Abstr. 2003;48(3):112–3.
Schleyer T, Eisner J. The computer-based oral health record: an essential tool for cross-provider quality management. J Calif Dent Assoc. 1997;22(11):57–64.
Schleyer TK, Spallek H, Bartling WC, Corby P. The technologically well-equipped dental office. J Am Dent Assoc. 2003;134(1):30–41.
Schleyer TK, Thyvalikakath TP, Spallek H, et al. Clinical computing in general dentistry. J Am Med Inform Assoc. 2006;13(3):344–52.
Sfikas PM. HIPAA security regulations protecting patients' electronic health information. J Am Dent Assoc. 2003;134:640–3.
Szekely DG, Milam S, Khademi JA. Legal issues of the electronic dental record: security and confidentiality. J Dent Educ. 1996;60(1):19–23.
Torres-Urquidy MH, Wallstrom G, Schleyer TK. Detection of disease outbreaks by the use of oral manifestations. J Dent Res. 2009;88(1):89–94.

Toth D. The best practice management software for your office. Dental Products Report. Dec 21. 2015. http://www.dentalproductsreport.com/dental/article/best-practice-management-software-your-office. Accessed 17 June 2018.

Tsui FC, Espino JU, Dato VM, et al. Technical description of RODS: a real-time public health surveillance system. J Am Med Inform Assoc. 2003;10(5):399–408.

US Department of Health and Human Services. HHS acting secretary declares public health emergency to address national opioid crisis. 2017. https://www.hhs.gov/about/news/2017/10/26/hhs-acting-secretary-declares-public-health-emergency-address-national-opioid-crisis.html. Accessed 17 June 2018.

Wagner MM, Moore AW, Aryel RM. Handbook of biosurvellance. Burlington: Elsevier Academic Press; 2006.

Wong WK, Moore A, Cooper G, Wagner M. WSARE: what's strange about recent events? J Urban Health. 2003;80(2 Suppl 1):i66–75.

Chapter 13
Knowledge Standardization, Management, and Integration

Miguel H. Torres-Urquidy, Valerie Powell, Franklin Din, Mark Jurkovich, and Valerie Bertaud-Gounot

13.1 Achieving Interoperability of Medical and Dental Records: Diagnostic Codes for Dentists

Healthcare is foundationally dependent on the use of specialized knowledge and very early, in their formative years, dentists and physicians learn to communicate and, more importantly, think in very specific ways. Given the complexity of the human body, its physiopathology, and the remedies to restore it to a natural state, clinicians had to develop a specific way to communicate. Just like different cultures, whether countries, cities, neighborhoods, or even generations, have developed different ways to describe their intrinsic realities, professions are forced (some more than others) to create their own languages. In the case of professions, this is primarily an outcome of their search for optimization. Conversely, these optimizations have other consequences or byproducts. Learning a new language takes effort, resources, and time. This creates a natural barrier, which separates those in the

M. H. Torres-Urquidy (✉)
Centers for Disease Control and Prevention, Atlanta, GA, USA
e-mail: miguel@forwardthinkingconcepts.org

V. Powell
Robert Morris University, Pittsburgh, PA, USA
e-mail: powell@rmu.edu

F. Din
FraudLens Inc., Arlington, VA, USA
e-mail: frank.din@fraudlens.com

M. Jurkovich
HealthPartners Institute, Minneapolis, MN, USA
e-mail: jurko003@umn.edu

V. Bertaud-Gounot
Psychiatric Hospital of Rennes, Rennes, France
e-mail: valerie.bertaud@univ-rennes1.fr

A. Acharya et al. (eds.), *Integration of Medical and Dental Care and Patient Data*, Health Informatics, https://doi.org/10.1007/978-3-319-98298-4_13

know from those who are not. Over time, other byproducts emerge such as gaining added value for knowing such new language, its proper use and interpretation. Possessing such knowledge and language, coupled with the ability to make proper decisions and implement procedures that restore health, lead to even more tangible added value.

Nonetheless, there is the risk that overspecialization can create unintended consequences. Dentistry and medicine, each with their own proprietary ways to communicate, have evolved into having different conventions and habits. A good example is how dentists do not routinely report diagnoses, whereas physicians not only report but are also reimbursed based on them. The reasons behind such differences have been attributed to cognitive factors (Bader and Shugars 1997; Torres-Urquidy 2012). Yet, such differences remain, although it seems this is starting to change.

The Centers for Medicare and Medicaid Services started requiring dentists to submit diagnostic information for reimbursement in selected states (Arizona, Iowa, Maine, Michigan, Nevada, Vermont) (California Dental Association 2015; Soderlund 2015). This has required procedural changes specific to the adoption of the International Statistical Classification of Diseases and Related Health Problems (International Classification of Diseases, or ICD for short) version 10 (ICD-10). It is anticipated that these changes will bring benefits such as the ability to epidemiologically better track the impact of diseases and, coincidently, the submission of diagnostic codes is related to those conditions that may have possible oral and systemic connections (Lepsky et al. 2015). What goes unsaid, however (Jurkovich 2017; Soderlund 2015), is the possible loss of professional hegemony for dentists (Starr 2017). The future remains uncertain, yet more changes are happening. SNOMED International announced the release of SNOMED CT General Dentistry in January 2018 (SNOMED International 2018). In addition, other diagnostic terminologies have also been widely implemented such as SNODDS (2016), which is an evolution of prior diagnostic terminologies such as SNODENT and the EZ codes (Manchir 2016).

The aforementioned developments are important given that, as we mentioned in the introduction, technological changes do not occur in a vacuum, and understanding what may drive or repulse the adoption of a particular technology is key to enduring change. Again, it remains to be seen what these developments will bring in the way dentists practice dentistry and how they will impact integration of care.

In terms of integration, we can foresee how diagnostic codes, using similar code sets, and aligning how dentists and physicians function, can foster interactions not currently possible. By recording information using a similar knowledge source (ICD-10, SNOMED, etc.) we can more easily make different information systems exchange information, not only between providers but also in much bigger contexts (biomedical research, health insurance, public health, etc.). Of course, there are more direct benefits: initially this would help avoid known pitfalls by preventing the loss of meaning or introduction of errors. Expediting the procedures can lead to improved outcomes, as well as reduced costs and respective savings.

Questions remain on what is the optimal way to adopt such unified ways of communicating. It seems that such ways continue to evolve organically. As a consequence, we can expect that the integration will occur following the principles of Constructal law (Bejan and Lorente 2010) where changes will happen as small, concurrent, modifications (some technology here, a policy there, incentives elsewhere) and those modifications that bring benefit will stay, while those that do not will be abandoned.

Now that you have been warned about the challenges that lie ahead, this chapter provides an in-depth exploration of standardization, knowledge management, and evolution of controlled terminologies, ontologies, and vocabularies.

13.2 The Role of Standards in the Integration of Patient Records

The development, use, and maintenance of standards will definitely play a role in the integration of medical and dental data. In this section, we will briefly review what standards are, as well as their strengths and weaknesses.

Standards are agreements between two or more parties to follow a given set of rules or principles given certain situations. The agreement allows the user of standards to know, in advance, what will occur when interacting with other parties that follow the same standard. More specifically, for healthcare, Jernigan et al. (2010) define data standards as the "…uniform use of common terms and common methods for sharing data…". Again, from this definition we can derive that agreement or shared understanding is fundamental for making standards useful.

We experience the use of standards every day. Driving on a particular side of the road, initiating a conversation with a greeting, or using currency to pay for a service are examples of situations in which a large number of people have agreed to use and follow the same set rules and/or procedures. Using standards brings benefits to those who decide to abide by them. For instance, having the appropriate regional currency allows a person to travel to different parts of the region and conduct transactions efficiently. On the other hand, the use of standards has its costs, either related to development or maintenance. In the case of the early days of currency, in Mesopotamia (Powell 1996), currency could be seen as the representation of grains and the currency value was linked not only to the grains themselves but to the ability to protect the grains or whether that protection was available. Thus, developing this standard had additional costs than just the simple agreement between trade parties. In modern days, the development, use, and maintenance of standards have costs that are not only financial but also cultural, technical, and/or political.

It is also important to discuss the objective of standards. Different healthcare data standards have been developed to suit different needs. Traditionally, standards have been divided into those tailored to represent knowledge or "content standards" and those that facilitate data communication or "interchange standards" (Hammond and Cimino 2006). The philosophies behind the development of these two types of standards are different, and their applications also vary. For instance, an example of content standards is the International Classification of Diseases (ICD). This classification or "system" lets clinicians in different environments know the diagnosis of the same patient. ICD was originally created to keep track of the reasons for mortality (Jernigan et al. 2010). The use of the standard evolved and the ICD is now used around the world to record not only mortality causes, but also diagnoses used in clinical operations, including documenting patient information and billing. Usually, these standards are referred to as nomenclatures, terminologies, or vocabularies. The difference between these names depends usually on the content and objective for which each standard was developed. For instance, Hammond and Cimino (2006) define a nomenclature as a "system of terms that is elaborated according to pre-established naming rules" while a terminology is a "set of terms representing the system of concepts of a particular subject field." Other naming conventions include classification systems, dictionaries, and ontologies. In a gist, these systems have the goal to represent knowledge in a structured way.

A different type of standard is used for the exchange of clinical information. Primary examples are the standards produced by the Health Level 7 group (http://www.hl7.org/). This group developed the HL7 Messaging Standard, which enables member organizations to utilize one format to send and receive communications between information systems.

Standards specifying appropriate storage structures for the data will also be important for the area of medical and dental data integration. An example of this type of standard is the ANSI/ADA Specification No. 1000—Standard Clinical Data Architecture for the Structure and Content of an Electronic Health Record (American Dental Association 2003), which was developed by the American National Standards Institute and the American Dental Association. The ADA continuously produces documents such as specifications and reports that support dental care. These activities are conducted by the Standards Committee in Dental Informatics. Like the ADA, there are several organizations participating in the development of standards.

Fortunately, there are several standards that are currently in use by both physicians and dentists, and a primary example is DICOM (Digital Imaging and Communications in Medicine) developed by the American College of Radiology and the National Electrical Manufacturers Association (Howerton Jr. and Mora 2008) which is used for the electronic exchange of image based information. It will be up to those interested in integrating medical and dental data to identify the appropriate choice of standards depending on the type of information that needs to be transmitted.

13.2.1 Challenges

Despite the advances in the development of standards, there are still challenges that need to be addressed when incorporating them. These can result in "unforeseen" issues that may prevent the proper use and transmission of data. For instance, when implementing standards it is necessary to consider issues such as the cultural background, context, costs, and other factors that can play a role in their success.

Figure 13.1 presents two signs, made to serve the same goal but based on different standards. Each sign is intended to ask drivers to "stop." Although both are in the same language (Spanish), different interpretations can lead to problems for a driver who is unfamiliar with the alternative sign.

In Fig. 13.1, we have a representation of two "STOP" signs written in Spanish that read "Alto" and "Pare". Both signs seek to convey the same message to their reader, which is "to decrease their speed until the vehicle is no longer moving." Yet, different countries have different conventions for which each sign is commonly used. In most cases, most drivers will understand what they are supposed to do even if they are visitors from a country that uses a different convention. However, in some instances, a driver unfamiliar with one of the words may not know how to interpret the sign, which could cause an accident. In this particular case, the word "Alto" in Spanish has also the meaning of the adjective "tall", adding to the possibility of confusion. Thus, in this case the cultural background plays a role in the interpretation of the standard.

Figure 13.2 presents the sign "Construction ahead", intended to warn drivers that they may encounter an area under construction when driving in the UK. Taken out of context, this sign can be jokingly interpreted as the "man with a broken umbrella." In this case, "context" plays a big role in defining meaning, actually changing it completely.

Another challenge with standards is the context in which they are used. We will illustrate this issue by referring to a road sign used in the United Kingdom, and depicted in Fig. 13.2. The sign is used to alert drivers of construction ahead.

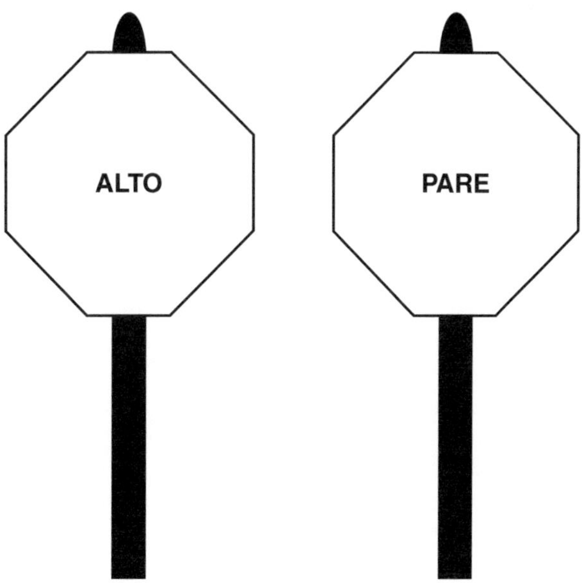

Fig. 13.1 Signs based on different standards

Fig. 13.2 The role of context in standards

However, the road sign is also known as "The man with a broken umbrella". If a driver sees the sign, he knows that soon he will encounter a construction area. However, if the same driver is in a party and one jokingly refers to the street sign, the driver understands that the sign's meaning is different than before.

The former and latter examples—the stop sign and the road sign—showcase that, even though an agreement was made to implement a standard, its interpretation still varies with the context or cultural background. Fortunately, there are solutions to address different interpretations. However, they are costly. In the case of the stop sign, the country or regional area could change all their signs for new and unambiguous ones. Afterwards, policy makers would have to retrain the population of the country or regional area to recognize the new sign. The implementation of this solution hinges on the resources the country or regional area has to be able to make this change. Another approach would be to educate all the visiting drivers on what the stop signs mean. In the case of "The man with a broken umbrella" authorities could forbid people misusing the meaning of the sign. Naturally, the problem with this solution is its legitimacy and the likelihood of enforcing the rule. Another issue with the sign example is that the signs themselves need to be maintained and someone needs to keep track of the location, use, and the structural condition of the sign.

It is also important to control "expectations" for those implementing standards. Given the issues above, it is possible that two systems that are standard compliant do not communicate. This can lead to misunderstandings and the eventual failure to adopt a particular standard. Yet the challenge here is not the standard itself, but the failure to adopt the appropriate procedures, policies, and cultural changes that are necessary to establish communication.

Despite all these issues, it is highly beneficial to adopt standards and accompanying technologies since the benefits usually surpass the initial costs of adoption. In other parts of this book we review specific aspects of integrating medical and dental data as well as the particular use of standards that lend themselves naturally to accomplish this integration.

13.3 Rationale for Data Standards and Coded Terminologies for Dentistry

Information Technology (IT) continues to change very rapidly. The speed with which information can be processed today has dramatically altered industries. Our financial system is a classic example.

The change to "on line banking", rather than writing checks, and the amazing accuracy of those financial exchanges, is a testament to standards and structure. Even our beloved "plastic" or credit cards are no longer needed at many merchants, as they simply use bar codes and other structured information tools to obtain and exchange information.

Health care has lagged in many areas where information technology may have provided some significant areas of improvement. Medicine and the allied health professions, including dentistry, have adopted IT in some areas quite robustly. However, until federal incentives for "meaningful use" were put into place, the major focus was on the financial systems for billing patients and insurance companies. Clinical systems, true electronic health records (EHRs), are still far from universal. This creates artificial limits on their overall utility.

Standards for use and development as well as structure, such as structured terminology, are critical to the successful development, deployment, and adoption of IT into our financial and retail sectors. They are equally important to successful use in health care.

Information technology (IT) standards have been successfully deployed and adopted in some areas of our health care system. An example is the ability to use electronic claims where our computer systems assist us in "sending" claims either directly to an insurance company or through a claims clearinghouse. These have proven to be efficient, accurate, and allow for bi-directional information exchange. Funds can be directly deposited, often within a day or two. Even attachments necessary with certain claims can now be sent and received electronically, thanks to the use of standards.

Though still in relatively early stages, data analytics, use of artificial intelligence (AI), and machine learning are being used by many industries today. The more structured is the information, the greater the utility of these tools. Structured data, particularly data with agreed upon standards, enhance the data quality and ability to both compare and exchange information. Using terminologies that are accepted and broadly used can provide a significant amount of structure to health care clinical records.

Studies are now regularly published in health care and IT journals that indicate improved patient care processes, improved patient outcomes, and corresponding care-cost reductions when EHRs are effectively designed, implemented, and used. These systems are critical in providing a clinician with the "right information, at the right place, and at the right time". Correct and timely information can add an important element to clinical decisions.

EHRs can provide the greatest set of tools when properly designed using structured data and data standards. This allows for analytics of historical data, comparison to current conditions, and development of decision support tools. Additionally, data structure and data standards can allow for information exchange across platforms (EHRs from different vendors, as an example) and data aggregation that may lead to a better understanding of care and outcomes.

13.3.1 Purpose

Once all the information in this paper is absorbed, it is hoped that the reader will understand:

1. The importance of data standardization, controlled vocabularies, and clinical terminologies to integration interoperability of dental and medical data.
2. The improvements to clinical care that result from proper use of the three elements (data standardization, controlled vocabularies, and clinical terminologies).
3. The need to integrate terminologies, fully, into decision support, allergy and drug contraindication alerts, and knowledge discovery processes.
4. The need for commercial off-the-shelf (COTS) software developers to plan for the use of such data elements, even if they are not used at the current time.
5. The need for dental opinion leaders to promote, continually, these three elements.

13.3.2 Understanding the Need: Data Standardization

While dentistry has come a long way towards using similar language or representations for similar care, there is still a great deal of variation when reviewing either paper clinical records or the "progress notes" recorded in our various software systems.

A hypothetical example of a relatively common dental treatment, an MO composite on an upper right first bicuspid, can begin to show us this variation:

#5 MO composite.
#5 MO COMP.
#5 MO tooth colored restoration.
#5 MO Filtek (or multiple other brand names).
#5 MO A3 Filtek Supreme.

The list can go on. In our software systems, some of this is already "forced" into being more standardized. For billing purposes, this becomes a specific tooth and specific surface(s) and material only. Billing is required to follow a standard for claims submission for insurance reimbursement to take place.

A dental clinician would readily recognize that each of these examples can mean essentially the same thing. A computer, however, would recognize this as five different treatments (except for the billing segment). Though Natural Language Processing

(NLP) within systems is becoming quite effective, the NLP still must be programmed to recognize all of these and many more variations as being "the same thing". It must also be updated frequently to account for the many brands and brand names that are added or changed. Furthermore, a clinician might use abbreviations or have a spelling error that would further confuse an electronic system, even one with great NLP capabilities.

To create data standardization, a software vendor might develop a data entry screen that offers fewer choices: (1) choose the tooth, (2) choose the surfaces, and (3) choose the material—composite, amalgam, porcelain, zirconium, glass ionomer, gold, etc.—but not a brand). Another software vendor might provide a list of terms, perhaps the same ones as above, and then "map" them to a specific equivalent term that would not necessarily be visible to the clinician. Other systems might use other techniques, but all would be creating sound standardization of the data to make it more useful for analysis and simple functionality (such as submitting a claim for payment).

13.3.3 Controlled Vocabularies

In the example above, we present several different phrases that essentially mean the same thing. These are considered "synonyms" and we discussed methods that software vendors might use to reduce the number of synonyms or create an easier method for a clinician to pick from the list of synonyms.

Another issue that the last example identifies is the specific product itself, the brand name. There is value in knowing this brand name because the content in other brands is likely a bit different and, over time, it may be possible to identify what content or product design provides the best performance in a specific situation. This is also valuable to forensic dentists.

Software vendors have at least a few methods for limiting the synonyms by separating or recording brand name in a different field. This effectively begins to "control" the vocabulary and makes our standardized data potentially easier to search and relate to other information or among other clinicians.

One of the promising methods for documenting brand names is something that is used every day in the retail world, bar coding. Hospitals have been using bar codes on pharmaceuticals to track use and which patient is receiving which medications. Clinicians scan the bar code on a patient's wristband or record, then scan the medication to be provided to the patient. This has been bar coded in the hospital pharmacy to include dosage, etc. and provides a way to verify the patient by comparing the pharmacy order to the scan of the patient's wristband. Many reports and journal articles suggest that this is significantly reducing medication errors in the hospital setting.

Many of our dental products already contain bar codes. It is likely that some vendors will simply allow us to scan in a bar code for the specific product while we are using our software to document the actual treatment or service. Product identifiers (bar codes) are already being used and further explored through standards development organizations.

Software vendors could also create a separate field from the procedure itself to document the brand name or product used. This would also effectively "control" the vocabulary and should provide another way of being able to search on the material used in a specific treatment for a specific patient. It is possible this workflow might be just as efficient clinically.

13.3.4 Clinical Terminologies

The EDR is now set up so that the dental clinician who wants to record a treatment of 'upper right bicuspid with an MO composite restoration' has a limited number of choices to describe the treatment and the computer only saves one description. So, all 'upper right first bicuspid with an MO composite restoration' are saved in the computer as '#5 MO COMP'. Aren't we done yet?

Within a specific system, then, data is now standardized and the vocabulary is controlled. It should be easy to search and locate the specific information on a specific patient for a specific treatment on a set day or search in many other ways on our set of structured and stored data. We can even do some (limited) data analysis on the set of patients, materials, etc. stored in the system. However, it may not be possible to effectively compare this information with that of other dental clinicians or aggregate the information so that we can gain a far greater understanding of what might work best for large populations of patients. It would also have greater potential to "individualize" care based on the data available from hundreds or even thousands of clinicians.

Further, if the information needed to be shared with another dental clinician (perhaps a general dentist sending information to another general dentist because a patient has moved cross country), it may not be "shareable" information.

If we wish to send the information of 'upper right first bicuspid with an MO composite restoration' to another dental clinician, we cannot be sure that the other software system can read and use the information that we sent. His or her EDR may not have standardized on the '#5 MO COMP'. The other software system may have settled on '#5 MO Composite' as the concept. If we send '#5 MO COMP', his software must try to interpret this string against his list of synonyms.

If '#5 MO COMP' is not in the synonyms list, we have failed to share information. With so many EDR vendors and so many ways of representing similar treatments or procedures, the ability to share information becomes exceedingly complex without the use of a "reference" terminology.

So, the controlled vocabulary is still insufficient for true integration and interoperability. One controlled vocabulary is as valid as another is and the harmonization between controlled vocabularies is not standardized. Further, the controlled vocabulary does not provide any information regarding how one concept relates to another. For instance, both caries and periodontal abscess are bacterial diseases, but nowhere in a controlled vocabulary is this information captured. Thus, it is not possible to perform logical analysis of dental terms using only a controlled vocabulary. Using the caries and periodontal abscess example, it is not possible for a computer to include both conditions in a frequency distribution of oral bacterial diseases.

To resolve this issue, we need to progress toward a reference terminology in which:

- *Specificity*: A single concept is established as the base against which all similar terms are equated. One concept with multiple synonymous terms.
- *Relatedness*: Each concept has an explicit relationship to other concepts. Generally, the main relationship that gives the reference terminology its structure is the "is a" relationship (commonly expressed as (type–subtype) or (parent–child)).

These terminologies are produced by Standards Development Organizations (SDO), like SNOMED International's terminology, SNOMED CT. Standards Development Organizations within their own well-defined domain of knowledge, construct a data set that can act as a universal representation of medical concepts. To make these concepts useable in any application, they all assign an alphanumeric code to each concept. These codes are the same anywhere in the world. So, if '#5 MO COMP' is coded '123', then any application throughout the world that understands this code system, will correctly identify '123' as '#5 MO COMP'. This, then, allows for data exchange and data aggregation, potentially unleashing the power Artificial Intelligence and data analytics might provide to help dental clinicians provide even better care for their patients.

The value of coding all concepts has added advantages in that an abstract alphanumeric, '123' is easier to process than a string in which a variant in the string may or may not change the meaning of the concept. We now have all the elements necessary to make EDRs interoperable.

13.3.5 We Have Terminologies in Dentistry: Look at CDT—Aren't They Good Enough or Do We Need More?

It is likely evident that coded terminologies and interoperable EDRs are essential for quality and can assist clinicians in providing the best possible care for their patients. What follows then, is a need to determine what information and tools are needed to make an EDR as effective as possible.

Up to this point, we have used the example of '#5 MO COMP' because the concept is easy for any dental clinician to understand. Further, any clinician knows that we already have a way to code this concept. Current Dental Terminology (CDT) allows us to code '#5 MO COMP' as a combination of the tooth number (which, by definition, is a terminology) '#5', the surface or surfaces 'MO' (part of some terminologies) and the concept of 'COMP' which is captured in the CDT codes of 'D2330–D2394.' (The computer system has captured the MO and recognizes it as two surface and correlates it with the material, composite, and the tooth number, 5, a posterior tooth, to select the proper CDT code, D2392.) But that is all we can do with this terminology. The code of '#5', 'MO' and 'D2392' provides no information about the diagnosis that led to the treatment, nothing about the signs and symptoms, nothing about co-morbidities, nothing about the patient's medical status, etc. In any dental record, we would like to capture all clinically relevant information. Tooth number, surface(s) and CDT code do not do that. At best, tooth numbering and CDT is incomplete.

Though not exclusively, CDT has been primarily designed to identify procedures. It is updated annually by a cross section of interested parties (general and specialty dentists, government, insurance industry, etc.) to make sure it is relevant and functional. Its use is virtually ubiquitous in the United States and, for some purposes, it is required, such as electronic claims submissions.

However, CDT does not provide dentistry with a method to record or document the other very important information introduced above. Other terminologies will be necessary to create the most robust and helpful EDR.

Since 2012, there has been increasing cooperation among several of the organizations with terminologies that can serve the dental profession. SNOMED International has developed cooperative agreements with LOINC and ICD. The American Dental Association and SNOMED have a cooperative agreement. SNODENT has become an American National Standards Institute (ANSI) standard. SNODENT is now a set of SNOMED CT terms that apply to dentistry and are referred to as "active" terms. All of SNODENT is included within SNOMED CT (or will be shortly). Many dental schools have used the Dental Diagnostic System (DDS codes). DDS is becoming a subset of SNODENT and thereby a subset of SNOMED CT. Within SNOMED CT, smaller sets, called "ref sets", have been developed to identify the most commonly used diagnostic terms in dentistry as well as another to properly populate an odontogram. All of this is important to dentistry because it provides a standards-based ongoing maintenance system (like CDT has), assuring a future of structured terms that dentistry needs, a reduction in potential "mapping" (a significant expense), and greater comfort and ease of use for vendors, making adoption more practical.

The first thing that needs to be decided is what kind of information should be captured in a complete dental record. In other words, what is a minimal level of information that must be captured in a dental record that allows another dentist to form a complete clinical picture just by reading the record? Secondly, can this set of information be captured in some coded terminology to meet the needs of an EDR and allow the information to be readily transferred and analyzed?

To answer these questions, let us examine a generic dental visit. The dentist conducts an examination, reviews the medical history, makes a diagnosis, treats the problem and evaluates the treatment for a prognosis. The dentist may also order a prescription and perhaps a lab test. Let us code this generic visit using some existing terminologies that are, or can be, used in dentistry.

Table 13.1 provides examples of coding for the initial "dental examination".

A patient history is a requirement of a good medical/dental record. Examples of coding a "medical history of liver disease" are shown in Table 13.2.

Once the examination has taken place, the signs and symptoms along with any descriptive qualifiers are noted. Things like "severe throbbing pain in the lower left

Table 13.1 Coding for dental examination

SNOMED	34343003 (plus multiple qualifiers)
CDT	D0120-D0180, specifying multiple types of exams
ICD	Z00 (and sub headings)

Table 13.2 Codes for medical history of liver disease

SNOMED	161535005
CDT	None
ICD	Can represent current disease but not a history of

Table 13.3 Coding for severe throbbing pain in the lower left jaw

SNOMED	29695002, throbbing pain; 76948002, severe pain; 255480002, lower left quadrant; 91609006 bone structure of mandible
CDT	None
ICD	No codes for clinical findings separated from diagnosis

Table 13.4 Coding for primary active dental caries into the middle third of dentin

SNOMED	733942006
CDT	None
ICD	K02.62 (dental caries into dentin)

Table 13.5 Coding for 19 DO amalgam

SNOMED	31196005, amalgam restoration, 2 surface, permanent; 245658003, mesial-occlusal; 89625000, mandibular left first molar
CDT	D2150 specification of tooth and surface require other terminologies)
ICD	none

Table 13.6 Coding for good prognosis

SNOMED	170968001
CDT	None
ICD	None

jaw." Such statements can be parsed into the individual important components like "severe," "throb", "lower left," "jaw." Each of these can be coded (see Table 13.3).

Table 13.4 shows how a diagnosis of "dental caries in the middle third of dentin" for the problem can be coded.

A decision is made to perform some procedure to correct the disease or abnormality. As noted in the introduction, treatments can be coded. For "#19 MO amalgam," the coding would be as shown in Table 13.5.

Once treatment is performed, there is some evaluation of the "prognosis" of the treatment. The coding would be as shown in Table 13.6.

A drug may be prescribed, like Amoxicillin, 500 mg tablets. The coding examples are shown in Table 13.7.

RxNorm is a terminology representing all medications and is widely used in the United States.

Table 13.7 Coding for amoxicillin 500 mg tablets

SNOMED	374646004
CDT	None
ICD10	None

Table 13.8 Coding for a PT or PTT test for bleeding control

SNOMED	42525009
CDT	None
ICD10	None for specific tests

LOINC is a terminology widely used worldwide to represent lab tests and other observables.

Table 13.9 Extensiveness of codes

History and exam	SNOMED
Diagnosis	SNOMED, ICD10
Procedure and Treatment	SNOMED, CDT
Prognosis	SNOMED
Medications	SNOMED, RxNorm
Labs	SNOMED, LOINC

Lab tests can be ordered. For example, a dentist contemplating an extraction may wish to order a PT, PTT, or INR for a patient with liver disease who may have a clotting problem (see Table 13.8).

So, if we include the patient's personal demographic information as well as the items above, medical history, signs and symptoms, diagnosis, treatment, labs, medications, and prognosis, we have all the needed information to understand the fullness of the office visit.

Now the second half of the issue, can these data be coded? Short answer yes, every data element can be coded as evidenced in the examples above. Table 13.9 is not definitive but is used merely to demonstrate that there is at least one terminology to cover an aspect of clinical information.

The names in the right-hand column are names of different terminologies. They are useful for coding a complete dental record. The fact that one or all of these are unknown to you is immaterial to this discussion. The important observation and conclusion from viewing this table is that there is a way to code every pertinent piece of clinical data.

13.3.6 Benefits of Terminologies and Data Standards

Okay, so terminologies and data standards are integral to a complete EDR. Assume that you have a complete EDR with all critical data elements properly coded via one or more terminologies. What is the benefit besides the ability to share the record with another dentist?

Let us start by assuming that a dentist has used a fully realized EDR with coded data elements everywhere for a year. What kinds of benefits accrue to this practitioner?

The best way to analyze this is to compare the fully coded EDR against a standard dental management application in which only CDT codes are maintained. The dentist can generate a lot of knowledge from the EDR data that is nearly impossible to generate from a dental management application. Examples are:

- We wish to analyze root canal treatment utilization. If we are using management software alone, we can do a count of the number of root canal treatments that were performed, the percentage of root canal treatment versus all other procedures, etc. However, there is no way to determine how many root canal treatments were the results of periapical abscess versus fractured tooth pulp exposure. With the complete coded EDR, such an evaluation is very straightforward.
- Is there a link between periodontal disease and heart disease? If there is a correlation, what type of periodontal disease at what severity is correlated with what type of heart disease? This analysis is nearly impossible with management software but straightforward with a full EDR. Just query the records in which the code(s) for heart disease and the code(s) for periodontal disease appear for the same patient.

How about proactive decisions? Suppose the patient has a complex medical history and is taking multiple medications. You have determined that multiple extractions are indicated. What precautions should the dentist take before the extractions, what alterations need to be made to the medication schedule (e.g., stop Coumadin treatment 3 days prior to extraction?), and is there a change in prognosis? Decision support that evaluates all these factors automatically would be a great patient safety check. Coded data makes decision support modules possible.

The terminologies used in the examples and in the chart are a mixture of medical, pharmaceutical, and dental terminologies. How do we determine which one we should use?

A quick look at the table and examples would suggest that dentistry adopt SNOMED CT and forget all the others. SNOMED CT can code most of dentistry. It is not a complete ontology (a structuring of knowledge about things according to their essential qualities) that can fully describe all of medicine and dentistry. Other, more focused terminologies, like LOINC for lab tests, are more comprehensive within a specific domain than SNOMED CT. Thus, one of the factors to consider is, "can we sacrifice details for simplicity without losing clinical information?" The true answer to this question requires a careful and detailed analysis of the data requirements for the individual clinical specialty. In our case, the domain is dentistry. This type of analysis is difficult, time consuming, and ultimately may not answer the question.

Since we recognize that every terminology has strengths and weaknesses, in a perfect world a better approach is to use whatever is best for a specific purpose. So, using LOINC over SNOMED CT is best for coding of laboratory tests. RxNorm is a better choice over SNOMED CT for drug information. SNOMED CT is the choice for coding of clinical findings. For coding of dental procedures, CDT is the logical choice. This strategy provides the most comprehensive way to code dental information.

However, we also must be practical and pragmatic. We recognize that there are costs and workflow limitations as well as specific government requirements. For instance, to submit an insurance charge for payment, we must use CDT for procedures and, if a diagnostic code is required by the insurance company or government entity, ICD10 for the diagnosis.

It is possible, and even likely, that software firms will add terminologies for use incrementally, as dental clinicians request the tools to do so. Effective and complete care documentation may be initially more important to clinicians than even decision support tools. While ICD10 provides a tool for documenting a diagnosis (at least a more generalized one) for payment purposes, it does not routinely include the findings, observations, and tests that led to the diagnosis. It also provides fewer relationships than other terminologies. These factors are possibly as important as the diagnosis itself. Thus, we may see a subset of the SNOMED CT terminology being adopted to document these areas in a coordinated manner that will allow for future development of decision support and quality analytics.

Outside of CDT and possibly ICD10, there are few EDRs that incorporate these terminologies. There is a lot of work to do. Many of the EDRs in use today were built on platforms or with data field structures that were developed long before we understood what should and could be documented and recorded. These systems adapted to dental workflows, some quite well, some less so. Though health care reform and the availability of funding through "meaningful use" dollars were meant to develop more structured and interoperable systems, they impacted only a minority of dental clinics due to their requirements. Thus, software vendors have continued to respond primarily to customer requests.

As medical insurers and medical care delivery systems begin to recognize the connection between oral and overall health, the drive towards "care-coordination" may be one of the strongest factors moving dentistry towards more structured data and more capability to exchange information with our medical colleagues. This may be one of the drivers moving dental software vendors into adding more terminology capability to their systems.

Change can be complex and difficult. This will mean change for software vendors and adaptation of workflows as just two of possibly many issues that need careful consideration. However, the value to patient care and outcomes may make this an opportune and necessary change.

Everything that preceded this section should have convinced you that clinical terminologies are useful and more importantly, inevitable. So EDRs, whether custom designed or commercial off-the-shelf (COTS) products, must begin to account for these terminologies in their products. This means that all future software must be designed to accept the coded entries even if the software is not yet prepared to use the coded data elements. In simple terms, the software must account for a clinician selecting a clinical condition and the associated code for that selection. And there must be fields within the database to store this data. The functionality to use this data can be added later. The important thing is to start collecting the coded data as soon as possible.

Workflow considerations are always important to dental clinicians and therefore, software vendors. Thankfully, dental clinicians are rarely required to remember the alphanumeric codes used in structured terminologies. Instead, they use terms they would normally use to describe something. This is referred to as a clinical interface (sometimes referred to as an interface terminology). An example would be a dental clinician selecting a diagnosis of localized chronic moderate periodontitis and not having to remember a SNOMED identifier of 715,286,003. Like the example of combining tooth 5 with surfaces MO and material composite to select the correct CDT code in the early example, the software system instantly "maps" the terms used by the clinician to the proper code and the clinician never sees this process.

The actual terminologies to be used are a matter for debate. This author prefers SNOMED CT as the choice for coding of clinical findings, diagnosis, and problem lists (medical conditions). CDT and ICD10 will continue to be required for filing of claims for reimbursement for procedures. Other terminologies possibly have less immediate utility to dentistry.

13.3.7 Do We Really Need to Share Dental Information with Our Healthcare Brethren?

Dentistry is not separate and distinct from the rest of healthcare. We need to be able to share information with medicine, pharmacy, etc. for patient safety, and treatment efficiencies. There is no reason for patients to have a medical history for a physician and one for a dentist, etc. This occurs because the two professions do not share patient information. In a world with a truly interoperable EDR, pertinent parts of a patient's EMR can be shared with his or her EDR. For instance, both a dentist and a physician need to know if a patient has liver disease. Having each capture and record such information is redundant and prone to errors.

Dentists often write prescriptions for their patients. Consider the advantages of an electronic prescription order versus a paper prescription. The advent of drug registries and the requirements in some states for health care clinicians to check these registries prior to prescribing is a function that can be integrated into an e-prescription that cannot be accomplished with paper. Further, some states are beginning to require e-prescribing.

As above, there is a time savings because the redundancy of entering demographics and medical history is avoided. The dental clinician and/or pharmacy can also run the prescription against a knowledgebase of drug-drug interactions prior to dispensing the drug, thus preempting potential harm to the patient.

13.3.8 Summary

Information technology and its ability to utilize "big data", apply artificial intelligence, and to more comprehensively review (structured) information is changing society in many ways. However, health care lags behind finance, retail, and many other industries.

Moreover, IT capabilities in dentistry lag seriously behind those of our medical colleagues. Patient expectations are greater than ever (who hasn't heard one of their patients complain about filling out medical histories time and again?). Increasingly, patients are using web-based tools to do health assessments. Dentistry needs to be able to respond and provide more knowledge-based individualized care that arises from aggregating and understanding the data collected. Dentistry needs to push the vendor community to add tools that will assist in reaching one of the key tenets of the new health IT, right information at the right place and at the right time.

13.3.9 Final Thoughts

Dental care delivery is changing substantially also. Far more technology is being used in every practice today from caries detection to crown construction. Further, we have seen much practice consolidation with larger "networks" of dental clinics working under similar umbrellas and often the same (and sometimes not very user friendly) EDR.

If dentistry continues to lag medicine in IT, there is an increasing risk that the economic footings of IT will be based on the medical model and possibly large medical care delivery systems. Their economics are so very different from those of dentistry, even from the large dental service organizations that exist today. This could lead to a substantially more expensive IT "solution" WHEN (not if) it becomes necessary for dentistry to adopt these significant changes. The solo and small group practices, so necessary to rural care delivery in particular, may need to absorb considerable costs that will be passed on to patients, making dentistry less affordable for more people. The sooner dentistry responds and starts adopting to change, the greater the opportunities available to the profession.

13.4 Knowledge Representation and Ontologies

13.4.1 Introduction

Intelligent beings are required to construct mental models about their reality since most things that exist are external to them. For instance, a clinician first needs to construct a mental model of the patient's problem before deciding on a particular diagnosis or treatment. This requires clinicians to gather data and make sense of it in a structured way. Depending on the complexity of the task, clinicians use different "tools" to generate this structure. If the problem at hand is relatively simple, they may just ask questions of a patient and store the answers in memory or on a sheet of paper. However, as problems have become more complicated, humans have invented tools to manage this complexity and increase their capability not only to store but also to make sense of large amounts of information. In the past century, the use of computers introduced the concept of electronic databases, and as our understanding of how to use these tools increased we discovered how important it is to correctly structure data and information. Part of this discovery process led to the adoption of several major approaches to meaningfully capture information. In this section we will review Ontologies as one of several approaches used to structure information. We will provide some definitions, historical background, and examples of ontologies that provide a good understanding of how this type of knowledge representation can pave the way for supporting medical and dental data integration.

13.4.2 Historical Precedents

Throughout history there have been many authors that explored the concept of knowledge representation. Representation of knowledge was one of the preoccupations during the early development of science. Greek philosophers dealt with the concept of being and the representation of knowledge and set precedents for those who would study the topic later on. Aristotle's Metaphysics described how a set of 'Categories' could classify most known entities at the time. In addition, he also pointed out that these categories were not 'composite', that is, "they need to be composed in order to make statements about the nature that can yield affirmation" (Sandholm 2005). Although these categories are debatable, they set the foundation for what is commonly known as the idea of "Concepts" to represent information.

Concepts or ideas are representations of certain things or elements. But what defines a concept? Campbell et al. (1998) provided a good description of what is called the Ogden and Richards (1923) semiotic triangle (Fig. 13.3). This triangle provides a framework for characterizing meaning by establishing the relationships between thought, symbols, and reality (thus defining a concept).

The Ogden-Richards Semiotic Triangle establishes the different elements that play a role in representing knowledge through concepts.

As described by Campbell et al., the semiotic triangle identifies the relationships between words, thoughts, and things. The triangle explicitly states the relationships where a word (symbol) corresponds to a thought. The word can trigger a thought, which is related to an object, and vice versa. With this simple diagram, we can determine how information is generally processed by humans and likely by other "smart" entities such as computers. Thus, this triangle can be seen as the basis for modern knowledge representation systems, especially those based on the use of concepts.

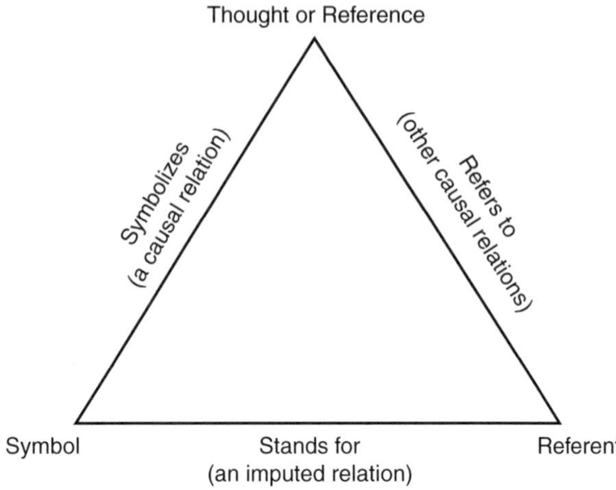

Fig. 13.3 Ogden-Richards semiotic triangle

As we will see next, modern Ontologies and Information Models draw extensively on this approach to handle knowledge representation.

13.4.3 Ontology

Ontology can be simply defined as a "formal conceptualization of a domain" (Gruber 1993). In simpler terms, we could define ontology as a group of ideas or concepts that are organized in a meaningful way or structure that can later be reused to explain or "reason" about a particular subject.

13.4.3.1 Definitions

More formally, the term "ontology" originates from the Greek root "ontos" (being) and "logos" (word) referring "to the subject of existence, i.e. the study of being as such" (Gasevic et al. 2006). Guarino (1998) defines an ontology as "a particular system of categories accounting for a certain vision of the world." They are also defined as "categories of things that exist or may exist in some domain" (Gasevic et al. 2006). Gruber (1993) states that an ontology is "an explicit specification of a conceptualization". In a nutshell, an ontology conceptualizes or defines concepts that represent the whole or a part of reality. Ontologies use concepts in different ways. On occasion, concepts represent not things, but relationships between things. Using this approach, ontologies manage to capture the meaning of reality in a manageable way. By manageable we refer to the ability to create, maintain, and use the knowledge stored in the ontology.

Currently, there are different views and even controversy on how ontologies should be categorized. In this section, we will have more of an applied perspective

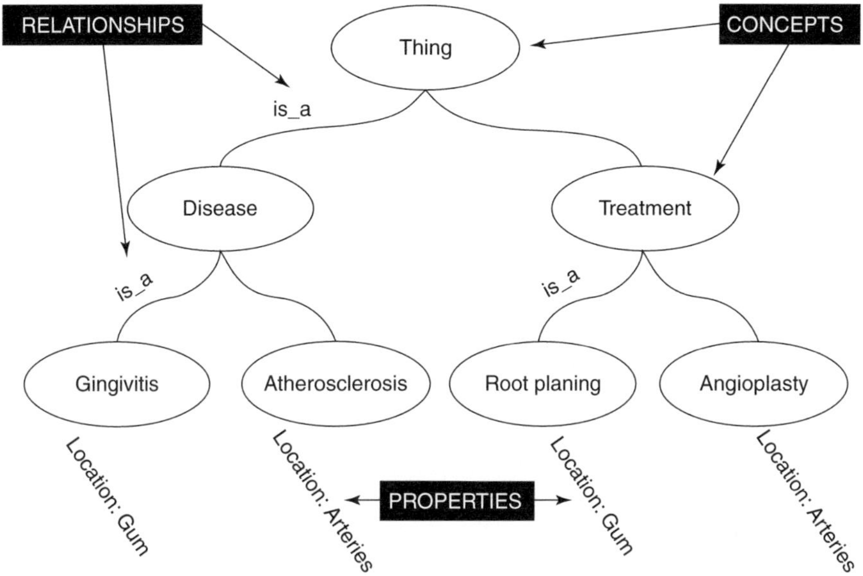

Fig. 13.4 Basic ontology representing clinical information in the form of concepts and their properties as well as the relationships between concepts

since the integration of dental and medical data will most likely require utilization of functioning applications that will enable making sense of information in different domains. For a comprehensive review of the different views on ontological work, including the philosophical aspects of knowledge representation, we recommend the reader to review the work of Smith (Smith 1998) and others (Staad and Studer 2009).

The functional view of ontologies divides them into two major types: (1) content-oriented ontologies, which are likely dealing with a particular area of knowledge and; (2) functional ontologies, which traditionally are linked to a particular application and/or are intended to assist solving a particular problem.

13.4.3.2 Components and Structure

Ontologies are primarily composed of concepts (Fig. 13.4). Another objective of an ontology is to capture not only the concepts that represent entities in the real world, but also the properties of those concepts. A third goal of an ontology is to represent the relationships between concepts. These relationships can also be concepts. Establishing these relationships alone does not necessarily enable information systems to understand the meaning behind those concepts (this would be a semantic network). To increase their sophistication, advanced implementations of ontologies utilize formal processes or logic to maintain the relationships between concepts valid and tractable. There are different approaches to do this and a popular method is the use of the Web Ontology Language "OWL" in combination with "Description Logics", which we will describe next.

13.4.3.3 Web Ontology Language (OWL)

OWL is a processing language intended to provide a framework in the form of eXtended Markup Language (XML) statements. With these statements it is possible to specify the entities that form the ontology and what the boundaries for each entity are. A way to understand OWL and how it helps in constructing and maintaining an ontology is by using the example of a picture puzzle. When beginning to solve a puzzle usually we do not know *where* pieces are supposed to fit. Yet we know *how* pieces are supposed to fit thanks to their shape. As we progress putting the pieces together, a picture starts to emerge and it becomes easier to add more pieces. OWL serves as the standard that defines the shape of the pieces allowing us to integrate concepts into the ontology, and, at the same time, making them remain consistent with one another. In other words, OWL assists us in maintaining knowledge integrity. OWL is intended to be machine-readable.

Technically, OWL is not used alone but in a combination of group of stacked technologies (World Wide Web Consortium (W3C) 2011). XML gives the language in which an ontology can be expressed. XML Schema lists a set of constraints in the type of documents and datatypes that can be expressed. The Resource Description Framework (RDF) gives an emphasis in semantics since it makes available a model for objects and relations. Finally, the RDF Schema allows for specifying the properties and classes.

OWL is known to be available in three "flavors." These flavors permit different levels of expressiveness. OWL *Lite* allows for primarily creating a classification and maintaining simple constraints. For example, this version of OWL is good when rapidly migrating an established thesaurus or classification into a formal ontology. OWL *DL* (Description Logics) allows for representing knowledge with "maximum expressiveness while retaining computational completeness (all conclusions are guaranteed to be computable) and decidability (all computations will finish in finite time)" (World Wide Web Consortium (W3C) 2011). We will talk more about Description Logics in the next section. OWL *Full* allows for "maximum expressiveness" yet without computational guarantees. Software is unlikely to support the features of this version of OWL.

13.4.3.4 Description Logics (DLs)

Description Logics (DLs) can be defined as "… formalisms for representing knowledge" as described by Baader et al. (2004). The purpose of these is to allow the construction of "intelligent applications" that are capable of uncovering the "implicit consequences of explicitly represented knowledge". In other words, they allow expressing the rules by which concepts will relate/operate with each other. Description Logics built from earlier developed systems for representing knowledge and reasoning such as logic-based formalisms and non-logic-based representations. Logic-based representations are powerful and good for handling general-purpose tasks. These systems rely on the use of a variant of first-order predicate calculus. The non-logic representations use ad hoc data structures such as semantic networks and frames. Modern ontologies rely heavily on the use of DLs. Our challenge is to make proper use of this tool to capture the clinical reality.

13.4.3.5 Ontologies in Practice

Ontologies are used for different purposes. Again, the intention of this section is to provide a practical view of ontologies. Next, we are going to provide functional examples, first from the medical perspective, and then examples from the dental domain. In the biomedical domain, ontologies are currently used for supporting research and clinical care. Rubin et al. (2008) provide examples relevant to biomedicine. Here, we mention those that are relevant for integration of medical and dental data:

- Searching for diverse data: biomedical literature is complex and filled with intricate descriptions of synonyms, acronyms, and abbreviations which make the retrieval of information difficult. Ontologies can serve as smart mechanisms to unify content. The classical example is the Gene Ontology (GO) which provides a method to uniquely identify functions, processes, and products related to gene activity making retrieval of information more coherent.
- Exchanging data: transferring information between healthcare entities or systems will be paramount as multidisciplinary teams seek to care for common patients. In biomedicine, an example of the use of ontologies for exchanging data is the handling of Microarray data. Microarrays primarily identify the expression levels of biomarkers for subsequent linkage with clinical conditions. This information is obtained using different platforms which can be represented using the Microarray Gene Expression Data (MGED) Ontology. The MGED Ontology provides a common set of concepts for describing the experimental design enabling the exchange of data.
- Integrating data: the modern healthcare environment is increasingly requiring the utilization of data across specialties, providers, and geographic domains. A natural choice for supporting this integration is the use of ontologies given their ability to "translate" information with similar meanings but expressed in different contexts. An example is the ontology developed by the Advancing Clinico-Genomic Trials (ACGT) on Cancer project (Smith and Brochhausen 2008) to integrate clinical and genetic data from different cancer studies conducted in several research centers. In this project ACGT Master Ontology was created for "integration for the domains of clinical studies, genomic research and clinical cancer management and care" (Smith and Brochhausen 2008).

13.4.3.6 Ontologies in Dentistry

The adoption of ontologies in dentistry is gaining traction primarily among dental researchers. There are several examples of ontologies developed with a specific goal in mind. These include addressing Sjögren syndrome (Long and Goldberg 2006) or for studying saliva (Ai et al. 2010). These two are good examples of how medical and dental data necessarily need to be integrated in order to support a comprehensive view when providing care and conducting research. In the case of Sjögren syndrome (Long and Goldberg 2006), this is an autoimmune disease that is known for destroying the ability to produce saliva and tears. Yet, the impact of this disease can be systemic, affecting other organs including kidneys and lungs. Thus, it is important to be able to retain information about the whole patient. The other example is the Saliva Ontology (Ai et al. 2010) which aims to support research activities including the development of saliva tests that monitor systemic health and specifically identify diseases. Thus, it is important to support a comprehensive view of the patient's health.

In the case of clinical dental practice, there are several terminologies with historical relevance (Leake 2002). The Current Dental Terminology (American Dental Association 1991), International Classification of Diseases-Dental Application (World Health Organization 1994), and the Uniform System of Codes and List of Services (Canadian Dental Association 2001) are used on a daily basis. Yet work needs to be done in order to utilize their content for integration. A preliminary example is the ontology developed by Torres-Urquidy and Schleyer (2009), which aims to incorporate not only canonical but also an empirical representation of dental knowledge. Their ontology is therefore more likely to bridge the gap between theoretical/textbook concepts and the practical notions used routinely for patient care. Another example of the use of ontologies in dentistry is the case of the Swedish Oral Medicine Web (SOMWeb) system (Falkman et al. 2008) which is intended to support a community of practice (CoP) aimed to improve the communication between experts. In the latter case, with the use of technology developments driven by ontological principles, the authors were able to provide better support for the activities and increase the adoption of evidence-based care.

Next, we are going to explore the process for building a Knowledge Base (an ontology) in dentistry. First, we are going to introduce some general procedural concepts, next we are going to review how some of these methods were used by colleagues (Bertaud-Gounot et al. 2010) to develop an Ontology for Dental Emergencies.

13.4.3.7 Building a Knowledge Base

When building a knowledge base, it is important to understand the processes that help us formalize knowledge. van der Lei and Musen (1995) introduce analysis at several levels:

- Knowledge level analysis of an application task specifies the behaviors that are required to solve a problem in the world.

- Symbol level analysis specifies the computational mechanisms needed to model the requisite behaviors.

Subsequently, Musen (1988) proposes six steps in the acquisition of expert knowledge when building an intelligent system:

- *Identification*, where the primary themes of the system are characterized;
- *Conceptualization*, in which the identification of ideas occurs. This includes concepts and their relationships. Newell (1982) identified this as the "knowledge-level analysis";
- *Formalization*, which identifies mechanisms for implementing an expert system and transfer the conceptualized knowledge into the rules and parameters of the eventual system;
- *Implementation*, in which the knowledge base used by a system informs or provides new knowledge in the form of advice;
- *Testing*, in which the system advice is validated by a domain expert and also the knowledge engineer;
- *Revision* of the system, since it is possible that the system does not "behave" as expected due to incorrect representation or modeling of the "facts" and concepts.

However, there is an important consideration that we should face before constructing a new knowledge base, and that is the "Knowledge Acquisition Bottleneck" (Musen 1988). He points out why building knowledge bases or "encoding expert knowledge" is difficult. Several reasons have been discussed including: (1) the inability of experts to communicate and/or (2) "introspect" which create "barriers" for translating and transferring experts' abilities and mental processes to a knowledge base. Thus, during the development process, it is important to remain attentive to issues arising from not establishing the proper communication with subject matter experts.

13.4.3.8 Building the Ontology

There are several approaches for building an ontology. While obtaining knowledge from a subject matter expert can follow the approach presented in the previous section, building an ontology can also be done by using the example of the picture puzzle that we presented before. When first including the content (concepts) that are going to be part of the future ontology we can see these concepts as pieces of a puzzle. In some instances, you may have all the pieces available before starting the assembly of the puzzle, while in others you may only have parts of the puzzle. In this case, the creators of an ontology may know specifically all the information that should be contained in the ontology (for instance, a pre-existing terminology), while in others, the incorporation of new concepts occurs as new information is discovered (this case would apply to the Gene Ontology). As we start assembling the puzzle, some pieces are relatively easy to place given their characteristics. For instance, in a picture puzzle of a map the position of a piece that contains information on a particular street intersection is almost self-explanatory, while the adjacent pieces should be more or less easy to discern whether they fit or not. On the other hand, if we have a puzzle piece that does not have clearly distinctive features, such as part of water or of a park, it will be difficult to identify its final position at the beginning. It will take the arrangement of several pieces before we can be more or less certain of where the piece should go. Similarly, when constructing an ontology and incorporating concepts and relationships between concepts, some concepts will have a clear starting position and others will have to be repositioned and their relationships reassessed as we incorporate more concepts. With the use of elements such as OWL and Description Logics, information systems help us in identifying the good fit of concepts, making sure that the overall structure of the ontology is consistent with reality. Going back to the puzzle example, OWL and DL serve to set the boundaries and shapes of puzzle pieces, thus making sure that we do not place a rounded piece in a squared segment.

Formally, ontologies can be constructed using a top-down or bottom-up approach, each with its own advantages and limitations. The top-down approach starts by identifying a predetermined hierarchy. This is useful when the content is already well identified and the structures that are necessary to represent the relationships are well understood. The limitation of this approach is that the incorporation of new or extraneous information may be very difficult since it may require restructuring the whole content.

The bottom-up approach starts by incorporating concepts individually without having predefined structures; the relationships appearing as new concepts are added. This approach provides for more flexibility. Yet, not having a predefined structure can cause the incorporation of new concepts in areas of the knowledge structure in a way which would not necessarily represent reality appropriately. Having little structure would also make discovering such inconsistencies more difficult.

When constructing the ontology, it is also important to define a preliminary structure that will support the integration of concepts. This definition process is accomplished by using predefined ontologies developed by scientists and philosophers who have worked on identifying what categorizations are applicable to specific types of knowledge. These ontologies are called "top level". Examples of top level ontologies include the Basic Formal Ontology (BFO) (Grenon et al. 2004) and the Descriptive Ontology for Linguistic and Cognitive Engineering (DOLCE) (Gangemi et al. 2002). These provide classifications for concepts according to their inner characteristics. For instance, BFO defines two major categories of concepts: "Continuant" and "Occurrent". A very simple definition for a "Continuant" concept is an entity, which exists independent of time. This can be a "heart valve" or a "broken tooth." The alternative would be an "Occurrent" in which concepts refer to entities that only exist with the progression of time, for instance, "pulmonary insufficiency" or "restoring oral function". The top level ontology provides insights into how things should be represented. In addition, the use of top-level ontologies allows for unification between disparate ontologies. When seeking to integrate knowledge from medical and dental databases it should be easier to make the inferences between both databases if the information in both databases use structures that follow ontological principles and both use the same top level ontology.

Note: It is important to clarify that it is possible to use a top level ontology for defining the structure of your "new" ontology and still use a bottom-up approach for constructing the ontology. The key here is that the approach refers to the way in which concepts are incorporated into the structure of the ontology and not necessarily to the structure itself.

The construction of the ontology usually follows the sequence: (1) defining the goal of the ontology; (2) deciding whether to use a top ontology; (3) incorporating concepts into the predefined structure and repeating this process until you are satisfied given the primary goal; (4) evaluating whether the ontology is consistent and satisfies the notion of knowledge representation required for the goal.

The construction process itself is usually done by using ontology editors such as Protégé (Noy et al. 2010) or OBO-Edit (Wächter and Schroeder 2010). These editors take care of incorporating the elements described before such as the use of OWL-DL. In addition, they provide graphical representations of the ontologies being created. Another feature of these editors is the ability to check for consistency and coherence. As ontologies evolve, the addition of a new concept may make sense when looking at the neighboring concepts and "local" relationships, yet it may be incongruent with reality or the tendencies previously set for the rest of the ontology. Finally, these editors also provide additional functionality such as the creation of forms or the ability to export the ontologies onto the Web (Noy et al. 2010).

Example: An Ontology for Dental Emergencies

Dr. Bertaud-Gounot and colleagues have studied disease representation and diagnostic classification using ontologies (Bertaud-Gounot et al. 2012) and developed an ontology (Bertaud-Gounot et al. 2010) using data collected from the literature and validated with the help of subject matter experts. Their goal was to create an ontology that captures information about dental emergencies. For their process, they obtained articles and extracted concepts that would then be approved by the experts so they would be included in the ontology.

Process

The investigators obtained articles from Medline and the Medical and Surgical Encyclopedia (http://www.em-consulte.com/produits/traites/od1#). Their search included the following keywords: dental emergencies, mouth disease, periodontal disease, pulpitis, and tooth disease. The investigators created summaries from the articles and identified concepts that are relevant for emergency dental care. Once the concepts were identified, they were validated by the clinicians. The investigators used Protégé (Stanford University, CA) as editor and integrated content in an iterative multistep process. In addition, they utilized the Pellet reasoner to check for consistency each time a new concept was aggregated.

Content

The ontology has 202 concepts divided by 28 capturing diseases (Fig. 13.5) and 174 representing findings (Fig. 13.6). The ontology also has 377 restrictions (relations). These relations were established between the diseases and their respective clinical findings. Figure 13.7 illustrates an example of disease "Reversible pulpitis" characterized by the relationships in the ontology.

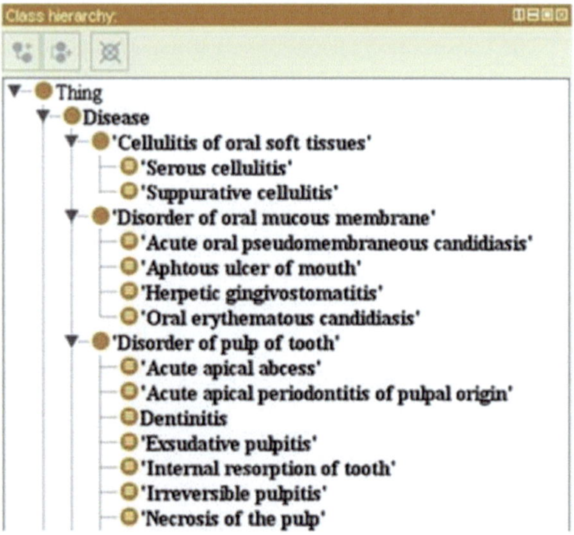

Fig. 13.5 Partial view of diseases represented in the ontology of dental emergencies

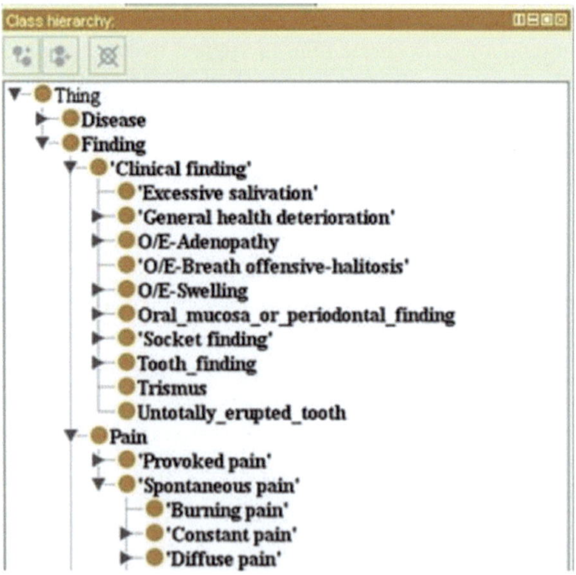

Fig. 13.6 Partial view of findings represented in the ontology of dental emergencies

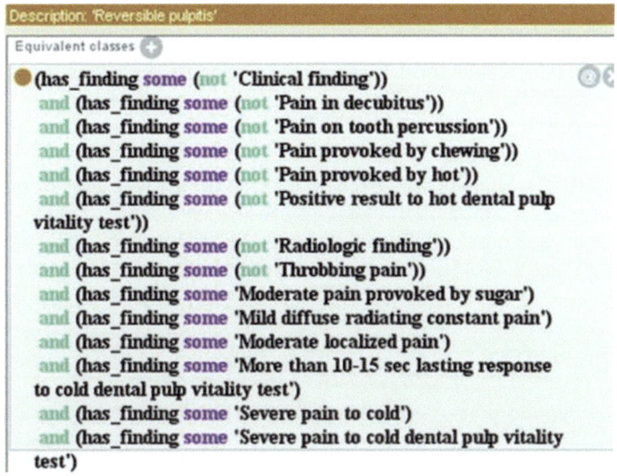

Fig. 13.7 Example of disease "Reversible pulpitis" characterized by the relationships in the ontology

Evaluation

The investigators evaluated the ontology by comparing the concepts and integration of content versus the occurrence of diagnoses found in regular clinical practice. Out of 32 cases, the clinicians' view fully differed from the ontology's in only one case. In addition, the investigators found that the clinicians had partially similar views in 11 cases and identical views in 20 cases of how the information was represented in the clinic and in the ontology.

13.4.3.9 Future of Ontologies in Medical/Dental Care

The need for better representation of patient data is likely to increase since we are now rapidly adopting information technology in all levels of healthcare. This will require making sense of large and disparate volumes of information. Thus, healthcare will have to embrace the adoption of technologies that seamlessly support data integration. Therefore, knowledge representation, and especially ontologies, will likely play a role in supporting this integration.

Disclaimer The views presented in this chapter are solely of the authors and do not necessarily represent the views of the US Government, Department of Health and Human Services and/or the Centers for Disease Control and Prevention.

References

Ai J, Smith B, Wong DT. Saliva ontology: an ontology-based framework for a Salivaomics knowledge base. BMC Bioinformatics. 2010;11:302.

American Dental Association. Current dental terminology. Chicago, IL: American Dental Association; 1991.

American Dental Association. ADA1000-2010D – ANSI/ADA standard clinical data architecture for the structure & content of an electronic health record. 2003. https://ebusinessadaorg/productcatalog/491/Informatics/ANSIADA-Standard-No-1000-for-Standard-Clinical-Data-Architec/ADA1000-2010D. Accessed 10 Jun 2018.

Baader F, Horrocks I, Sattler U. Description logics. In: Handbook on ontologies. Berlin: Springer; 2004. p. 3–28.

Bader JD, Shugars DA. What do we know about how dentists make caries-related treatment decisions? Commun Dent Oral Epidemiol. 1997;25(1):97–103.

Bejan A, Lorente S. The constructal law of design and evolution in nature. Philos Trans R Soc Lond B Biol Sci. 2010;365(1545):1335–47.

Bertaud-Gounot V, Richard F, Le Moing C, Duvauferrier R. Ontology of dental emergencies for diagnostic classification. Cape Town: Medinfo; 2010.

Bertaud-Gounot V, Duvauferrier R, Burgun A. Ontology and medical diagnosis. Inform Health Soc Care. 2012;37(2):51–61.

California Dental Association. Diagnostic code changes approaching. Sacramento, CA: California Dental Association; 2015. https://wwwcdaorg/news-events/diagnostic-code-changes-approaching. Accessed 10 Jun 2018

Campbell KE, Oliver DE, Spackman KA, Shortliffe EH. Representing thoughts, words, and things in the UMLS. J Am Med Inform Assoc. 1998;5(5):421–31.

Canadian Dental Association. Uniform system of codes and list of services. Ottawa, ON: CDA; 2001.

Falkman G, Gustafsson M, Jontell M, Torgersson O. SOMWeb: a semantic web-based system for supporting collaboration of distributed medical communities of practice. J Med Internet Res. 2008;10(3):e25.

Gangemi A, Guarino N, Masolo C, Oltramari A, Schneider L. Sweetening ontologies with DOLCE. In: Gómez-Pérez A, Benjamins VR, editors. Knowledge engineering and knowledge management. Ontologies and the semantic web, 13th international conference. EKAW 2002. Siguenza: Springer; 2002. p. 166–81.

Gasevic D, Djuric D, Devedzic V. Model driven architecture and ontology development. 1st ed. Berlin: Springer; 2006.

Grenon P, Smith B, Goldberg L. Biodynamic ontology: applying BFO in the biomedical domain. In: Pisanelli DM, editor. Ontologies in medicine. Amsterdam: IOS Press; 2004. p. 20–38.

Gruber TR. A translation approach to portable ontology specifications. Knowl Acquis. 1993;5(2):199–220.

Guarino N. Formal ontology in information systems. In: Guarino N, editor. Proceedings of the first international conference (FOIS'98). Trento: IOS Press; 1998. p. 3–15.

Hammond WE, Cimino JJ. Standards in biomedical informatics. In: Shorliffe EH, Cimino JJ, editors. Biomedical informatics: computer applications in healthcare and biomedicine. New York, NY: Springer; 2006.

Howerton WB Jr, Mora MA. Advancements in digital imaging: what is new and on the horizon? J Am Dent Assoc. 2008;139(Suppl):20S–4.

Jernigan DB, Davies J, Sim A. Data standards in public health informatics. In: O'Carroll PW, Yasnoff WA, Ward ME, Ripp LH, Martin EL, editors. Public health informatics and information systems. New York, NY: Springer; 2010. p. 213–38.

Jurkovich M. Dentistry and diagnostic coding. DrBicuspidcom. 2017. https://wwwdrbicuspidcom/indexaspx?sec=sup&sub=pmt&pag=dis&ItemID=321486. Accessed 10 Jun 2018.

Leake JL. Diagnostic codes in dentistry–definition, utility and developments to date. J Can Dent Assoc. 2002;68(7):403–6.

Lepsky S, Jurkovich M, Jönzzon K. ICD-10-CM for the dental industry. Workgroup for electronic data interchange. 2015. https://wwwwediorg/forms/uploadFiles/6D70900000026tocWEDI_ICD_10_CM_Module_II__11122015__FINALpdf. Accessed 10 Jun 2018.

Long JJ, Goldberg L. Diagnostic criteria of Sjögren's syndrome: a study in knowledge transfer. Orlando, FL: ADEA/AADR/CADR Meeting & Exhibition; 2006. p. 1461.

Manchir M. Newly approved standard enables electronic capture of patient diagnoses. ADA News. 7 Dec 2016. https://www.ada.org/en/publications/ada-news/2016-archive/december/newly-approved-standard-enables-electronic-capture-of-patient-diagnoses. Accessed 10 Jun 2018.

Musen M. Generation of model-based knowledge-acquisition tools for clinical-trial advice systems. Stanford, CA: Stanford University; 1988.

Newell A. The knowledge level. Artificial Intelligence. 1982;18(1):87–127.

Noy N, Tudorache T, Nyulas C, Musen M. The ontology life cycle: integrated tools for editing, publishing, peer review, and evolution of ontologies. AMIA Annu Symp Proc. 2010;2010:552–6.

Ogden DK, Richards IA. The meaning of meaning: a study of the influence of language upon thought and of the science of symbolism. New York, NY: Harcourt Brace; 1923. 1930

Powell MA. Money in Mesopotamia. J Econ Soc Hist Orient. 1996;39(3):224–42.

Rubin DL, Shah NH, Noy NF. Biomedical ontologies: a functional perspective. Brief Bioinform. 2008;9(1):75–90.

Sandholm T. The philosophy of the grid: ontology theory – from Aristotle to self-managed IT resources. Report no.: technical report TRITA-NA-0532. Stockholm: Royal Institute of Technology; 2005.

Smith B. The basic tools of formal ontology. In: Guarino N, editor. Formal ontology in information systems. Amsterdam, Oxford, Tokyo, Washington, DC: IOS Press (Frontiers in Artificial Intelligence and Applications); 1998. p. 19–28.

Smith B, Brochhausen M. Establishing and harmonizing ontologies in an interdisciplinary health care and clinical research environment. Health Technol Inform. 2008;134:219–34.

SNODDS. SNODDS dental diagnostic system. 2016. http://dentaldiagnosticterminology.org/. Accessed 10 Jun 2018.

SNOMED International. SNOMED CT General Dentistry Diagnostic refset package Release Notes – Jan 2018. https://confluence.ihtsdotools.org/display/RMT/SNOMED+CT+General+Dentistry+Diagnostic+refset+package+Release+Notes+-+January+2018. Accessed 10 Jun 2018.

Soderlund K. ADA assists members in transition to ICD-10. ADA News Aug 11 2015. https://wwwadaorg/en/publications/ada-news/2015-archive/august/ada-assists-members-in-transition-to-icd-10. Accessed 10 Jun 2018.

Staad S, Studer R. Handbook on Ontologies, Springer; 2nd ed. Berlin: Heidelberg; 2009.

Starr P. INTRODUCTION, The Social Origins of Professional Sovereignty. In: Starr P. The Social Transformation of American Medicine: The rise of a sovereign profession and the making of a vast industry. 2nd ed. New York: Basic Books; 2017. p. 3–29.

Torres-Urquidy MH, Schleyer T. Formal conceptualization of dental diagnoses: status report. In: Okada M, Smith B, editors. Proceedings of the second interdisciplinary ontology meeting. Feb–Mar: Tokyo; 2009. p. 17–23.

Torres-Urquidy MH. Characterization of the Cognitive Structures Used by Dentists. Pending Dissertation: University of Pittsburgh; 2012.

van der Lei J, Musen MA. The separation of reviewing knowledge form medical knowledge. Methods Inf Med. 1995;34(1–2):131–9.

Wächter T, Schroeder M. Semi-automated ontology generation within OBO-edit. Bioinformatics. 2010;26(12):i88–96.

World Health Organization. Application of the international classification of diseases to dentistry and stomatology ICD-DA, vol. 3. Geneva: World Health Organization; 1994.

World Wide Web Consortium (W3C). OWL web ontology language overview. 2011. http://wwww3org/TR/owl-features/. Accessed 30 May 2011.

Chapter 14
American National Standards for Health Data Integration

Mark Diehl†, Ted Klein, and Valerie Powell

14.1 Introduction to American National Standards

At the 1996 annual meeting of the American Dental Association a resolution was adopted by the House of Delegates stating a vision where a continuum of patient health data, unencumbered by boundaries dictated by profession, specialty or discipline improves the quality of health outcomes, patient safety, and economy of care delivery.[1] With this resolution, the American Dental Association became the first and remains the only major health care professional organization to endorse whole-patient integration of patient health data. The Association considers the electronic health record to be a complete collection of patient data, a compilation of an individual's lifetime health conditions and health care from conception through post-mortem. This body of patient data is in automated form (i.e., electronic form) rather than an automated conversion of conventional physical paper documents.

The American Dental Association's Standards Committee on Dental Informatics (SCDI) subsequently created a number of standards that implement the House of Delegates 1996 Resolution. Specification 1039 presents a conceptual data model for clinical care. Specification 1000 presents a logical data model for health care data.

[1] The American Dental Association House of Delegates Resolution 92H-1996 states this vision of seamless accessibility of health information throughout all aspects of health care, independent of profession, discipline or specialty, or care delivery environment.

† (Deceased)

M. Diehl
Health Informatics Program, Misericordia University, Dallas, TX, USA

T. Klein
Klein Consulting Informatics, LLC, Star Valley Ranch, WY, USA
e-mail: kci@tklein.com

V. Powell (✉)
Robert Morris University, Pittsburgh, PA, USA
e-mail: powell@rmu.edu

A. Acharya et al. (eds.), *Integration of Medical and Dental Care and Patient Data*, Health Informatics, https://doi.org/10.1007/978-3-319-98298-4_14

Both are American National Standards approved by the American National Standards Institute (ANSI) and both address whole-patient data and cross the professional and specialty boundaries traditionally separating medicine, dentistry, and other health care professions. When taken together, along with the companion implementation guide, these standards provide a blueprint for the construction of databases containing whole-patient health data and provide the foundation for semantic interoperability in the exchange of health information. Both the Specification 1039 and 1000 apply to the data tier of health information systems, providing the conceptual and logical data structures for persisting[2] the patient's health data.

The Specifications 1000, 1039, and related publications are based on current state and federal medico-legal requirements for health records, application of information theory, and the data requirements to support clinical processes and care outcomes. These standards are the only American National Standards that focus on the patient or health care recipient rather than on the management of health records, data exchange, or the encounter or business aspects of care delivery.

At the heart of these standards are models that conform to standard information modeling best practices.[3] These standards include a progression of standard information models from a clinical conceptual process model and a clinical conceptual data model to a clinical logical data model. The data entities and attributes presented in these standards are those needed to operationalize the processes identified in the process model. Because these data models are derived from a comprehensive, whole-patient clinical process model, the data likewise applies uniformly across professional and specialty boundaries.

Information modeling is an appropriate technique to develop a comprehensive understanding of healthcare processes and the data supporting these processes. The American Society for Testing and Materials (ASTM) standard E2145 for information modeling best practices defines a model as a representation in any form of real or envisioned things or events. Models provide a means to understand structures, processes, and concepts where size and complexity renders human perception or comprehension difficult or impossible. Models are valuable tools to explain, analyze or predict processes and structures, which currently exist, have existed in the past, or may exist in the future. The size, scope, and complexity of the health care delivery environment, along with the complexity of health knowledge and health care processes, makes information models an ideal vehicle to assist human understanding.

14.2 Modeling Process

As noted in ASTM E2145, information models progress from a description of processes through increasingly detailed descriptions of the data needed to enable these processes. As illustrated in Fig. 14.1, the data description depends upon a description of the processes that use these data, and the models provide a means to efficiently and effectively describe both processes and data.

[2] Storing data in the long term.

[3] ASTM 2145-07 Standard Practice for Information Modeling. Available from www.ASTM.org

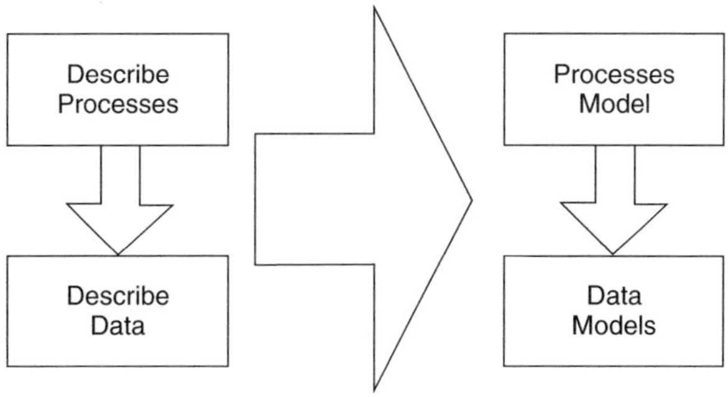

Fig. 14.1 Overview of the modeling process

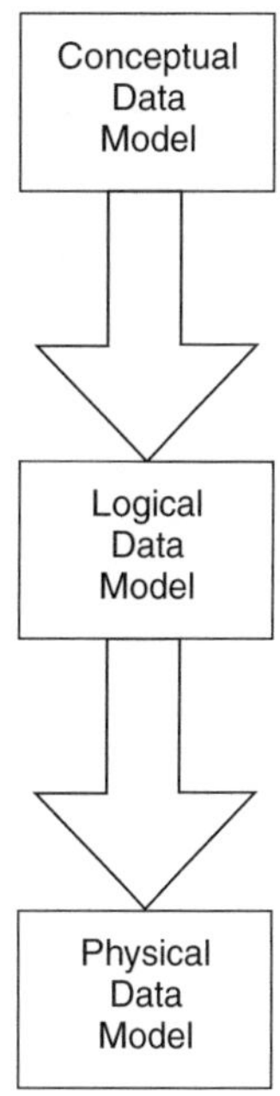

Fig. 14.2 Sequence of models generated to reach a comprehensive representation of healthcare activities

This approach predates information system and information theory, going back to the fundamental teachings of the architect Louis Sullivan, "form ever follows function."[4] The *process model* describes the processes and provides the starting point for a conceptual data model. The *conceptual data model* then identifies the fundamental data items and relationships used by the processes. The conceptual data model is the origin of one or more *logical data models* that expand upon and detail the conceptual data. The logical data models then become the origin of the *physical data model*—a description of the structure of persistent data to be deployed on a specific technology (Fig. 14.2).

[4] Louis H. Sullivan regarded excessively decorative elements as superfluous. Likewise in information modeling, excessive detail and ornamentation contribute little to understanding, rather these serve to complicate design, inhibit comprehension, and ultimately defeat the purposes of information modeling. See http://www.famousquotesandauthors.com/authors/louis_h_sullivan_quotes.html and http://en.wikipedia.org/wiki/Louis_Sullivan

This progression of models ensures that the data structure implemented in the system accurately and effectively meets the needs of the processes it supports.

The original Specification 1000 standard was adopted in 2001 and contained a description of the process model and data models. The Specification 1039 standard expanded upon this description and formalized the process model and derivation of the clinical conceptual data model. Both Specifications employ a structured description using the ANSI standard IDEF notation, IDEF0 for process modeling and IDEF1X for information modeling.[5] The IDEF notation has been successfully used in healthcare activity and data modeling the public and private sector organizations for well over a decade.[6,7]

14.3 ANSI/ADA Specification 1039[8]

The Specification 1039 establishes a shared understanding of the structure and content of data needed to support healthcare processes. It is the foundation for a variety of more detailed data representations of clinical information. Specification 1039 also determines the structure and content of clinical data presented in the various types of electronic health and patient records. The Specification document provides descriptions and graphic depictions of those activities and data structures specific to clinical healthcare and population health services. It presents a view of the mainstream of individual and population health and care delivery processes found in the United States, drawing generalities from the activities shared among practitioners and providers. Non-clinical processes and data structures (e.g. administrative, financial, supply chain, etc.) are addressed if they directly relate to personal and population health, and directly support healthcare delivery processes. Important to the reader is that this Specification does not address or establish standards for clinical care. It does not establish standards for the quality, efficacy or effectiveness of clinical practice, the conduct of clinical research, or informatics standards for manufacturing processes in the healthcare supporting industries.

In order to best support healthcare delivery, independent of technology, healthcare profession or specialty, or care delivery environment, the Specification of the clinical conceptual data model applies the "form follows function" approach. This

[5] IDEF methodology described by the National Institute of Standards and Technology, Federal Information Processing Standards Publications 183 Integrated Definition for Function Modeling (IDEF0) and 184 Integrated Definition for Information Modeling (IDEF1X), 23 December 1993. IDEF0 aims at capturing "decisions", "actions" and "activities" and IDEF1X has the goal of modeling data for using it as a resource. These use graphical representations as part of the modeling process.

[6] Bourke, M. K. Strategy and Architecture of Health care Information Systems. New York: Springer. 1994.

[7] United States Department of Defense, Military Health System (MHS) IDEF Process and Data Models used in the MHS Functional Area Model–Activity (FAM-A), and MHS Functional Area Model–Data (FAM-D), various dates.

[8] Available from the American Dental Association, Department of Standards Administration, 211 E. Chicago Ave., Chicago, IL 60611.

Table 14.1 Diagnostic therapeutic cycle

Human decision process	Equivalent healthcare decision process
Observation	Data acquisition
Reasoning	Diagnosis
Planning	Treatment plan
Action	Treatment

approach first analyzes the fundamental activities shared throughout the delivery of healthcare services.

This analysis creates a *clinical conceptual process model* as a high level structured analysis of the activities shared by care providers in the delivery of health care services. The component detail of the process model is such that it is possible to identify the principal types of data needed to support these activities, but it is only specified until activities of health care providers diverge. The model does not reach the depth of detail where the differences in clinical and business practices require differences in the description of activities and supporting data content and structure. The conceptual process model therefore establishes a clinical foundation for the conceptual data model that directly ties the data structure to clinical process.

All healthcare providers share a common, rational process in performing clinical services, the Diagnostic-Therapeutic Cycle.[9] This process is identical to that employed in other human decision processes, consisting of observation, reasoning and action, as illustrated in the table below (Table 14.1):

In IDEF0 notation, the Clinical Process or Diagnostic-Therapeutic Cycle appears in the Specification reflects the four fundamental processes performed in clinical care, and in many other service roles like automotive repair. The first process is to gather information about the case at hand. Component tasks may include performing a physical or clinical examination, use of imaging and physiologic instrumentation, performing histopathology and clinical chemistry studies, etc. Collectively, these produce a body of information that the doctor uses to determine one or more diagnoses and etiologies, as performed in the diagnosis, or data analysis process. One of the possible outcomes of the diagnostic process is the need for additional data, such as a radiographic referral. A differential diagnosis (e.g. Multiple myeloma 0.85, MGUS 0.11, plasmacytoma 0.04) may be the result of the diagnosis process, though commonly providers work from only a single diagnosis. A treatment plan process establishes the intervention plan to address the diagnosis. In complex cases, especially involving coordinated care among multiple professions and specialties, this plan may be constructed in multiple steps, may be revised as needed, and may indicate the need for acquisition of additional diagnostic data or performing a subsequent diagnosis step. In the treatment process those interventions identified in the treatment plan are performed. An important note is that outcome assessment is a subsequent performance of this process, where the assessed outcome is the product of the diagnostic process and may indicate the need for subsequent care.

[9] This Diagnostic-Therapeutic Cycle is variously known by a variety of terms and is widely cited in the medicine texts used in first-year professional education; this is also noted in Van Bemmel, J., and M. A. Musen (Eds.). Handbook of Medical Informatics. first edition. Springer. 1997.

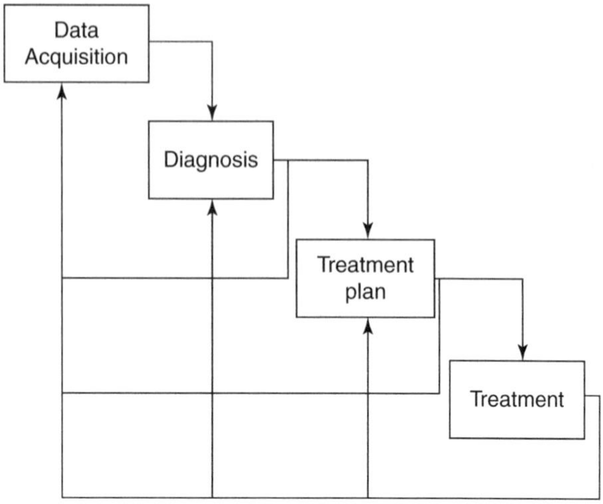

Fig. 14.3 Clinical process as recursive activities

IDEF0 identifies the individual activities and illustrates the relationships among these without showing the sequence in which these are performed. For the clinical process, this is important since the progression of these activities is rarely a single waterfall path, but rather a cascade with branches to previous activities as shown below (Fig. 14.3).

The extensive recursion illustrated above reflects clinical events where a provider may need to return to a previous activity to develop additional data, for example, where during diagnosis the need for data from additional clinical tests becomes evident. This clinical process is continuously repeated over a period of time until the course of care is completed.

The arrows in the IDEF diagram are called ICOMs, standing for *Inputs*, *Controls*, *Outputs*, and *Mechanisms*. *Controls* are those things that are employed to regulate or constrain the activity. *Inputs* are what is consumed or changed by the activity, and *Outputs* are newly created or modified things produced by the activity. Data or information under this notation is always an output or a control—it can never be an input since it the original data or information is never altered or destroyed. The ICOMs, especially the outputs and controls define categories of data to be represented in the conceptual data model. These also approximate the major subject areas in the logical data model derived from the conceptual data model.

As shown in the Fig. 14.4, the Specification 1039 conceptual data model is centered on the individual, a single person or other living thing.[10]

In this model (Fig. 14.4), every individual has one or more health conditions, defined as their state of health and well-being. As noted in the process model diagram shown above, an output of the Obtain Patient Health Data activity is Health Service Information including the body of Health Facts. The data model diagram shows the connection between the Individual and one or more Health Facts gener-

[10] Other conceptual models are centered on the provider, the procedure, or the encounter.

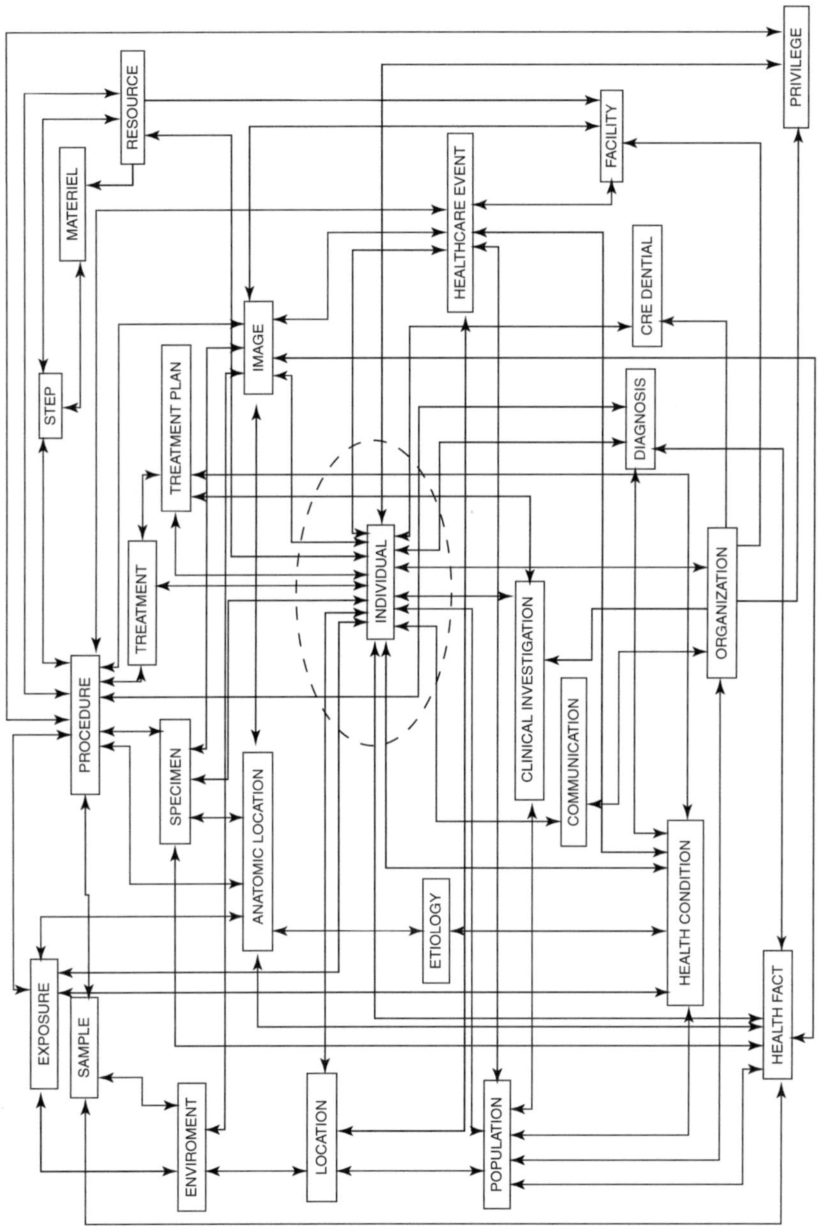

Fig. 14.4 Model showcasing the interactions of the individual with different elements supporting the healthcare delivery process

ated by that activity. The care provider operates on the assembled body of facts to determine a diagnosis and etiology, and the patient and care provider determine the course of care as a Treatment Plan. This plan may be linked to a desired or intended Health Condition as an expected outcome.

In both the process model and the data model, neither the activities nor data are siloed or compartmentalized by profession or specialty. This conceptual data model serves as the starting point for a clinical logical data model, in the Specification 1000, and becomes one span of the bridge linking the clinical database to the clinical processes it supports.

14.4 ANSI/ADA Specification 1000

The ANSI/ADA Specification 1000 was approved as an American National Standard by ANSI on 2 February 2001. This standard was initiated in response to the American Dental Association House of Delegates Resolution 92H-1996 previously cited. The origin of this work was the Computer-based Oral Health Record concept model in the mid-1990s. The standard was the culmination of a work effort that created a standard health care logical data model based on the COHR Concept Model, and conducted protracted public review of its component subject areas from 1997 through 2000. A revision and updating of the standard and its logical data model began consensus review in 2008 and was approved by ANSI on 22 February 2010.

The Specification 1000v2 logical data model was developed by expanding upon the Specification 1039 conceptual data model. The numerous 'many-to-many' relationships were broken, additional entities created, and attributes added to the entities to provide detail. Several new subject areas were added to reflect expanding interest in the application of the logical model to health care practice, management, and regulation. The Specification logical data model now contains 32 subject areas as identified below:

Individual	Organization healthcare materiel item
Individual characteristics	Provider healthcare materiel
Population	Patient health facts
Population characteristics	Patient specimen
Organization	Patient object
Location	Population health facts
Location associations	Patient health condition diagnosis
Location characteristics	Population health condition diagnosis
Communication	Patient treatment plan
Health care event	Treatment plan expected outcome
Health services provider	Population outcome reference
Provider credentials and privileges	Patient health service
Healthcare services	Clinical investigation
Health services objects	Clinical investigation design
Health care materiel	Codes and nomenclature
Healthcare materiel item	Reference tables

The concept of 'individual' is used rather than separate entities for patient or care recipient, provider, other interested party, etc. These component roles are type coded in other subject areas and are consistent with the entity-role designation in other standards such as the Health Level Seven Reference Information Model. The term Individual also allows for application to non-human recipients of health services, as in veterinary medicine. Where other industry standard and common data models in medicine and health care are usually from the context of the heath care encounter, the healthcare procedure, or its reimbursement, the context of the Specification 1000 logical data model is the individual and their condition of health and well-being. The Individual subject area is, therefore, the key and essential focal point of the Specification. This subject area establishes a standard data structure for the identification of all participants in the health care process.

14.5 Subject Area Descriptions

The Individual subject area provides a standard structure for the human name that is independent of cultural, geographic tradition, or language constraints. The same data structure is applicable to represent names in the individual's own preferred form. Thus a person's native Spanish or Asian name structure and content can be represented with the same data structure as readily as with a Western name structure.

Recognizing there is no uniformity internationally regarding the application of a national patient identifier, the Specification allows for a system-assigned identifier or a national identifier is applicable. Any number of alternate patient identifiers, such as motor vehicle operator number or another government-assigned identification number, can be represented. This data structure, where the individual's identification, name, associated detail and characteristics, and health data are in separate entities, readily enables deidentification of health care data for purposes such as research or to implement data privacy and confidentiality provisions.

The Individual Characteristics subject area presents a structure to record the essential characteristics of an individual as used in patient registration, demographic and epidemiology applications. An Individual may have one or more characteristics represented through a subtyping into eight separate entities by Race, Ethnicity, Language, Religion, Sex Characteristic, Taxonomy, Living Arrangement, and Physical Characteristic. Sex Characteristic is preferred over terms such as Administrative Sex, to allow for multiple characteristics to be presented (e.g. anatomic sex, sex preference, etc.). The Taxonomy enables consistent classification of non-human living things.

The Living Arrangement and Physical Characteristic are new entities added in this revision. The Living Arrangement contains data, such as noting whether an individual lives alone, that may be of importance when planning a course of care. The Physical Characteristic is a collective entity used to contain any number of data items, such as hair color, body mass index, etc., that are not generally considered a health fact.

The Population Characteristics subject area has much the same data structure as the Individual Characteristics, allowing for comparison of an individual with one or more populations in which that individual is a member. This relationship provides a data structure that also enables a key and essential element of evidence-based practice where expected outcome is predicted by experience in the appropriate population.

The Organization subject area establishes a standard data structure for the identification of organizations, the relationships among these organizations, and the relationships between the organizations and individuals participating in the health care process. The Location subject area provides a data structure that identifies, names and positions a specific location (geographic, not anatomic) as well as linking that location to individual and organizational occupants.

The Communication subject area creates a standard data structure for communications among individuals and organizations involved in the health care process. This data structure and its reference values are consistent with the Health Level Seven 2.X standards. The Health Care Event subject area reflects that the traditional view of the health care encounter or episode is being challenged by increasing emphasis care delivered outside of the health care facility and the impact of telemedicine and information technology. This subject area reflects that all such health care events share a common set of characteristics, being the junction of all participants of health care services at a point in time, unconstrained by physical co-location.

The Health Services Provider subject area identifies providers, classifies these as either individual providers (doctor, nurse, etc.) or an organizational provider (hospital, clinic, private practice, etc.), and associates the provider with locations and one or more professional specialties performed at a location.

The Provider Credentials and Privileges subject area establishes a standard data structure to identify and characterize the level of a healthcare professional's expertise obtained through formal training along with any other credentials obtained by that individual. This subject area contains data items used to assign credentials and privileges for both accreditation and certification. It also identifies and characterizes those services and procedures that a healthcare provider is authorized by an organization or other individual to deliver or perform and contains data that characterize a provider such as used in enrollment and credentialing transactions.

The Health Services Objects subject area contains object data, such as video images, of healthcare services and their components such as procedures and steps. These objects may be associated with individuals or organizations, such as a procedure associated with a particular hospital or practitioner. This subject area also provides a data structure to enable a detailed audio/video training module, such as for administration of an anesthetic block or performing a specific incisional biopsy.

The Health Care Materiel subject area establishes a standard data structure for those materiel items used in healthcare processes, where the Healthcare Materiel Item subject area links that data with a specific procedure for an individual. The Organization Healthcare Materiel Item subject area contains data structures required to track materiel items within an organization, such as in keeping an inventory of healthcare materiel at clinical locations, routing these items to the point of delivery of care services, and the subsequent recovery and disposition of those items. The Provider Healthcare Materiel subject area contains data structures to enable documentation of a provider's selection of specific materiel items to perform a procedure, reflecting the professional desires of that provider.

Another essential concept in this Specification is the representation of clinical knowledge about the case at hand. The Patient Health Facts subject area creates a structure for patient information that identifies and describes an individual's health facts at a date and time. The term fact as a collective term containing all relevant information items is preferred over separate terms such as finding, observation, symptom, etc., that are subtypes of the parent Fact entity.

The Patient Specimen subject area provides the data structure to document surrogates for that patient, such as excreta, secreta, blood and blood components, tissue, and tissue fluids that have been collected from an individual. The Patient Object subject area presents a data structure to link an image or other representation of an individual's physical structure or process, and handled as a large data stream with associated processes needed to reconstruct the object.

The Population Health Facts subject area presents a structure that organizes and structures population health information as the basis for comparison to an individual's health facts.

The Patient Health Condition Diagnosis subject area establishes a standard data structure for the determination of an individual's health conditions supporting the diagnostic processes performed by a care provider.

The Population Health Condition Diagnosis subject area provides a data structures [sic] serving as an evidence-basis or reference for the diagnostic processes used by a care provider to determine an individual's health condition.

The Patient Treatment Plan subject area presents data structures required to support the planning of health care services, presentation to the care recipient, and informed consent by the care recipient. The Treatment Plan Expected Outcome subject area enables the documentation of the desired or expected outcome on which the treatment plan is based. The Population Outcome Reference subject area presents a data structure reference to support the evidence-based logical processes. For example, this could be used to determine the probability of achieving an outcome for an individual, if this is known for the population of which that individual is a member and which presents those same health facts and diagnoses.

The Clinical Investigation subject area provides a data structure supporting clinical investigations in health care research, identifying the participants in a clinical investigation (e.g. investigators, organization, etc.), the type of study population (e.g. control population), and specifies the hypothesis. This can also link the investigation to another study. The Clinical Investigation Design subject area contains data that identifies and details the study methodology or protocol along with specific materiel to be used. This subject area also identifies the subjects participating in the investigation and associates those individuals with the study population.

The Codes and Nomenclature and Reference Tables subject areas are essential to provide reference data for the implementing subject areas, such as individual and population characteristics, clinical components and the supporting services. The Codes and Nomenclature subject area provides a standard data structure to identify, characterize, and track over time those reference codes and nomenclature used in the health care process, present these independent of language, and relate codes both within a code system and to codes in other code systems.

14.6 ANSI/ADA Specification 1027

Implementation of this Specification is addressed in the ANSI/ADA Specification 1027 Implementation Guide. This document shows how to forward engineer the logical data model, optimize the physical data model, and create a functioning database that is Specification 1000 compliant. The importance of compliance lies in the benefits of seamless, Standards-compliant data. Such data provides the semantic interoperability that along with the syntactic interoperability of standards such as promoted by Health Level Seven, enables individuals to share thought. Without this semantic interoperability a concept may not be totally understood when conveyed from one person to another, even though the physical communication may have succeeded.

14.7 Anticipating Oral Health Inclusion in Mainstream Standards

What this section is about are the social-technical issues in including oral health in standards. As standards have been prepared for the development of health information technology, the question arose as to whether dental records should be explicitly included. In the 1990s Schleyer and Eisner (1994) envisioned "Dental Interface Objects" which would "communicate patient information between computer systems of physicians, dentists, dental specialists, and other partners in the healthcare team."

Schleyer (2004) cited the ADA House of Delegates resolution 92H-1996, calling for "the seamless availability of patient health information across health care professions, specialties and care delivery environments." (American Dental Association 1996) Schleyer felt that what was then called the National Health Information Infrastructure (NHII) could not only address "missed health care opportunities," but could also "facilitate collaboration among general dentists and specialists." Schleyer recommended an educational campaign to help dentists understand the potential benefits of NHII. He mentioned ANSI/ADA Specification No. 1000 and the dental extensions to DICOM as "essential building blocks." Schleyer felt that dentistry should "become an active participant" in the NHII. Diehl (2002) states that "cross-enterprise data integration removes the barriers that prevent timely access to accurate and professionally meaningful health information."

Farman (2002) pointed out that the DICOM (Digital Imaging and Communications in Medicine) standard, at that time, could support intraoral radiography, panoramic radiography, cephalometric radiography, CT, intraoral cameras, and other modalities of interest in oral healthcare. He reports that the American Dental Association (ADA) became a member of the DICOM standards committee in 1996. In 1998 and 1999, respectively, supplements to the DICOM standard were approved covering radiography and visual light imaging used in dentistry. According to Farman, in 2000 the ADA first "suggested" and then formally recommended DICOM implementation for the communication of images in dentistry.

In order to avoid unanticipated vocabulary problems, the HL7 standard attempts to be as agnostic as possible as to vocabulary content. In fact, in the upcoming HL7 version 2.8 (under very active development), all vocabulary items that are not internal HL7-only structures (like those that describe the types of technical acknowledgments, etc.) are being removed from the normative part of the standard precisely because those who do not read the standard carefully treat the lists of 'suggested values' as the normative values that must be used. This is erroneous, and leads to under-specified vocabulary. These suggested values will be explicitly identified as values that some using HL7 have found useful, and should not be considered as mandatory for use.

In all cases when using standards, the latest version should be consulted (even if an earlier version is being implemented). Over the years, all standards include new material in later releases that are often useful for understanding best practice for using the standards, and even may provide useful hints for piecemeal extensions when an existing older version doesn't quite meet all the requirements, but business conditions mandate that a complete newer version cannot be fully used.

If the designers of a healthcare-related standard are not working from a goal of serving "all of healthcare," including oral health, and if the example of HL7 is not followed, there is a risk of over-constraining vocabulary by confining vocabulary to that in specific lists. An example could be a list of provider degrees or clinical credentials. Obviously if such a list (as a reference table in a relational database) contains the role designations MD, DO, DNP, and RN, but not DDS, DMD, or RDH, then dentistry would be excluded. Another kind of improper constraint could arise from misuse of a Role-Based Access Control (RBAC) matrix, where dental provider role categories are entered as not being permitted to prescribe or administer medications. These two examples are based on discovered instances involving incorrect interpretations of standards or of following outdated standards documents. Any method for specification of anatomic sites that precludes use of the anatomic site representation and identification necessary for dental care (such as uniquely numbering deciduous, permanent, and supernumerary teeth) would be incapable of supporting integration of medical and dental records. At the Society for Imaging Informatics in Medicine (SIIM) conference in 2010, PACS (Picture Archiving and Communication System) vendors pointed out that DICOM-compliant PACS technology for veterinary practices already supported integration of medical and dental care and patient records (DICOM 2006). Another risk is not achieving the same level of specificity in the content dimension in standards for oral health as for other domains of healthcare.

References

American Dental Association. Council on dental practice: supplemental record 1 – seamless electronic patient record. Supplement to annual reports and resolutions. Chicago, IL: American Dental Association; 1996. p. 282–3.

DICOM. DICOM correction item CP-643, add veterinary identification tags. 2006. ftp://medicalnemaorg/MEDICAL/Dicom/Final/cp643_ftpdf. Accessed 10 Jun 2018.

Diehl M. What data integration means to the practicing dentist. Dent Clin N Am. 2002;46:606–15.

Farman AG. Use and implication of the DICOM standard in dentistry. Dent Clin N Am. 2002;46:565–73.

Schleyer TKL. Should dentistry be part of the national health information infrastructure? J Am Dent Assoc. 2004;135(12):1687–95.

Schleyer T, Eisner J. The computer-based oral health record: an essential tool for cross-provider quality management. CDA J. 1994;22:57–64.

Chapter 15
Economics of Clinical Data Integration

Stephen Foreman, Joseph Kilsdonk, and Kelly Boggs

15.1 A Cost Benefit Analysis of Expanding Dental Insurance Coverage

15.1.1 Introduction

Dental health insurance coverage in the United States (US) is either nonexistent (Medicare and the uninsured), spotty (Medicaid) or limited (most employer-based private benefit plans) (HealthCare.gov 2018). More than 114 million Americans do not have dental insurance at all (NADP Dental Plans 2018). A recent survey found that 18% of adults in the US were unable to access dental care based on cost (Federal Reserve System 2017). Perhaps as a result, there is lack of dental health utilization in the United States. What public policy makers may not appreciate is that the lack of dental health care access in the US increases medical care cost expenditures. Improving dental benefits will likely decrease the overall health care costs by an amount that is greater than the cost of the improved benefits (ADA News 2018).

Given the current debate over repeal of the Affordable Care Act, it would appear to be politically and economically difficult or impossible to expand dental insurance

S. Foreman (✉)
Health Economics, Robert Morris University, Pittsburgh, PA, USA
e-mail: foreman@rmu.edu

J. Kilsdonk
Office of Medical Education, Aspirus Healthcare Systems, Wausau, WI, USA
e-mail: joseph.kilsdonk@aspirus.org

K. Boggs
Network Engagement, Aspirus Network Inc., Wausau, WI, USA

Joseph Kilsdonk and Kelly Bogg were formely with Marshfield Clinic.

A. Acharya et al. (eds.), *Integration of Medical and Dental Care and Patient Data*, Health Informatics, https://doi.org/10.1007/978-3-319-98298-4_15

coverage (Sommers et al. 2017). Health insurance costs have been rising at double digit rates (Amadeo 2016). Employers have been limiting or dropping health care coverage rather than expanding it. In 2012, 50.1% of employers offered a health insurance benefit while in 2015, it was 45.7% (Vistnes et al. 2015). Lack of dental coverage has remained as a barrier for the required care, hence expanding dental insurance coverage would improve access to affordable care especially for geriatric people and people with disabilities. Medicaid funding is a major source of state government spending. Many states suffer budget challenges from their Medicaid commitments. Expanding Medicaid dental coverage during times of budget challenge would meet substantial political resistance as well. Addressing issues related to provider payment and shortages are critical.

A report estimated that $42 trillion dollars will be spent between 2016 and 2030 to treat chronic conditions (Masterson 2017). What may well be unknown to the public, and to policy makers, is that strong and increasing evidence suggests relationships between oral health and a range of chronic illnesses. Such findings show correlations between periodontal inflammatory conditions and diabetes, myocardial infarction, coronary artery disease, stroke, preeclampsia, and rheumatoid arthritis and other chronic conditions (Eke et al. 2015; Firestein 2003; Mealey and Oates 2006; Xu et al. 2017). This suggests that improved oral health may well have the potential to reduce the incidence of chronic diseases as well as their complications. If chronic disease incidence is alleviated it will be possible to avoid medical care costs. It would be important to know more about the extent to which improved oral health could reduce health care costs and improve lives.

Further studies are necessary for costs and benefits of providing Medicare and Medicaid dental benefits, or the cost of providing dental insurance to the uninsured. Few studies have indicated that periodontitis increases medical care costs (Chalmers et al. 2017; Glurich et al. 2017; Ide et al. 2007; Sato et al. 2016). A controlled study to assess the benefit of providing dental coverage through a government payer system will provide comprehensive information. For a preliminary inquiry, one can consider work already done and using some cost and benefit estimates, determine whether it is possible that benefits of extending dental coverage outweigh costs.

15.1.2 Dental Insurance and Coverage in the United States

The failure of traditional Medicare to cover dental care has engendered some (albeit not much) public debate (Willink et al. 2016). The expense of the Medicare prescription drug program and the controversy surrounding its enactment may well have eroded public support for expanded Medicare coverage (Oberlander 2015). While there has been no shortage of effort paid to improving Medicare, the one common theme in all of the initiatives is that dental care has been conspicuously omitted. As a result, 55.5 million Medicare recipients continue to have no dental insurance coverage through Medicare (Henry J Kaiser Family Foundation 2015).

Medicaid dental coverage is an optional benefit that states may or may not elect to provide. Forty-six states and the District of Columbia provide dental coverage under Medicaid (Chazin 2015). Of the 46 states, 13 states provide dental emergency services (examples: relief of oral/dental pain), 17 states provide limited coverage as defined by the ADA and 17 states provide "extensive" coverage (Chazin 2015). However, even where coverage has been provided, barriers to care are so high and payments to dental providers have often been so low as to make it difficult or impossible for Medicaid beneficiaries to obtain adequate dental care (USDHHS 2016).

Finally, the term "dental insurance" is actually a misnomer. Private dental policies cover routine treatments, offer discounts for more complex treatment, and impose a low yearly cap on total payments. In fact, dental insurance has been called "part insurance, part prepayment, and part large volume discount" (Rubinstein 2005). Effectively, many (if not most) people who have dental insurance find coverage to be quite restrictive. For example, many plans impose a yearly cap ($1500 is common) or large coinsurance amounts (50% for orthodontia) (Rubinstein 2005). Even with discounts it is easy for many people to exceed the annual limit.

Given the lack of dental insurance coverage, it is not surprising that the status of oral health in the US is not particularly good. In 2011–2014 approximately 21.8% of people under the age of 20, 31.6% of adults between the ages of 20 and 44, 27.2% of adults between the ages of 45 and 64, and 21.8% of adults 65 and older had untreated caries (Dye et al. 2015). Of adults 30 and older, 46% have periodontal disease while it was 64.1% for adults 65 years and older (Eke et al. 2015). If these levels of untreated disease were found for systemic diseases, there would be public outcry.

15.1.3 Relationship Between Dental Problems and Chronic Illness

The evidence of relationships between dental disease, particularly periodontal disease, and chronic illnesses is now voluminous. The "two-way" relationship between periodontal disease and diabetes is clear. Clinical trials have demonstrated that treatment of periodontal disease improved glycemic control in diabetics (Casanova et al. 2014). Recent studies have found associations between periodontitis, all-cause mortality, and chronic kidney disease (Ricardo et al. 2015). A meta-analysis of the relationship between periodontal disease and hypertension found that periodontal diseases are associated with a higher risk of hypertension, particularly for severe periodontitis (Martin-Cabezas et al. 2016).

Bokhari and colleagues (Bokhari et al. 2015) used a meta-analysis to investigate the association between periodontal disease and various systemic biomarkers and systemic conditions of heart disease, stroke, and hypertension in Southern Asia. A study of patients with rheumatoid early arthritis and first degree rheumatoid arthritis measuring dental plaque and periodontal pocket depth found that patients with rheumatoid arthritis and periodontal disease "share pathophysiological mechanisms that explain how greater periodontal plaque index and periodontal pocket depth are directly related to indices of clinical activity of the joint disease (Giraldo 2016)." Investigations into the association between periodontitis and chronic obstructive pulmonary disease recognize that periodontal disease is associated with a number of lung conditions including chronic obstructive pulmonary disease and pneumonia (Madalli et al. 2016).

15.1.4 Implications for Health Policy

The implications of these findings about oral and systemic associations are profound. Professionally, evidence suggests that managing patients with chronic illness and periodontal disease will require teamwork and a deeper knowledge base for dentists and for physicians (Elangovan et al. 2014). Dentists should be alert for early signs of chronic illness among their patients and physicians should be alert for signs of dental disease. Dentistry and medicine have operated as professional silos in the past. The relationship between dental disease and chronic medical conditions suggests that continued separation is detrimental to patient centered care.

Policymakers are beginning to understand the implications of improved dental care as a method of holding down health care costs for chronic systemic disease. Grant Makers in Health, a nonprofit support group that helps foundations and corporate donors direct their charitable giving to improve health, has sponsored a program advocating integration of medical and dental care (Council on Foundations 2018). The case for integration included better opportunity to spot disease precursors both for dental and medical conditions as well as raise patients' awareness of the importance of oral health. Other reasons to integrate medical and dental care include increasing the effectiveness and efficiency of disease prevention, improving chronic disease management, overcoming patient specific barriers to accessing services, and providing cost savings (Council on Foundations 2018).

Health insurers are beginning to understand the importance of integrating medical and dental health. Aetna (2018) is now offering integrated medical and dental insurance. Kaiser Permanente has opened an integrated medical and dental clinic based on its review of the body of evidence that such integration reduces health care costs and reduces inequities (Roniger 2017). UnitedHealth Optum studied members who had medical insurance and dental insurance, looking at members who used dental services and those who did not. Members with chronic disease who received dental care averaged $1037 per year less in health care costs than members who did not use dental care. Large cost savings were seen for members with diabetes and members with renal disease (UnitedHealthCare 2013). The association of dental disease and chronic systemic disease produces extremely important health policy concerns. As evidenced in the UnitedHealth care study, if treatment of periodontitis and other dental problems leads to reduced incidence of chronic illness, fewer complications from chronic diseases, and reduced morbidity among chronically ill patients, increased access to dental services will reduce health care costs.

15.1.5 The Cost of Chronic Disease in the United States

The prevalence of chronic disease and per capita costs are growing at an alarming rate. In 2012 half of American adults, 117 million, had one or more chronic conditions (CDC 2018) The number of people with chronic conditions is expected to increase by 1% per year for the foreseeable future. The most common chronic conditions include hypertension, disorders of lipid metabolism, upper respiratory disease, joint disorders, heart disease, diabetes, cardiovascular disorders, asthma, and chronic respiratory infections (Anderson 2010).

One in four Americans has multiple chronic conditions (CDC 2018). It is estimated that about 69% of adults have two or more chronic conditions while it is approximately 35% for adults with four or more chronic conditions (Sambamoorthi et al. 2015). Seventy-eight percent of private health insurance spending is attributable to the 48% of privately insured persons with chronic conditions. Seventy-three percent of healthcare spending for the uninsured is for care received by the one third of uninsured people who have chronic conditions (Anderson 2010). For Medicare beneficiaries over 65, per capita spending for beneficiaries who have no chronic conditions is $2668 annually, for two or three chronic conditions it is $8562, for four or five chronic conditions spending rises to $17,050 per person and for six or more annual spending is a staggering $42,446 (Chartbook 2012). The cost associated with diabetes has increased from $245 billion in 2012 to $327 billion in 2018 (American Diabetes Association 2018). A report by UnitedHealth finds that more than 50% of adult Americans could have diabetes (15%) or prediabetes (37%) by 2020 (Allen 2010). These estimates conclude that diabetes and prediabetes will account for 10% of total healthcare spending in 2020 (Allen 2010).

With respect to cardiovascular disease, of the 55.5 million Medicare beneficiaries, 58% of them have high blood pressure, 45% have high cholesterol, 31% have ischemic heart disease, 29% have arthritis, 28% have diabetes, 16% have heart failure, and 15% have chronic kidney disease (Henry J Kaiser Family Foundation 2015). The Centers for Medicare and Medicaid Services (2012) estimates that 86% of Medicare beneficiaries (47.7 million) have two or more chronic conditions. Among this population 52.9% (25.2 million) have high cholesterol and high blood pressure with an annual cost to Medicare of $13,825 per person (CMS.gov 2013). Thirty-six percent have high cholesterol and ischemic heart disease (17.3 million) at a per person cost of $20,529. Thirty-two percent of beneficiaries had two or more chronic conditions at a cost of $18,043 per person. Five low incidence dyads had annual costs exceeding $45,000 per beneficiary: stroke and chronic kidney disease (2% of multiple chronic) at $51,715, stroke and COPD (1.4%) with an annual per person cost of $49,025, stroke and heart failure (2.3%) at $47,568 per person, stroke and asthma (0.4%) at $46,913 per person, and COPD and chronic kidney disease (4.9% at $45,011 per person (Dad and Weiner 2015)..

15.1.6 Potential Benefits of an Aggressive Dental Treatment Plan

The potential for large health care cost savings through an active and aggressive program of dental care is so large that such studies are clearly indicated. Suppose, for example, that 10% of all medical care costs required for treating diabetes, cardiovascular disease, and arthritis could be avoided through an active aggressive program of dental care.[1] And, if greater proportions of costs can be saved or if the estimates of costs are low, potential benefits will be even larger. Once again, it would be important to know whether aggressive dental care could produce such savings and how much.

15.1.7 Costs of an Aggressive Dental Treatment Plan

How much would an aggressive dental treatment plan cost? What do we mean by an aggressive dental treatment plan? Examples include dental insurance provided to all Medicare beneficiaries and Medicaid beneficiaries at the level of current private dental insurance coverage and strongly encourage beneficiaries to receive dental treatment, providing dental coverage in order to reduce their costs. More examples would include health insurance companies, understanding the benefits from dental care, requiring their private employer customers to cover the costs of dental care. How much would all of this cost? How would it compare to the benefits that may be available?

In order to estimate the potential costs of providing enhanced coverage for dental care we use the ADA estimate of the number of people without dental insurance, 114 million people. Willink and colleagues (2016) estimated the cost of providing dental care to Medicare beneficiaries. They determined per beneficiary cost to be $540 per year for coverage up to a $1500 cap. If dental care were to be provided to all 114 million uninsured persons the total annual cost would be $68 billion.

Of course, as noted a number of times above, these estimates are based on providing full "universal" dental insurance coverage at levels equivalent to current benefit levels for private dental insurance. It may be that an appropriate package of dental services that deals specifically with periodontitis can be provided for less than the full cost of private dental insurance. Once again, further research should provide better information.[2]

15.1.8 Comparing Costs and Benefits

If the cost of diabetes, cardiovascular disease, and arthritis is $1.4 trillion, then 10% ($140 billion) of medical care costs can be "saved" through improved dental care, by a $68 billion investment. Much of the savings would be derived by Medicare and Medicaid since health care costs for these programs are higher per capita than private health insurance.

---

[1] Ide and colleagues (2007) found that people with severe periodontitis incurred 21% higher health care costs than those who were free of periodontal disease. Additional studies of this nature would be important to support a measured approach to expanding dental coverage.

[2] It is also possible that dental care for persons with greater incidence of chronic illness as is the case with Medicare beneficiaries may require even higher levels of spending per beneficiary. Again, it would be good to know, scientifically, if this is the case.

Moreover, these estimates do not consider indirect costs in the form of lost wages or premature death. These costs are externalities to the health insurance programs. To the extent that they represent a social benefit that a national dental insurance program might internalize, it would be appropriate to consider their impact in the cost-benefit analysis.

In any event, better understanding of the potential for deriving savings in health insurance costs related to chronic diseases like diabetes, cardiovascular disease, and arthritis would be crucial to any determination whether to expand insurance coverage for dental care.

15.1.9 Expanded Dental Insurance Coverage

Heretofore, the case for expanding Medicare coverage to include dental care has taken the form of "benefit" to patients rather than benefit to health insurance programs and society and has been cast in emotional and political terms. In truth, there is no commitment to providing oral health access to any age group, much less the elderly. Rubenstein notes that "at least one commentator has suggested that the dental profession should join with senior citizen groups when the time is right to ask Congress to expand Medicare to cover oral health (Rubinstein 2005)". Rubinstein (2005) emphasizes that "calls for action" are "mere words" unless they are accompanied by political actions that health policy professionals and the dental profession must help promote. Another commentator suggested that "as soon as the debate over Medicare prescription drug coverage ends, the debate to provide dental care coverage for the elderly should begin" (Manski et al. 2015). Rubenstein et al. further suggests that "the dental community must convince Americans, and particularly aging boomers, that oral health is integral to all health, and for that reason, retiree dental benefits are an important issue."

There has been little if any discussion regarding the need to add dental benefits to health insurance sold through the exchanges created by the Affordable Care Act. Moreover, little attention has been given to Medicaid dental coverage. It would be good for policy makers to consider the potential savings that could occur by expanding dental benefits in these programs.

In truth, a decade of deficit spending and public distaste for out of control program costs in the Medicare and Medicaid programs as well as the unpopularity of the process that was used to provide Medicare prescription drug coverage (with perceived abuses by the health insurance and drug lobbies) and national health reform makes it unlikely that the public would be willing to approve expansions in insurance coverage for dental care "for its own sake" or "as the right thing" or to "benefit seniors." What this political climate has produced is an arena in which a good idea that could provide appropriate return on investment for society might well be rejected out of hand based on the political history of health insurance coverage. As a result, it is incumbent on policymakers, medical and dental research scientists, and health economists to investigate and confirm the potential savings that expansion of dental insurance coverage has the potential to produce and to develop hard evidence regarding potential costs of the expansion prior to, not as a part of, political efforts aimed at dental coverage expansion. A responsible, well informed effort to expand dental coverage may well go far to restore public confidence in the health policy process.

15.2 Management of Health Care Resources

The adage of "putting your money where your mouth is" is often referenced when being challenged about public statements or claims. In this instance, we use it literally. There have been numerous reports on health disparities, the burden of chronic diseases, increasing healthcare costs, and the need for change. Long-term economic benefits associated with the cost of care are dependent upon integrating oral health with medicine. This is particularly true as it relates to the management of those conditions which impact the economics of healthcare the most. Effective management of health care resources and information are critical to the economic well-being of our healthcare system. We can no longer afford to manage care in isolation. Integration of care between medicine and dentistry holds much promise in terms of reducing the cost of care and an integrated Medical-Dental Electronic Healthcare Record (iEHR) is the vehicle that will lead to downstream cost savings.

15.2.1 Economics of Integrated Decision Making

In the US, the Centers for Medicare & Medicaid Services (CMS) have conducted demonstration projects around chronic disease management. Section 121 of the Benefits Improvement and Protection Act of 2000 mandated CMS to conduct a disease management demonstration project (Bott et al. 2009). On 1 April 2005, in an effort to reduce the cost of care and improve quality associated with chronic diseases, CMS partnered with ten premier health systems to effectively manage chronic diseases in a Medicare Physician Group Practice Demonstration (PGP).

It was the first pay-for-performance initiative for physicians under the Medicare program (Kautter et al. 2007) It involved giving additional payments to providers based on practice efficiency and improved management of chronically ill patients. Participants included ten multispecialty group practices nationwide, with a total of more than 5000 physicians, who care for more than 200,000 Medicare beneficiaries (Frieden 2006). The chronic diseases that were targeted were based on occurrence in the population and included diabetes, heart failure, coronary artery disease, and hypertension (Frieden 2006). The CMS joined together to form partnership and the partners selected included Billings Clinic, Billings, Montana; Dartmouth-Hitchcock Clinic, Bedford, New Hampshire; The Everett Clinic, Everett, Washington; Forsyth Medical Group, Winston-Salem, North Carolina; Geisinger Health System, Danville, Pennsylvania; Marshfield Clinic, Marshfield, Wisconsin; Middlesex Health System, Middletown, Connecticut; Park Nicollet Health Services, St. Louis

Park, Minnesota; St. John's Health System, Springfield, Missouri; and University of Michigan Faculty Group Practice, Ann Arbor, Michigan.

Under the PGP, physician groups continued to be paid under regular Medicare fee schedules and had the opportunity to share in savings from enhancements in patient care management. Physician groups could earn performance payments which were divided between cost efficiency for generating savings and performance on 32 quality measures phased in during the demonstration as follows: year 1, 10 measures, year 2, 27 measures, and years 3 and 4 having 32 quality measures. For each of the 4 years only the University of Michigan Faculty Group Practice and Marshfield Clinic earned performance payments for improving the quality and cost efficiency of care. A large part of the success of this project was attributed to being able to extract, evaluate, and monitor key clinical data associated with the specific disease and to manage that data through an electronic health record (Table 15.1).

Table 15.1 shows some of the quality measures from the PGP initiative that was incorporated at Marshfield Clinic for Diabetes, congestive health failure, coronary artery disease and preventive care.

During the third year of the demonstration project Marshfield Clinic, using a robust electronic health record, succeeded in saving CMS $23 million dollars; that's one clinic system in 1 year. As a result of such demonstration projects and as of this writing, CMS is looking to establish Accountable Care Organizations (ACO) as the medical front runners to new care delivery methods for quality and cost control. ACOs is a term used to describe partnerships between healthcare providers to establish accountability and improved outcomes for patients (Song 2014).

In a CMS workshop on 5 October 2010, Don Berwick, the administrator of CMS, stated "An ACO will put the patient and family at the center of all its activities…" An emerging model of an ACO is the patient-centered medical home (PCMH) (Greene et al. 2012). PCMH is at the center of many demonstration projects. ACOs were derived from studies piloted by CMS. Since funds provided by CMS do not cover routine dental care as part of the patient management or quality and cost objectives, CMS ACO studies are limited if they become models for the PCMH, due to the exclusion of dental. Figure 15.1 illustrates an example of a model with a patient-centered approach and multiple entities involved in collaborative care model.

More recently, organizations representing the major primary care specialties—the American Academy of Family Practice, the American Academy of Pediatrics, the American Osteopathic Association, and the American College of Physicians have worked together to develop and endorse the concept of the "patient-centered medical home," a practice model that would more effectively support the core functions of primary care and the management of chronic disease (American College of Physicians 2007). In 2011, Geisinger Health System, Kaiser Permanente, Mayo Clinic, Intermountain Healthcare, and Group Health Cooperative announced they will be creating a project called the Care Connectivity Consortium (Consortia-pedia 2012). This project was intended to exchange patient information across the organizations of the Care Connectivity Consortium. Although progressive in their approach their project did not include dental.

Table 15.1 Quality measures from the PGP initiative

Diabetes	HbA1C management HbA1C control Blood pressure management Lipid measurement LDL cholesterol Urine protein testing Eye exam Foot exam Influenza vaccine Pneumonia vaccine
Congestive heart failure	Left ventricular function assessment Left ventricular ejection fraction testing Weight measurement Blood pressure screening Beta blocker therapy ACE inhibitor therapy Warfarin therapy for patients HF Influenza vaccine Pneumonia vaccine Heart failure patient education
Coronary artery disease	Antiplatelet therapy Drug therapy for lowering LDL cholesterol Beta-blocker therapy—prior MI Blood pressure management Lipid profile ACE inhibitor
Preventive care	Blood pressure screening Blood pressure control Blood pressure control plan of care Breast cancer screening Colorectal cancer screening Patient education Pneumococcal vaccine Influenza vaccine

According to a 2010 Surgeon General Report it is widely accepted across the dental profession that oral health has a direct impact on systemic health, and increasingly, medical and dental care providers are building to bridge relationships that create treatment solutions. National Institute for Dental and Craniofacial Research (2010) For example CMS has been involved in developing initiatives aimed at addressing dental access amongst children. Similarly, the US Department of Human and Health Services (USDHHS) along with other federal agents are developing a framework that builds upon improving oral health access and eliminating oral health disparities (U.S. Department of Health and Human Services Oral Health Coordinating Committee 2016). The case for medical and dental professionals' co-managing patients has been suggested for almost the past century. In 1926 William Gies reported that "The frequency of periodic examination gives dentists exceptional opportunity to note early signs of many types of illnesses outside the domain

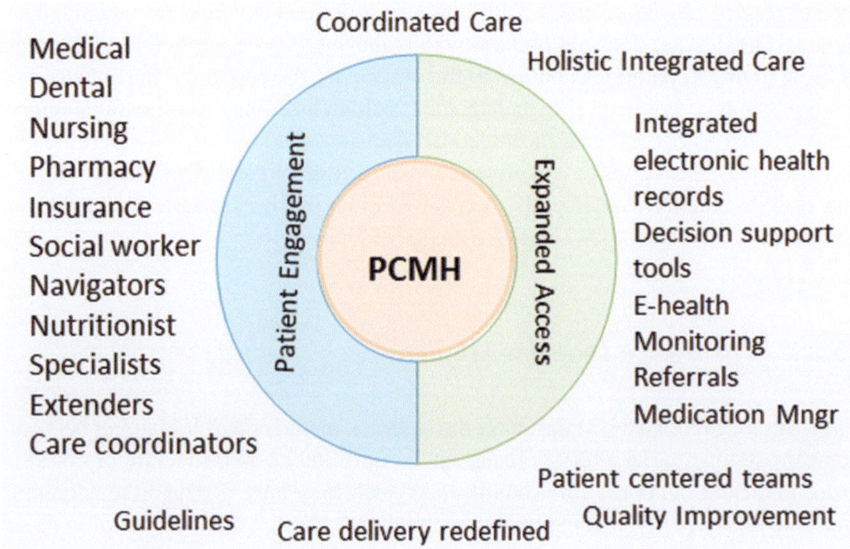

Fig. 15.1 Example of patient-centered approach and multiple entities involved in collaborative care model

of dentistry" (ADEAFGIES Foundation 1926). As described by Dr. Richard Nagelberg, D.D.S. "The convergence of dental and medical care is underway. Our patients will be the beneficiaries of this trend. For too long, we have provided dental care in a bubble, practicing – to a large degree – apart from other health-care providers. Even when we consulted with our medical colleagues, it was to find out if premedication was necessary, get clearance for treatment of a medically compromised patient, or find out the HbA1c level of a diabetic individual, rather than providing true patient co-management. We have made diagnoses and provided treatments without the benefit of tests, reports, metrics, and other information that predict the likelihood of disease development and progression, as well as favorable treatment outcomes. We have practiced in this manner not due to negligence, but because of the limitations of tools that were available to us" (Dental Economics 2011).

Integrated medical/dental records need to be a tool in a provider's toolbox. In the case of Marshfield Clinic, dental was not included in their past CMS demonstration project as dental was not a CMS covered benefit, and thus was not a part of the demonstration. However, as a leader in healthcare, Marshfield Clinic recognized the importance of data integration for both increased quality and cost savings. "Marshfield Clinic believes the best health care comes from an integrated dental/medical approach," said Michael Murphy, director, Business Development for Cattails Software. Integration enhances communication between providers and can ultimately lead to better management of complex diseases with oral-systemic connection, avoidance of medical errors, and improved public health (Acharya 2016).

While the CMS PGP and other demonstration projects along with independent studies have been shown to improve quality and reduce costs through integration, greater results may be afforded if studies are not done in isolation from dental data. In fact, if healthcare does not find a way to manage the systemic nature of reservoir of more than 120 pathogens known to the oral cavity the economic impact and cost savings around chronic disease management will hit a ceiling. The economic opportunity of having clinical data for integrated decision making is readily identified by the insurance industry. The effective management of clinical data around chronic and systemic oral and medical disease as part of an iEHR is the greatest healthcare cost savings opportunity associated with such a tool.

15.2.2 Insurance Industry Studies

The insurance industry sustains itself through risk management [obtaining best outcomes] using actuarial analysis [data] and controlling costs [reduction of costs] in order to ensure coverage [profitability]. As such they have pursued the economic and outcome benefits of integrated medical/dental clinical decision making. As an example, in 2009 there was a study conducted by the University of Michigan, commissioned by the Blue Cross Blue Shield of Michigan Foundation (Dental Care News 2009), the study included 21,000 Blue Cross Blue Shield of Michigan members diagnosed with diabetes who had access to dental care, and had continuous coverage for at least 1 year. With regular periodontal care, it was observed that diabetes related medical costs were reduced by 10%. When compounding chronic health complications were also examined, the study showed a 20% reduction in cost related to the treatment of cardiovascular disease in patients with diabetes and heart disease, a 30% reduction in cost related to treatment of kidney disease for patients with diabetes and kidney disease, and a 40% reduction in costs related to treating congestive heart failure for patients with diabetes and congestive heart failure. According to a joint statement by lead researchers, and Blue Cross Blue Shield of Michigan executives, "Our results are consistent with an emerging body of evidence that periodontal disease … addresses quality of care and health care costs for all Michigan residents."

Also, at the Institute for Oral Health conference in November 2007 Joseph Errante, D.D.S., Vice President, Blue Cross Blue Shield of MA reported that the 2003 Blue Cross Blue Shield of Massachusetts claims data showed medical costs for diabetics who accessed dental care for prevention and periodontal services averaged $558/month, while medical costs for diabetics who didn't get dental care were about $702/month (Errante 2010). Similarly insured individuals with cardiovascular diseases who accessed dental care had lower medical costs, $238/month lower than people who did not seek dental treatment (Errante 2010). The cost is $144 less per visit for those diabetics who accessed prevention and periodontal services. Those savings could be translated into access to care or additional benefits for more individuals.

In the case of neonatal health there is similar research. Over 9.85% of all births in the US were delivered preterm, with many infants at risk of birth defects

(Martin et al. 2018). According to a January 2006 statement issued by Cigna, announcing their CIGNA Oral Health Maternity Program, "the program was launched in response to mounting research indicating an increased probability of preterm birth for those with gum disease. These research-based, value-added programs are designed to help improve outcomes and reduce expense" (Inside Dentistry 2006). The program was initially designed to offer extended dental benefits free of charge to members who were expectant mothers, citing "research supporting the negative and costly impact periodontal disease has on both mother and baby." According to research cited by CIGNA, expectant mothers with chronic periodontal disease during the second trimester are seven times more likely to deliver preterm (before the 37th week), and the costs associated with treating premature new-borns is an average of 15 times more during their first year, and premature new-borns have dramatically more healthcare challenges throughout their life. CIGNA also cited the correlation between periodontal disease and low birth weight, pre-eclampsia, and gestational diabetes as additional rationale to support extended dental benefits to expectant mothers. Six months later CIGNA initiated Well Aware for Better Health, an extended benefits, free of charge, program for diabetic and cardiovascular disease patients aimed at "turning evidence into action by enhancing dental benefits for participants in disease management" programs. It is interesting to note, not only does CIGNA offer extended dental benefits to targeted groups, they also reimburse members for any out-of-pocket expenses associated with their dental care (co-pays, etc.)

Aetna initiated the Dental/Medical Integration (DMI) Program in 2006. Aetna's DMI program offers enhanced benefits in the form of free-of-charge extended benefit dental care to Aetna's 37.2 million Indemnity, PPO, and Managed Choice medical plan members, specifically targeting members deemed at-risk, including those who are pregnant, diabetic, and/or have cardiovascular disease and have not been to a dentist in 1 year. As a result of various outreach methods a 2013 report showed that implementing the DMI program resulted in (1) Lowering the medical cost of patients involved in DMI by an average of 17%; (2) Improve the glycaemic control by 45%; (3) Forty two percent of the patients used less major and basic dental services and (4) Only about 3.5% required few hospital admissions as compared to 5.4% for non-members (Aetna 2013).

Delta Dental of Wisconsin understands the connection between oral and systemic health and has created a program that is designed to offer members with certain chronic health conditions the opportunity to gain additional benefits. More than 2000 groups now offer Delta Dental of Wisconsin's Evidence-Based Integrated Care Plan (EBICP) option (Delta Dental of Wisconsin 2018). EBICP provides expanded benefits for persons with chronic systemic diseases that have oral health implications. Oral health benefits include increased frequency of cleanings and/or applications of topical fluoride and managing the oral health challenges faced by the patients. EBICP offers additional cleanings and topical fluoride application for persons who are undergoing cancer treatment involving radiation and/or chemotherapy, persons with prior surgical or nonsurgical treatment of periodontal disease, women who are pregnant, persons with chronic medical conditions, and persons with suppressed immune systems.

The iEHR provides the insurance industry in partnership with the healthcare industry an integrated tool to facilitate these health, and subsequently economic, outcomes across medicine and dentistry.

15.2.3 Increased Efficiency and Patient Safety Through Integrated Electronic Health Records

In addition to the anticipated savings through better outcomes using integrated clinical data (Jha et al. 2009), an example of a positive economic outcome associated with an integrated record as related to increased efficiency and patient safety is found in the United States Veterans Administration (VA) hospitals and clinics. The VA is one of the few institutions that have implemented the shared electronic medical/dental record successfully that provides the ability to be the "one stop shop" for their patients. An April 2010 press release published on the Department of Veterans Affairs website highlighted the success of the VA's health information technology in terms of cost reductions and "improvements in quality, safety, and patient satisfaction" (Dark Daily 2011).

The press release spotlighted a study conducted by the public health journal, Health Affairs, which focused on the VA's health IT investment from 1997 to 2007. The study confirmed that while the VA has spent $4 billion on their technology initiative, a conservative estimate of cost savings was more than $7 billion. After subtracting the expense of the IT investment, there was a net savings of $3 billion for the VA during the 10 years covered by the study (Dark Daily 2011). Furthermore, the study estimated that "more than 86 percent of the savings were due to eliminating duplicated tests and reducing medical errors. The rest of the savings came from lower operating expenses and reduced workload." Independent studies show that the VA system does better on many measures, especially preventive services and chronic care, than the private sector and Medicare. VA officials say "its [integrated] technology has helped cut down hospitalizations and helped patients live longer"(U.S. Department of Veterans Affairs 2010)

The Journal of Obstetrics and Gynecology reported on a tragic loss of life due to the systemic nature of oral health. A study found oral bacteria called Fusobacterium nucleatum was the likely culprit in infecting a 35-year-old woman's fetus through her bloodstream (Carroll 2010). The doctors determined that the same strain of oral bacteria found in the woman's mouth was in the deceased baby's stomach and lungs. Integrated records would have provided critical data to the obstetrician including oral health issues and when the patient had her last dental exam. How does one measure the economic impact of a life not lived and another derailed by such tragedy?

In a randomized controlled study, Lopez et al. determined that periodontal therapy provided during pregnancy to women with periodontitis or gingivitis reduced the incidence of preterm and of low birth weight infants (López et al. 2005). The

Institute of Medicine and National Academies estimate that preterm births cost society at least $23 billion annually (March of Dimes 2014). Data integration of the iEHR enables the effective management between the dentist and obstetrician to ensure proper periodontal therapy has been provided during pregnancy. Such management based on the Lopez et al. study, will have direct impact in reducing the prevalence per preterm births leading to reduced health care costs.

There have also been studies indicating a correlation between poorer oral hygiene or deficient denture hygiene and pneumonia or respiratory tract infection among elderly people in nursing homes or hospitals (Rosenblum 2010; Scannapieco 2006). Lack of access is certainly a key factor to consider. However, lack of available data respective to the interrelationship between oral health and systemic health also contributed to the apathy in these cases.

As identified above, complications are correlated to cost. As conditions compound, costs go up. Marshfield Clinic, as part of their iEHR is creating a shared problem list that identifies both oral and medical conditions, a history of recent visits, and a medication lists for monitoring at the point of care [be it a medical or dental visit]. Enabling the clinical data sharing and care management milestones serves as a tool to prevent conditions from compounding and escalating costs such as those described above.

15.2.4 Other Areas of Economic Impact Relative to iEHR Clinical Data

Several other areas of economic impact will be seen as iEHR's become broadly deployed. Some of these are listed below:

- Medication management. A great deal of provider and allied support time is spent obtaining medication information between dentistry and medicine [and vice versa] including current medications, contraindications, tolerances, etc. Marshfield Clinic Cattails software has created a dashboard that readily identifies this for both the medical and dental providers. Not only is time saved, but chances for complications or escalation of conditions is reduced [both of which impact cost]. For example an integrated record allows medical providers treating respiratory infections to include or exclude oral flora as the possible source of the infection which would lead to more knowledgeable prescribing decisions on the antibiotics used.
- Coordination of care has a direct impact on cost for the system and the patient. For example, in 2008 55.6% of the US population aged 2 years and older that was diagnosed diabetes had been to the dentist in the past year (The Office of Disease Prevention and Health Promotion n.d.; USDHHS 2000). The US government's program Healthy People 2020 includes an initiative to increase the proportion of people with diagnosed diabetes who have at least an annual dental examination. The American Diabetes Association recommends that diabetic patients be seen semi-annually and more frequently if bleeding gums or other oral issues are present. The American Diabetes Association also recommends the

consultation between the dentist and physician to decide about possible adjustments to diabetes medicines, or to decide if an antibiotic is needed before surgery to prevent infection. The target from Healthy People 2020 is a 10% improvement at 61.2%. Integrated medical/dental records could allow for the coordination of efforts between providers to include communication of treatment plans and services leading to quicker resolution, increased patient compliance, less patient time away from work or home, and potentially less travel.

- The iEHR that includes medical and dental records create a platform to integrate clinical appointing between medicine and dentistry. As such, combative patients or severely disabled patients needing anaesthesia in order for care to be delivered can be treated with one hospital sedation vs. multiple sedations. Family Health Center of Marshfield, Inc. (FHC) Dental Clinics shares an iEHR with Marshfield Clinic and uses its integrated scheduling feature to complete dental care, lab work, ENT care, woman's health, and preventive studies, all in one visit.
- Follow up care management can be more focused and coordinated. For example, without the knowledge of dental conditions, medical providers could spend months attempting to control diabetes with periodontal disease. However, with access to an iEHR, the practitioner or allied care manager can determine a patient's oral health status immediately to determine the possible influence of periodontal disease.
- The iEHR with a shared patient data dashboard brings to light history and physical examination data without having to have patients be the historian to their physician on their last dental visit or for the dentist to have to rely on the patient's recall of medications or medical diagnoses. For example, if an integrated record saved providers 5 min per hour of patient care, that would be 40 min per day. Imagine giving a physician or dentist 40 min more a day. In a capitated system, this allows for more patients to be seen in a day for roughly the same amount of expenditure. In a production based clinic this allows more patients to be seen and more charges per day. In either case, the investment into informatics is covered. In an underserved area, more patients get care more quickly, which creates the opportunity for quicker resolution, which can lead to a healthier society, which in turn may lead them back to a productive livelihood sooner.
- An iEHR results in one comprehensive system for acquisition, orientation, training, and support. PC based owners who also own a Mac and Mac owners who also have to operate a PC can relate. Need we say more? Imagine if your PC functioned just like a Mac [or your Mac functioned just like a PC]. No cross learning of software quirks. Not having to purchase two separate units to begin with reduced costs and increased space. Not having to jump from one computer to the other computer to get data from one to another to create a report. Not having to call two separate computer companies for service or updates.
- Third party coordination. Having an iEHR creates a platform for interfacing with third party payers. A common system and language for timely reimbursement, in part the result of an iEHR, is driving the diagnostic coding for dentistry. Such an integrated interface provides a tool to bridge with healthcare payors that historically kept payment as segregated as the oral and medical health professions. The iEHR overcomes that limitation. Timely payment, consolidation of payment, expansion of covered patient and provider benefits based on clinical integration,

and a viable system for interfacing are all potential economic benefits of iEHR clinical data.

- The iEHR creates new horizons for research that will lead to cost saving discoveries. As an example, knowing the benefits of research, Marshfield Clinic Research Institute (MCRI) has created an Oral and Systemic Health Research Project (OSHRP). The creation of OSHRP, led by Dr. Murray Brilliant, allows MCRI to capitalize on its existing and growing strengths in the areas of complex disease interactions and Personalized Health Care (PHC) to advance oral health and the health of the rest of the body. The OSHRP has three specific goals:
  - Understand the connections between oral and systemic health (diabetes, heart disease, pre-term births).
  - Understand the causes of oral diseases and determine the effect of genetics, diet, water source (well/city + fluoridation), and microbiome.
  - Understand how improving oral health aids systemic health (comparative effectiveness) and bring Personalized Health Care (PHC) to the dental arena.
- The OSHRP research resource will be unique in the nation. As MCRI has done with other projects, it will share this resource with qualified investigators at other academic institutions both within and outside of Wisconsin. OSHRP will advance scientific knowledge, improve healthcare and prevention, reduce the cost of oral healthcare, and create new economic opportunities. Such knowledge will have a direct economic impact on the cost of care and care management.
- The iEHR creates an ability to have an integrated patient portal to comprehensively maintain their health records. Portals are becoming more and more popular in the healthcare industry as a means to help maintain compliance with care management recommendations and preventative procedures. This web-based patient health portals allows improving both quality and access to care (Shimpi et al. 2018). Portals provide patents a tool with which to stay up to date on their care and recommendations.
- Portals can take iEHR clinical data, adapt it through programming, and provide creative visual reinforcement for patients as they monitor their health status. The more patients engage in owning their health status, the more preventative services are followed through with. The more medicine and dentistry can leverage the prevention potential [which insurance companies have come to realize] the more likely costly conditions can be avoided.

15.3 Conclusion

The link between oral health and systemic health is well documented. The separation of dental and medical is not a sustainable model in modern healthcare delivery. A new model of integrated care is necessary. Aristotle said, "The whole is greater than the sum of its parts." Increased access to combined medical and dental histories and diagnoses at the providers' fingertips makes vital information available. Shared diagnoses between medical and dental providers could aid in formulating interventions and to accelerate decision making abilities by allowing for the prioritizing of medical/dental procedures. Clinical management and treatment of the patient would be expedited with immediate access to both records. Quality could be improved through a complete picture of the patient through the dashboard. All of these will have a direct or indirect economic benefit.

The iEHR will be the tool that facilitates such delivery and the studies and scenarios described in these pages point to significant economic benefits to patients, payors, and providers. Increased access, multi-provider monitoring, and shared problems lists with enhanced decision making abilities from iEHR could reduce healthcare costs. The greatest cost reduction will be found with using the iEHR to manage chronic diseases. A combined dental/medical electronic record with a shared data informatics platform is most likely to yield the best long-term economic solution while maintaining or enhancing positive patient outcomes.

References

Acharya A. Marshfield Clinic Health System: integrated care case study. J California Dent Assoc. 2016;44(3):177–81. http://www.ncbi.nlm.nih.gov/pubmed/27044239

ADA News. Study: dental benefits can help employers improve workforce, their bottom line. 2018. https://www.ada.org/en/publications/ada-news/2018-archive/january/study-dental-benefits-can-help-employers-improve-workforce-their-bottom-line. Accessed 16 Jun 2018.

ADEAFGIES Foundation. William J. Gies and the Gies Report. 1926. http://www.adea.org/ADEAGiesFoundation/William-J-Gies-and-Gies-Report.aspx. Accessed 16 Jun 2018.

Aetna. Aetna's dental medical integration program may help lower costs and result in better health – the health section. 2013. https://news.aetna.com/news-releases/aetnas-dental-medical-integration-program-may-help-lower-costs-and-result-in-better-health/. Accessed 17 Jun 2018.

Aetna. Dental-Medical Integration Program. Aetna Dental. 2018. https://www.aetnadental.com/professionals/dental-overall-health/dental-medical-integration-program.html. Accessed 16 Jun 2018.

Allen J. Diabetes: half of U.S. adults at risk by 2020, says United Health Group – ABC News. 2010. https://abcnews.go.com/Health/Diabetes/diabetes-half-us-adults-risk-2020-united-health-group/story?id=12238602. Accessed 16 Jun 2018.

Amadeo K. Rising health care costs: causes, by year. 2016. https://www.thebalance.com/causes-of-rising-healthcare-costs-4064878. Accessed 16 Jun 2018.

American College of Physicians. Nation's top primary care physician organizations release guidelines for patient-centered medical home recognition programs. ACP Newsroom. ACP. 2007. https://www.acponline.org/acp-newsroom/nations-top-primary-care-physician-organizations-releaseguidelines-for-patient-centered-medical-home. Accessed 17 Jun 2018.

American Diabetes Association. The cost of diabetes: American Diabetes Association®. 2018. http://www.diabetes.org/advocacy/news-events/cost-of-diabetes.html. Accessed 16 Jun 2018.

Anderson G. Chronic care: making the case for ongoing care – RWJF. 2010. https://www.rwjf.org/en/library/research/2010/01/chronic-care.html

Bokhari S, Khan A, Leung W, Wajid G. Association of periodontal and cardiovascular diseases: South-Asian studies 2001-2012. J Ind Soc Periodontol. 2015;19(5):495–500. https://doi.org/10.4103/0972-124X.157876.

Bott D, Kapp M, Johnson L, Magno L. Disease management for chronically ill beneficiaries in traditional medicare. Health Aff. 2009;28(1):86–98. https://doi.org/10.1377/hlthaff.28.1.86.

Carroll L. Mother's gum disease linked to infant's death – health – oral health. NBC News. 2010. http://www.nbcnews.com/id/34979552/ns/health-oral_health/t/mothers-gum-disease-linked-infants-death/. Accessed 17 Jun 2018.

Casanova L, Hughes F, Preshaw P. Diabetes and periodontal disease: a two-way relationship. BDJ. 2014;217(8):433–7. https://doi.org/10.1038/sj.bdj.2014.907.

CDC. Chronic disease overview. Publications. Chronic disease prevention and health promotion. CDC. 2018. https://www.cdc.gov/chronicdisease/overview/index.htm#ref1. Accessed 16 Jun 2018.

Centers for Medicare and Medicaid Services, Chartbook: 2012 Edition (2012). https://www.cms.gov/Research-Statistics-Data-and-Systems/Statistics-Trends-and-Reports/Chronic-Conditions/Downloads/2012Chartbook.pdf.

Chalmers N, Wislar J, Boynes S, Doherty M, Nový B. Improving health in the United States: oral health is key to overall health. J Am Dent Assoc. 2017;148(7):477–80. https://doi.org/10.1016/j.adaj.2017.04.031.

Chartbook. Chronic conditions among medicare beneficiaries. 2012. https://www.cms.gov/research-statistics-data-and-systems/statistics-trends-and-reports/chronic-conditions/downloads/2012chartbook.pdf

Chazin S. Supporting efforts to advance adult dental coverage and access in medicaid - CHCS blog. 2015. https://www.chcs.org/health-affairs-grantwatch-blog-supporting-efforts-advance-adult-dental-coverage-access-medicaid/. Accessed 16 Jun 2018.

CMS.gov. Medicaid incentives for prevention of chronic diseases grants. 2013. https://www.cms.gov/Newsroom/MediaReleaseDatabase/Fact-sheets/2011-Fact-sheets-items/2011-09-13.html. Accessed 17 Jun 2018.

Consortia-pedia. Care connectivity consortium (CCC) – consortiapedia. 2012. http://consortiapedia.fastercures.org/consortia/ccc/. Accessed 17 Jun 2018.

Council on Foundations. Grantmakers in health. 2018. https://www.cof.org/content/grantmakers-health. Accessed 16 Jun 2018.

Dad T, Weiner D. Stroke and chronic kidney disease: epidemiology, pathogenesis, and management across kidney disease stages. Semin Nephrol. 2015;35(4):311–22. https://doi.org/10.1016/j.semnephrol.2015.06.003.

Dark Daily. VA uses integrated health informatics to produce $3 billion in savings. 2011. https://www.darkdaily.com/va-uses-integrated-health-informatics-to-produce-3-billion-in-savings-12811/

Delta Dental of Wisconsin. Medical conditions. Delta Dental of Wisconsin. 2018. https://www.deltadentalwi.com/your-health/medical-conditions. Accessed 17 Jun 2018.

Dental Care News. U and M study links good oral care to lower diabetes cost. 2009. https://bcbsm.com/content/dam/public/Providers/Documents/newsletters/dcn-2009-oct.pdf. Accessed 17 Jun 2018.

Dental Economics. The convergence of dental and medical care – Dental Economics. 2011. https://www.dentaleconomics.com/articles/print/volume-101/issue-4/practice/the-convergence-of-dental-and-medical-care.html. Accessed 15 Jun 2018.

Dye B, Thornton-Evans G, Iafolla T. Dental caries and tooth loss in adults in the United States, 2011-2012. NCHS Data Brief. 2015;197:197. http://www.ncbi.nlm.nih.gov/pubmed/25973996

Eke P, Dye B, Wei L, Slade G, Thornton-Evans G, Borgnakke W, et al. Update on prevalence of periodontitis in adults in the United States: NHANES 2009 to 2012. J Periodontol. 2015;86(5):611–22. https://doi.org/10.1902/jop.2015.140520.

Elangovan S, Hertzman-Miller R, Karimbux N, Giddon D. A framework for physician-dentist collaboration in diabetes and periodontitis. Clin Diabet. 2014;32(4):188–92. https://doi.org/10.2337/diaclin.32.4.188.

Errante. Institute for Oral Health – DentistryIQ. 2010. https://www.dentistryiq.com/articles/2010/07/institute-for-oral.html. Accessed 16 Jun 2018.

Federal Reserve System. The fed – economic preparedness and emergency savings. 2017. https://www.federalreserve.gov/publications/2017-economic-well-being-of-us-households-in-2016-economic-preparedness.htm. Accessed 16 Jun 2018.

Firestein G. Evolving concepts of rheumatoid arthritis. Nature. 2003;423(6937):356–61. https://doi.org/10.1038/nature01661.

Frieden J. CMS Projects focus on chronic illnesses. Caring Ages. 2006;7(8):22–3. https://doi.org/10.1016/S1526-4114(06)60225-4.

Giraldo. Annual European congress of rheumatology – PDF. 2016. http://docplayer.net/48932734-Annual-european-congress-of-rheumatology.html. Accessed 16 Jun 2018.

Glurich I, Nycz G, Acharya A. Status update on translation of integrated primary dental-medical care delivery for management of diabetic patients. Clin Med Res. 2017;15(1–2):21–32. https://doi.org/10.3121/cmr.2017.1348.

Greene S, Tuzzio L, Cherkin D. A framework for making patient-centered care front and center. Permanente J. 2012;16(3):49–53. http://www.ncbi.nlm.nih.gov/pubmed/23012599

HealthCare.gov. Dental coverage in the health insurance marketplace. 2018. https://www.healthcare.gov/coverage/dental-coverage/. Accessed 16 Jun 2018.

Henry J Kaiser Family Foundation. Total number of medicare beneficiaries. 2015. https://www.kff.org/medicare/state-indicator/total-medicare-beneficiaries/?currentTimeframe=0&sortModel=%7B%22colId%22:%22Location%22,%22sort%22:%22asc%22%7D. Accessed 16 Jun 2018.

Ide R, Hoshuyama T, Takahashi K. The effect of periodontal disease on medical and dental costs in a middle-aged Japanese population: a longitudinal worksite study. J Periodontol. 2007;78(11):2120–6. https://doi.org/10.1902/jop.2007.070193.

Inside Dentistry. Dentistry at large: CIGNA launches oral health maternity program. 2006. https://www.aegisdentalnetwork.com/id/2006/02/dentistry-at-large-cigna-launches-oral-health-maternity-program. Accessed 15 Jun 2018.

Jha A, DesRoches C, Campbell E, Donelan K, Rao S, Ferris T, et al. Use of electronic health records in U.S. hospitals. N Engl J Med. 2009;360(16):1628–38. https://doi.org/10.1056/NEJMsa0900592.

Kautter J, Pope G, Trisolini M, Grund S. Medicare physician group practice demonstration design: quality and efficiency pay-for-performance. Health Care Fin Rev. 2007;29(1):15–29. http://www.ncbi.nlm.nih.gov/pubmed/18624077

López N, Da Silva I, Ipinza J, Gutiérrez J. Periodontal therapy reduces the rate of preterm low birth weight in women with pregnancy-associated gingivitis. J Periodontol. 2005;76(11s):2144–53. https://doi.org/10.1902/jop.2005.76.11-S.2144.

Madalli R, Kheur S, Reddy M, Kheur M, Mahalle A. Assessment of role of Porphyromonas gingivalis as an aggravating factor for chronic obstructive pulmonary disease patients with periodontitis. Dent Hypotheses. 2016;7(3):100. https://doi.org/10.4103/2155-8213.190485.

Manski R, Hoffmann D, Rowthorn V. Increasing access to dental and medical care by allowing greater flexibility in scope of practice. Am J Public Health. 2015;105(9):1755–62. https://doi.org/10.2105/AJPH.2015.302654.

March of Dimes. Premature babies cost employers $12.7 billion annually. 2014. https://www.marchofdimes.org/news/premature-babies-cost-employers-127-billion-annually.aspx. Accessed 17 Jun 2018.

Martin-Cabezas R, Seelam N, Petit C, Agossa K, Gaertner S, Tenenbaum H, et al. Association between periodontitis and arterial hypertension: a systematic review and meta-analysis. Am Heart J. 2016;180:98–112. https://doi.org/10.1016/j.ahj.2016.07.018.

Martin J, Hamilton B, Osterman M, Driscol A, Drake P. Births: final data for 2016. Nat Vital Stat Rep. 2018;67:53. https://www.cdc.gov/nchs/data/nvsr/nvsr67/nvsr67_01.pdf

Masterson, L. Skyrocketing chronic diseases will cause major healthcare spending spike. Healthcare Dive. 2017. https://www.healthcaredive.com/news/skyrocketing-chronic-diseases-will-cause-major-healthcare-spending-spike/443853/. Accessed 16 Jun 2018.

Mealey B, Oates T. Diabetes mellitus and periodontal diseases. J Periodontol. 2006;77(8):1289–303. https://doi.org/10.1902/jop.2006.050459.

National Institute of Dental and Craniofacial Research, Oral health in America: report of the surgeon general (2010). https://profiles.nlm.nih.gov/ps/access/NNBBJT.pdf.

NADP Dental Plans. NADP – National Association of Dental Plans. 2018. http://www.nadp.org/. Accessed 16 Jun 2018.

Oberlander J. The political history of medicare. american society on aging. J Am Soc Aging. 2015. http://www.asaging.org/blog/political-history-medicare

Ricardo A, Athavale A, Chen J, Hampole H, Garside D, Marucha P, Lash J. Periodontal disease, chronic kidney disease and mortality: results from the third National Health and Nutrition Examination Survey. BMC Nephrol. 2015;16:97. https://doi.org/10.1186/s12882-015-0101-x.

Roniger L. Kaiser Permanente premiers integrated medical-dental clinic. 2017. https://www.drbicuspid.com/index.aspx?sec=log&itemID=321032. Accessed 16 Jun 2018.

Rosenblum R. Oral hygiene can reduce the incidence of and death resulting from pneumonia and respiratory tract infection. J Am Dent Assoc (1939). 2010;141(9):1117–8. http://www.ncbi.nlm.nih.gov/pubmed/20807912

Rubinstein H. Access to oral health care for elders: mere words or action? J Dent Educ. 2005;69(9):1051–7.

Sambamoorthi U, Tan X, Deb A. Multiple chronic conditions and healthcare costs among adults. Expert Rev Pharmacoecon Outcomes Res. 2015;15(5):823–32. https://doi.org/10.1586/14737167.2015.1091730.

Sato M, Iwasaki M, Yoshihara A, Miyazaki H. Association between periodontitis and medical expenditure in older adults: a 33-month follow-up study. Geriatr Gerontol Int. 2016;16(7):856–64. https://doi.org/10.1111/ggi.12569.

Scannapieco F. Pneumonia in nonambulatory patients. The role of oral bacteria and oral hygiene. J Am Dent Assoc (1939). 2006;137(Suppl):21S–5S. http://www.ncbi.nlm.nih.gov/pubmed/17012732

Shimpi N, Schwei K, Cooper S, Chyou P, Acharya A. Understanding patients' oral health information needs. Findings of a survey on use of patient portals in dentistry. J Am Dent Assoc. 2018; https://doi.org/10.1016/j.adaj.2017.09.051.

Sommers B, Gawande A, Baicker K. Health insurance coverage and health — what the recent evidence tells us. N Engl J Med. 2017;377(6):586–93. https://doi.org/10.1056/NEJMsb1706645.

Song Z. Accountable care organizations in the U.S. Health Care System. J Clin Outcomes Manag. 2014;21(8):364–71. http://www.ncbi.nlm.nih.gov/pubmed/25960631

The Office of Disease Prevention and Health Promotion. About healthy people. Healthy people 2020. n.d. https://www.healthypeople.gov/2020/About-Healthy-People. Accessed 19 Mar 2018.

U.S. Department of Health and Human Services Oral Health Coordinating Committee. U.S. Department of Health and Human Services Oral Health Strategic Framework, 2014–2017. Public health reports (Washington, D.C.: 1974), vol. 131. Thousand Oaks, CA: SAGE Publications; 2016. http://www.ncbi.nlm.nih.gov/pubmed/26957659

U.S. Department of Veterans Affairs. Veterans Health Administration 2010 facility quality and safety report - patient satisfaction. 2010. https://www.data.va.gov/dataset/veterans-health-administration-2010-facility-quality-and-safety-report-patient-satisfaction. Accessed 17 Jun 2018.

UnitedHealthCare. Medical dental integration study. 2013. https://www.dentistryiq.com/articles/2010/07/oral-health-america.html. Accessed 16 Jun 2018.

USDHHS. Oral health in America: a report of the surgeon general. NIH publication no 00-4713. 2000. https://profiles.nlm.nih.gov/ps/retrieve/ResourceMetadata/NNBBJT/

USDHHS. OIG 2015 work plan. Medicare (United States). Medicaid. 2016. https://www.scribd.com/document/245771221/OIG-2015-Work-Plan. Accessed 16 Jun 2018.

Vistnes J, Davis K, Miller G. STATISTICAL BRIEF #477: results from the 2014 MEPS-IC private-sector national tables. 2015. https://meps.ahrq.gov/data_files/publications/st477/stat477.shtml. Accessed 16 Jun 2018.

Willink A, Schoen C, Davis K. Dental care and medicare beneficiaries: access gaps, cost burdens, and policy options. Health Aff. 2016;35(12):2241–8. https://doi.org/10.1377/hlthaff.2016.0829.

Xu S, Song M, Xiong Y, Liu X, He Y, Qin Z. The association between periodontal disease and the risk of myocardial infarction: a pooled analysis of observational studies. BMC Cardiovasc Disord. 2017;17(1):50. https://doi.org/10.1186/s12872-017-0480-y.

Chapter 16
The Need for Interprofessional Medical-Dental Education

Casey Hein and Joseph Kilsdonk

16.1 Interprofessional Medical–Dental Education

16.1.1 Introduction

There is a growing appreciation of the need to address patient care systemically and holistically. Although *Oral-Systemic Medicine* has already been translated into consumer publications and mainstream media, the unfortunate truth is that it has not been included in the education, training or clinical practice of non-dental healthcare providers (HCPs) (Gorman et al. 2004; Hein 2006; Kiefer 2008; Oz and Levine 2013). Consumers may have an increased awareness of the importance of oral health; however, this body of evidence has not been widely translated into patient care outside of dentistry and dental hygiene. Today, we know that HCPs generally practice the way they were trained. Accordingly, the medical and nursing professions (in addition to other non-dental healthcare disciplines), must address oral-systemic health in both pre-licensure and continuing education.

In considering why non-dental HCPs lack this important body of knowledge, the general assumption has been that content specifically related to oral diseases and conditions as well as the potential effect on the rest of the body does not substantially exist in the curricula of the undergraduate programming of medical, nursing, and pharmacy students, nor undergraduate students of allied healthcare professions

C. Hein (✉)
International Center for Oral-Systemic Health, College of Dentistry, University of Manitoba, Winnipeg, MB, Canada

Rady Faculty of Health Sciences, University of Manitoba, Winnipeg, MB, Canada
e-mail: casey.hein@umanitoba.ca

J. Kilsdonk
Office of Medical Education, Aspirus Healthcare Systems, Wausau, WI, USA
e-mail: joseph.kilsdonk@aspirus.org

A. Acharya et al. (eds.), *Integration of Medical and Dental Care and Patient Data*, Health Informatics, https://doi.org/10.1007/978-3-319-98298-4_16

in general. A study conducted at the College of Dentistry of the University of Manitoba and published in 2010 (Hein et al. 2011) attempted to determine the extent of this gap in knowledge, how non-dental healthcare educators view the importance of oral-systemic science in preparing future generations of HCPs, current teaching practices, curriculum delivery methods and content as well as interprofessional education programs that focus specifically on oral-systemic health. The *Oral-Systemic Health Educational Curriculum Survey*, specifically created for this investigation, was circulated on-line to poll associate or academic deans from medical, nursing and pharmacy schools, in universities across Canada, the United States, Europe, Asia, Australia, and New Zealand. The survey queried the magnitude of oral-systemic science that was being taught in undergraduate curricula. The survey yielded an overall response rate of 23%; 65% in the United States, 17.1% in Canada, 9.8% in Australia, 4.9% in Great Britain, and 24% in New Zealand, with 41.5% from schools of pharmacy, 39% from nursing, and 19.5% from medicine. Close to 54% of the respondents ranked the inclusion of oral-systemic science as somewhat important and 51% reported there were not any requirements to incorporate oral health education within curricula. The investigation found that the majority of students were not being taught to examine the mouth nor were they being instructed on how to perform an oral examination. Less than 5% considered the inclusion of oral-systemic content as "not at all helpful" and 60% rated their current curriculum in oral-systemic health as predominately "less than efficient" (inadequate). Further findings and conclusions of the study follow below:

- The disciplines of medicine, nursing, and pharmacy were in agreement that the inclusion of oral-systemic health in undergraduate curriculum is important.
- Deficiencies in curricula of these non-dental healthcare professions regarding the inclusion of oral-systemic health were identified.
- There were no requirements at that time to incorporate oral-systemic health in the curriculum of undergraduate students of medicine, nursing, and pharmacy in many universities in the United States, Canada, Great Britain, Australia, and New Zealand.
- The majority of undergraduate students from these three disciplines were not being taught to examine the mouth nor were they instructed on how to perform an oral examination. However, of those who did receive some education and training on how to examine the oral cavity, medical and nursing students received instruction more often than did students of pharmacy.
- Administrators strongly agreed that courses about oral-systemic health for non-dental health care students would be utilized.
- There were a number of obstacles which must be overcome to enlist the support of non-dental academics in collaborative development of courses that focus on the oral cavity and on the importance of oral health in ensuring overall health.
- Topics related to oral-systemic health that were perceived by the disciplines of medicine, nursing, and pharmacy to be the most important are related to the most prevalent diseases of the oral cavity, specifically periodontal disease and caries. The relationship between periodontal disease and systemic diseases such as respiratory diseases and atherosclerosis may be of high priority.

- Of those topics that were ranked as low in importance, the perception was that many of these topics were adequately covered with basic science courses, and/or various topics were not perceived as clinically relevant to the non-dental health-care disciplines.
- Despite the calls for inclusion of this knowledge base in disciplines outside of dentistry and dental hygiene, there were a number of factors, such as internal constraints, the absence of competencies and other professional requirements of students which presented a challenge to integration of this content into current curricula.

In a separate study conducted amongst primary care providers (PCPs) practicing in a regional health care system in Wisconsin, USA, only 3% of the PCPs reported lack of oral health training during their health-related schools (Shimpi et al. 2016b). Notably, half of the participants in this study indicated the incorporation of oral health into medical practice.

However, there is very few evidence of incorporation of education around oral-systemic connection in the medical or dental practices. Until there are curriculum dedicated to educating non-dental HCPs about oral-systemic health integrated into undergraduate education and continuing education of non-dental HCPs, the oral cavity will continue to be isolated from the other systems of the body. Consequently, failure to educate non-dental HCPs about oral-systemic interrelationships will continue to compromise the potential for optimal patient outcomes. This realization has sparked calls for curriculum reform in undergraduate education of HCPs to include oral-systemic health as a foundational base of knowledge in the interprofessional, collaborative care of patients at risk for diseases and conditions related to the oral cavity.

16.1.2 Call for Curriculum Reform

In 2000, then Surgeon General David Satcher led the ground-breaking report, *Oral Health in America*, bringing to the forefront the important message that "oral health is integral to overall health (USDHHS 2000)." The report pointed out some glaring gaps in knowledge-to-action and access to dental care. In addition, the report also cited the need to change non-dental HCPs' perception of the importance of oral health, and challenged medical and dental HCPs to "be ready, willing, and able to work in collaboration to provide optimal health care for their patients". As a prerequisite to collaboration, *Oral Health in America* advocated for educational reform that provided for curriculum changes and multidisciplinary training in oral health and disease topics. Following below are statements taken directly from the Report:

- **Too little time is devoted to oral health and disease topics in the education of non-dental health professionals**. Yet all care providers can and should contribute to enhancing oral health.
- Having informed health care professionals will ensure that the public using the health care system will benefit from interdisciplinary services and comprehen-

sive care. **To prepare providers for such a role will involve, among other factors, curriculum changes and multidisciplinary training**.

Seven years after the publication of *Oral Health in America*, 12 year-old Deamonte Driver, from Prince George's County, Maryland, died from an avoidable brain infection associated with untreated dental disease—an extreme example of what Satcher called a "silent epidemic" of untreated oral disease. This is a tragic yet compelling reminder of the disparity in access to dental care that currently exists (Pyle and Stoller 2003). This left many wondering how the healthcare system failed here, and how educating non-dental HCPs to screen and appropriately triage patients for oral diseases may make a difference in lives of many, many people like Deamonte Driver.

In 2006, the Josiah Macy Jr. Foundation funded a grant to the Columbia University Center for Community Health Partnerships, with assistance from the Association of American Medical Colleges (AAMC) and the American Dental Education Association (ADEA) to convene a panel to explore the subject of curriculum and clinical training in oral health for physicians and dentists (Campus News Columbia University 2004). The subsequent report, *Curriculum and Clinical Training in Oral Health for Physicians and Dentists: Report of a Panel of the Macy Study* (Formicola et al. 2008), emphasized the importance of common medical and dental curricula in oral-systemic health, and highlighted the need and opportunities for interprofessional collaboration in this area. In this report, the panel identified a number of attitudes and values to support clinical practice that would bring attention to oral-systemic health; many of which are listed below:

- Using and updating foundational basic and clinical science knowledge in oral and systemic health
- Including an oral health history in the medical history
- Including an oral examination when performing a complete physical examination
- Recognizing and responding to behavioral factors in health care (including habits affecting oral health such tooth brushing, flossing)
- Working collaboratively in the care of patients' oral and systemic health
- Utilizing both medical and surgical approaches for disease management (for example, in the treatment of dental caries)

The Macy Study also outlined specific content areas that are foundational knowledge and clinical skills pre-requisite to addressing oral-systemic connections in collaborative patient care. The panel recommended that educational strategies should be designed so that medical and dental students can have access to the type, breadth, and depth of information required by their respective profession. A synopsis of the educational sequences that were proposed to address oral-systemic connections in collaborative patient care, specifically related to the clinical presentation of major diseases and conditions (including oral manifestations of systemic diseases or other oral-systemic interactions), and clinical skills recommended by the panel (Formicola et al. 2005, 2008) are presented below. For optimal impact on patient care, the panel reasoned that it is reasonable for these recommendations to be expanded beyond medicine and dentistry to be included in the education and training of the entirety of allied healthcare.

Foundational knowledge of major diseases and conditions necessary to address oral-systemic connections in medical and dental collaborative patient care included:

- Hypertension and cardiovascular diseases
- Diabetes and association with periodontal disease (PD)
- Obesity, including increased risk for dental caries and PD
- Eating disorders (oral and systemic manifestations and conditions)
- Hematological disorders, including bleeding diatheses, Leukemia, and lymphomas—presentation in head, neck, and oral areas
- Oral and pharyngeal cancers
- Dental caries
- Periodontal Disease (PD)
- Sexually transmitted diseases, including oral manifestations
- Impact of medications and other therapies on oral health (e.g., radiation, transplantation, immune suppression, anticoagulation, etc.)
- HIV-AIDS and other immune disorders, including oral manifestations and Sjögren's syndrome
- Other infectious diseases and common oral pathology (thrush, herpes, varicella, leukoplakia, lichen planus, etc.)
- Common mental health conditions, including depression, and the oral impact of medication
- Substance abuse (alcohol, tobacco, drugs, and related oral conditions, e.g., "meth-mouth")
- Abuse/violence and trauma, including child abuse and neglect (especially oral and craniofacial manifestations)
- Pain syndromes (tooth pain, temporomandibular joint dysfunction)
- Human development across the life span—special issues for children and the elderly
- Issues in the medical and dental care of patients with disabilities and special needs

Clinical skills necessary to address oral-systemic connections in medical-dental collaborative patient care include:

- Interviewing patients across the life cycle, including cultural and linguistic competency and the correct use of interpreters
- Obtaining a medical history, including sexual history and gender orientation
- Obtaining an oral and dental health history
- Performing appropriate portions of the general physical examination, including vital signs, and assess general habits
- Performing head and neck examinations, including oral examinations (dental exam, recognition of caries, periodontal diseases, dental erosion from eating)
- Recognizing disorders, cleft palate and other anomalies, mucosal changes, signs of oral cancer)
- Assessing basic mental health status of patients

- Providing patient education and health counseling (e.g., use motivational interviewing or other techniques for patient behavioral change in nutrition, substance use, or oral hygiene habits)
- In addition, skills are needed that relate to the appropriate use of laboratory data and to decision making and treatment planning with patients and their families so practitioners can:
  - Ordering appropriate laboratory, radiographic, and other diagnostic tests as indicated, including biopsy of suspicious oral lesions
  - Integrating critical information from physical exam, history, and laboratory, radiographic, and other data to arrive at a differential diagnosis
- Formulating treatment options for the patient and discuss those options with patients, including risks and benefits of the proposed treatment plans as well as risks and benefits of not pursuing the treatment options available, and obtain related informed consent (or parental permission for a child)

In 2008, the AAMC issued the report, *Contemporary Issues in Medicine: Oral Health Education for Medical and Dental Students; Medical School Objectives Project* (Association of American Medical Colleges 2008), which adopted the recommendations of the Macy Study (as discussed above). Subsequent to the Macy Study, the AAMC and ADEA formed a partnership to expand MedEdPORTAL (an online peer-reviewed repository for educational and teaching resources) to include oral health and dental education content (AAMC 2017). This partnership was designed to facilitate broad access to educational and instructional materials in order to foster interdisciplinary education. However, to date, there is a paucity of content related to oral-systemic health that has been posted at this electronic portal (www.aamc.org/mededportal) (AAMC 2017). Although MedEdPORTAL may provide a vehicle for worldwide dissemination of content related to oral health, relying upon the individual contributions of content experts instead of a comprehensive approach that establishes an inter professionally vetted curriculum in oral-systemic medicine that is easily integrated into undergraduate programming of non-dental HCPs may fall short in fulfilling the robust recommendations outlined in reports such as *Contemporary Issues in Medicine: Oral Health Education for Medical and Dental Students; Medical School Objectives Project, Oral Health in America* (Association of American Medical Colleges 2008; USDHHS 2014), and the position of the American Dietetic Association (Touger-Decker et al. 2003).

In 2007, the American Dietetic Association published its first position paper (Touger-Decker et al. 2013) on nutritional and oral health, which acknowledged nutrition as an integral component of oral health, and supporting the integration of oral health with nutrition services, education, and research. Below are statements illustrated directly from the paper:

- "Collaboration between dietetics and dental professionals is recommended for oral health promotion and disease prevention and intervention."
- "Scientific and epidemiologic data suggest a lifelong synergy between nutrition and the integrity of the oral cavity in health and disease."
- "Practitioners of both disciplines must learn to provide screening, baseline education, and referral to each other as part of comprehensive client/patient care."

- "Dietetics practice requires registered dietitians to provide medical nutrition therapy that incorporates a person's total health needs, including oral health."
- "Inclusion of both didactic and clinical practice concepts that illustrate the role of nutrition in oral health is essential in both dental and dietetic education programs."
- "Collaborative endeavors between dietetics and dentistry in research, education, and delineation of health provider practice roles are needed to ensure comprehensive health care."
- "Given the functional and sensory structures of the head, neck, and oral cavity in diet and nutrition, basic physical assessment education (for dieticians) and training should include screening examination of the head, neck, and oral cavity."
- "Proactive prevention and co-management of nutritional status of older adults, remedying impaired intake of foods and nutrients associated with persistent oral health problems, compromise dental function, and as a result Quality of Life."
- "Aggressive co-intervention of oral and nutritional status of patients with head and neck cancer undergoing radiotherapy is important."
- "There must be collaborative reinforcement of the importance of the beneficial effect of high intake of vegetables and fruit in reducing the risk for oral and pharyngeal cancer, particularly in heavy smokers and alcohol drinkers."
- "Proactive co-management of immunocompromised patients is essential."

The Academy of Nutrition and Dietetics published a subsequent position paper in 2013 (Touger-Decker et al. 2013), which reiterated the importance of collaboration between dietetics practitioners and oral health professionals, proposing specific didactic and practice components for designing a curriculum for dietetics and dental education programs.

Another study investigated internal medicine trainees' level of knowledge and orientation of oral health, specifically in regard to periodontal disease and adverse health events. The study concluded that medical schools should provide more comprehensive training in oral/periodontal health (Quijano et al. 2010). There currently exist standards in medicine, (United States Licensing Examinations, Steps 2, 3 (USMLE 2018a, b)) that support the inclusion of oral-systemic health learning objectives in the pre doctoral curriculum. Further, a preliminary inquiry of Canadian non-dental HCPs conducted through electronic survey suggests that 88% of physicians, and 92% of pharmacists believe they do not have enough information on oral-systemic interrelationships (MdBriefCase 2009).

As pre-licensure and continuing education in non-dental healthcare disciplines becomes enriched by inclusion of oral-systemic science, one can expect that the healthcare community at large will increasingly integrate this body of knowledge in their critical assessment of patients, and factor into case management the implication of oral health thus impacting a positive patient outcome. Appropriate education and training to physicians, nurses, pharmacists, dieticians, speech pathologists and other non-dental HCPs could impact the epidemiologic trends in serious and often debilitating oral diseases and conditions. If non-dental practitioners were trained to screen and triage patients for oral conditions it could significantly facilitate access to oral healthcare in underserved populations and will influence a number of life threatening illnesses (e.g. cardiovascular disease, diabetes) known to be complicated by oral infections (Freeman et al. 2017). Non-dental HCPs have an important role to play in prevention and emergency management of oral trauma, sustaining the oral health of immunocompromised patients and special needs patients, managing the oral complications of eating disorders and gastric conditions, adjusting pharmaceutical therapies to ensure the integrity of the oral cavity, addressing the oral aspects of sleep apnea and other airway management issues, and properly attending to special medical precautions related to the oral cavity. Non-dental HCPs can also be enlisted as valuable members of interprofessional teams in prevention and health promotion—producing oral health rather than restoring oral health. Various cases such as patients with cardiovascular disease, those undergoing chemo- and radiation therapy, and implant and organ transplant recipients require collaboration and coordination between non-dental HCPs and oral HCPs to provide integrated medical and oral health care. Non-dental HCPs in long-term and geriatric care facilities may be the principal sources of oral health care given to residents.

Given the inequitable distribution of dentists and dental hygienists and the well supported need to expand access to dental care, non-dental HCPs are also well positioned to provide basic oral health care in homeless populations, refugee camps and low resource countries, in addition to many other oral health services that have been traditionally provided by oral HCPs.

16.1.3 Curricula Planning and Development

The Curriculum Project developed by the University of Manitoba is a classic example of curriculum development. Under the leadership of Casey Hein and others, Curriculum in Oral-Systemic Health for Non-Dental HCPs was developed in 2007 (ICOSH 2007). In 2007, at the University of Manitoba, the planning phase included appointment of an advisory board that comprised of internal and external group of 50 experts, representing the fields of academia, research, and clinical practice, from a wide range of disciplines including Dentistry, Dental Hygiene, Pharmacy, Dietetics and Human Nutritional Science, Nursing, Physician Assistants, Respiratory Therapy, Medicine, Occupational Therapy, Speech and Language Pathology, Psychology and Aging, and Community Health Science and Gerontology. After 14 months of members' input and exhaustive review, the blueprint for the *Curriculum in Oral-Systemic Health for Non-Dental Healthcare Providers*, was produced.

The Advisory Board played an important role in identifying barriers to knowledge translation and challenges associated with non-dental healthcare professions' willingness to integrate the *Curriculum in Oral-Systemic Health for Non-Dental Healthcare Providers* into curricula already beyond capacity.

During the planning phase, key aspects to be integrated into this curriculum, specifically to ensure that the curriculum has a novel content included:

- Influence the way non-dental healthcare students perceive the relationship of the oral cavity to the rest of the body.

- Provide clinical pathways for appropriate integration into the practice of relevant non-dental healthcare disciplines.
- Challenge both students and practitioners to build collaborative relationships with dental practitioners that ensure optimal overall healthcare for their patients.
- Provide the requisite knowledge base for interprofessional clinical placement/emersion experiences.
- Stimulate collaboration and innovative thinking on how to transcend professional boundaries to integrate clinical protocols that include application of oral-systemic medicine in everyday patient care.
- Provide the scientific justification for collaborative, interprofessional models of care that have overlapping boundaries centered on prevention and treatment of interrelated oral-systemic diseases and conditions which are largely driven by prolonged inflammation.
- Inculcate a philosophy of practice that embraces shared accountability for clinical outcomes related to oral-systemic diseases/conditions.
- Stimulate innovative thinking of new models of care which rely upon interprofessional teams and transdisciplinary care.
- Be driven by isolating the most important aspects of oral-systemic interrelationships that are relevant to non-dental healthcare students from every discipline, including less obvious disciplines.
- Ensure content is globally relevant, including applicability of content to second and third world countries.
- Ensure learning objectives are appropriate, congruent and clinically applicable to the scopes of practice of a range of healthcare disciplines, including allied health professions.
- Identify what non-dental practitioners can/should do with this knowledge in terms of clinical application (i.e., patient education, perform risk assessment, screening, and referral).
- Provide useful tools to assist non-dental HCPs in screening and appropriately referring patients at risk for oral diseases and conditions.
- Provide interprofessional education (IPE) capstones to learning by introducing relevant simulated case studies which would require learners to apply knowledge base and critical thinking skills in collaborative management of patients at risk for oral-systemic diseases/conditions.
- Solicit content experts from dentistry and dental hygiene, as primary authors, for the creation of manuscripts specific to the individual modules, and solicit the input of practitioners from disciplines appropriate to the subject matter prior to completion of the manuscript.
- Provide extensive peer review of content to ensure accuracy, relevancy, and applicability to the wide range of non-dental healthcare professions.
- Keep current of the best practices, credible evidence, and evolving models of care in oral-systemic health, to assist future revisions of the curriculum.

In summation, these activities substantially increased the interest and commitment to advance education in oral-systemic science in non-dental healthcare disciplines and stimulated ideas for interprofessional research in oral-systemic science within the University of Manitoba.

16.2 A Move Towards Integrated Educational Models

16.2.1 Overview

This section reinforces the 1995 Institute of Medicine (IOM) report titled "Dental Education: at the Crossroads (Field and Jeffcoat 1995)." To quote Yogi Berra, a baseball sage: "When you come to a fork in the road, take it (Psychology Today 2011)." The report includes a summary and recommendations of the IOM report and three transitional reports that followed: the 2000 Surgeon General's report identifying oral health as a silent epidemic (USDHHS 2000), the Josiah Macy Foundation report (Formicola et al. 2005), and a "Pipeline" study funded by both the Robert Wood Johnson and the California foundations (Andersen et al. 2005).

The implication being that dental education must take action and move beyond its crossroads. The title was apropos as the authors' analysis concluded: (1) economics surrounding dental education was unsustainable; (2) student service learning opportunities and access to care for patients were limited; and (3) new dental schools were not replacing those forced to close due to the economic climate. The IOM report additionally proposed key recommendations to reform dental education and service delivery. Fifteen years later, we remain at "the crossroads" as these issues remain largely unresolved. Furthermore, these recommendations have retained their validity. Their implementation would directly impact structures and services for contemporary models of dental education in the future.

The following IOM recommendations (Field and Jeffcoat 1995) are intrinsic to the proposed dental education reform:

Recommendation 2: To increase access to care and improve the oral health status of underserved population.

Recommendation 3: To improve the availability of dental care in underserved areas and to limit the negative effects of high student debt.

Recommendation 5: To prepare future practitioners for more medically based modes of oral health care and more medically complicated patients, dental educators should work with their colleagues in medical schools and academic health centers. Some of the important considerations towards integrating basic science education for dental and medical students proposed were:

- Provide for dental students at least one rotation, clerkship, or equivalent experience in relevant areas of medicine, and offer opportunities for additional elective experience in hospitals, nursing homes, ambulatory care clinics, and other settings.
- Continue and expand experiments with combined M.D./D.D.S. programs and similar programs for interested students and residents.
- Increase the experience of dental faculty in clinical medicine so that they, and not just physicians—can impart medical knowledge to dental students and serve as role models for them.

Recommendation 6: To prepare students and faculty for an environment that will demand increasing efficiency, accountability, and evidence of effectiveness, the committee recommends that dental students and faculty participate in efficiently managed clinics and faculty practices in which the following occurs:

- Patient-centered, comprehensive care is the norm.
- Patients' preferences and their social, economic, and emotional circumstances are sensitively considered.
- Teamwork and cost-effective use of well-trained allied dental personnel are stressed.
- Evaluations of practice patterns and of the outcomes of care guide actions to improve both the quality and the efficiency of such care.
- General dentists serve as role models in the appropriate treatment and referral of patients needing advanced therapies.
- Larger numbers of patients, including those with more diverse characteristics and clinical problems, are served.
- In summary, the IOM report identified that:
  – An outdated curriculum continues to be retained which reflects past dental practice rather than current and emerging practice and knowledge.
  – Clinical education does not sufficiently incorporate the goal of comprehensive care, with instruction focusing too heavily on procedures.
  – Medical care and dentistry are not integrated.
  – The curriculum is crowded with redundant material, often taught in disciplinary silos.

The 1995 IOM's Report was followed by the Surgeon General's Report on Oral Health in 2000 and a subsequent supplement by the Surgeon General in 2003 called "The National Call to Action" (USDHHS 2014). Five significant findings and recommendations from the Surgeon General's Report(s) that have implications pertaining to the envisioned structure and services of new models for dental education include:

1. Changing the perception of oral health so that it will no longer be considered separate from general health.
2. Improving oral health care delivery by reducing disparities associated with populations whose access to dental treatment is compromised by poverty, limited education or language skills, geographic isolation, age, gender, disability, or an existing medical condition.
3. Encouraging oral health research, expanding preventive and early detection programs, and facilitating the transfer of knowledge about them to the general population.
4. Increasing oral health workforce diversity, capacity, and flexibility to overcome the underrepresentation of specific racial and ethnic groups in the dental profession. In this regard, the National Call to Action urged the development of dental school recruitment programs to correct these disparities and to encourage part-time dental service in community clinics in areas of oral health shortage.
5. Increasing collaboration between the private sector and the public sector to create the kind of cross-disciplinary, culturally sensitive, community-based, and community-wide efforts to expand initiatives for oral health promotion and dental disease prevention.

Spurred by the 1995 IOM report and the 2000 Surgeon General's report, the Josiah Macy Foundation conducted a study entitled "New Models of Dental Education (Pyle 2012)." The study was prompted by concerns about declines in dental school budgets and the difficulties experienced by schools in meeting their educational, research, and service missions. The solutions 'must involve basic structural changes in the way dental education is financed and organized' (Bailit et al. 2008). This statement is supported by the fact that in the past 25 years more dental schools have closed than opened. Specifically eight schools have closed, whereas to date a couple has opened and handfuls are pending. Curriculum relevance was also a focus of the study (Formicola et al. 2005). Findings concluded that "changing the curriculums in dental schools to allow students to spend more time in community venues would be highly beneficial to both society and student. Society benefited from having underserved patients cared for while students were assessed as being 5–10 times more productive, more proficient, more confident, more technically skilled and more competent in treating and interacting with minority patients (Bailit 2010)". Macy study (Formicola et al. 2005) outcomes represented significant and foundational guideposts for assessing and planning any future models for dental education. Their report led to the Robert Wood Johnson Foundation Pipeline Study (Bailit 2010), a major research study funded by the Robert Wood Johnson Foundation and The California Endowment. The goal of the Dental Pipeline Program was to reduce disparities in access to dental care. The Pipeline study provided over $30 million for the startup or expansion of 15 schools and student clinical programs that incorporated services to underserved extramural clinical settings (primarily community health centers).

The following recommendations from the Surgeon General's report structured the goals of the Pipeline's initiative:

1. Increase the number of under-represented minority and low-income students enrolled in the dental schools participating in the Pipeline Program so that there would be a voice of minority and low-income students at all the funded schools.
2. Provide dental students with courses and clinical experience that would prepare them for treating disadvantaged patients in community sites.
3. Have senior dental students spend an average of 60 days in community clinics and practices treating underserved patients. Increasing the community experience of dental students was expected to have an immediate impact on increasing care to underserved patients. This third point is pivotal to future success of dental curricula and dental education economics.

In the 2009 supplemental volume of the Journal of Dental Education the Pipeline study reported the following outcomes (Andersen et al. 2009):

- Minority recruitment of low-income students increased by 27%.
- The rate of recruitment for under-represented populations was almost twice that of non-pipeline schools.
- The length of time dental students spent in extramural rotations increased from a mean of 16 days to a mean of 39 days over a period of 4 years.
- Procedural proficiency increased compared to that of their non-extramural peers.
- Of the 15 Pipeline-funded programs, only four schools achieved the goal of 60 days of extramural rotations; Through extra funding from TCE, the four schools extended extramural rotations to an average of 198 days.

- Based on this publication, it appears that only a handful of pipeline schools definitely plan to sustain their extended extramural rotations. Financial concerns were highlighted as the major problem in sustaining future recruitment and placement of students beyond the timeframe of the study.
- A survey of program seniors indicated a mean of 26% [range of 14–60% by school] were planning to devote > =25% of their practice to serving minority patients. Only 9% [range of 3–22% by school] were planning to practice at community clinics.

In the context of these outcomes, discussion indicated that the unwillingness of students to practice in underserved settings was based on several factors:

- Students that participated were already enrolled in traditional programs and were not necessarily seeking a pipeline experience or a future in community service.
- Concern over future reimbursement as a provider in a community setting.
- Limited time spent in underserved settings.
- Limited loan forgiveness scholarship opportunities.

The fact that the large majority of pipelines were unsustainable was attributed to lack of productivity in the school clinics while the students were on rotation at community based clinics. Schools generate meager, yet necessary, revenue streams on intramural student clinical activity to support the costly clinical and faculty infrastructure. Currently, similar economic constraints involved with outsourcing students to serving rural and underserved populations impacts the ability of traditional dental schools to participate in sustained outreach programs.

The Pew Center on the States National Academy for Health Policy released "Help Wanted: A Policy Makers Guide to New Dental Providers ("Help Wanted | The Pew Charitable Trusts, 2009)". This report provided an excellent summary outlining workforce needs, access issues, and strategies for dental-related services to help states and institutions develop creative ways to solve oral health access and care issues. The Guide proposes the following relevant components and trends for consideration in development of future sustainable school models:

- Dental colleges are willing to bear a large and disproportionate share of the burden in terms of access to care, particularly during a time of incredibly scarce resources.
- Expanded, extensive, and/or creative extramural rotations have been developed in recent years under the conceptual umbrella of service-learning. These often involve clinics providing direct or indirect payment to dental schools or clinics managed in some way by dental schools.

16.2.2 Current Status: Economics, Equity, and Education Converge

Dental education has certain obligations. First, education must adhere to accreditation standards with the goal of producing competent practitioners. Second, education must remain responsive and impact the societal need for care. Lastly, the delivery of dental education must be economically sustainable. The Macy, RWJF,

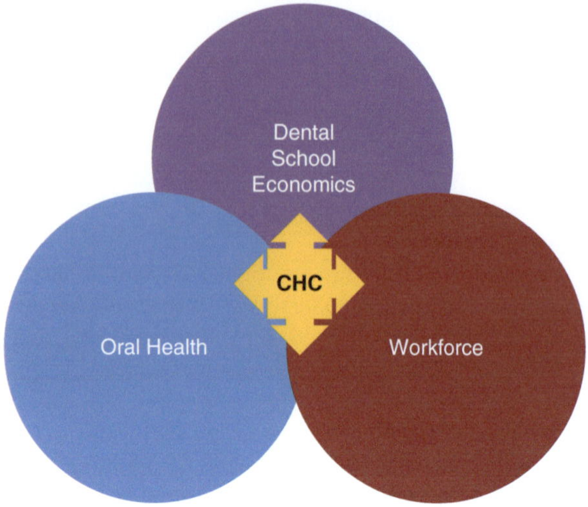

Fig. 16.1 Illustrates the synergy between access to care, student competency, and financially sustainable dental education converge around CHC/FQHCs

and IOM reports note that improved oral health, sustainable dental education economic models, and competent workforce pipelines converge around Community Health Centers (CHC). Figure 16.1 illustrates the synergy between access to care, student competency, and financially sustainable dental education converge around CHC/FQHCs.

Piskorowski et al. (2012) reaffirm this conclusion in an evaluation of an ongoing 7-year program, stating that: (the CHC model) is self-sustaining and can be used to increase service to the underserved and increase the value of students' clinical educational experiences without requiring grant or school funding, thus improving the value of dental education without increased cost.

Self-sustaining contracts with seven Federally Qualified Health Centers (FQHCs) have resulted in win-win-win-win outcomes: win for the underserved communities, which experienced increased access to care; win for the FQHCs, which experienced increased and more consistent productivity; win for the students, who increased their clinical skills and broadened their experience base; and win for the school in the form of predictable and continuing full coverage of all program costs (Piskorowski et al. 2012).

However, unlike medicine that outsources their students to clinical sites; dental education programs retain the majority of the student time within their own "clinical laboratories". As documented by the aforementioned studies, this limits students' exposure to extramural experiences. Costs to operate such intramural clinical programs are ever increasing and many schools' clinical operations run deficits. If that component can be outsourced to community-based resources such as a CHC, then the burden of cost is shifted away from the school. An example would be A.T. Still University's Arizona School of Dentistry and Oral Health (ASDOH), which matriculated its first class in 2003. At the prompting of the State's community based clinics, ASDOH designed a program that placed students into community-based settings for up to 6 months, an unprecedented length of time for an extramural rotation.

They also saw this as an opportunity to use an adjunct centric faculty that significantly reduced traditional education overhead. Through this innovation, the school was able to develop a program that was sustained by "fair market" value tuition and trained students where community needs were greatest for up to 6 months (which was then unprecedented). Conversely, if the CHC can rely on student service-learning to care for patients, the cost of care is reduced. Other schools are also advancing with innovative education and care delivery.

Although several schools are expanding with an aim of solving the existent access supply and demand issues, it is observed that even with all the startups and expansions, graduation numbers will not approach the output of schools in the late 1970s and early 1980s.

These creative models establish the foundation for a sustainable clinic structure by generating self-sustaining revenue through student service-learning, which, unlike medical student services, are billable. Simultaneously these new models provide access to care for the needy and student exposure to clinical experiences that are often not available in academic patient pools. These models also shift some of the cost of providing clinical education from the dental college to community-based clinics.

However, this innovation is not without criticism. Schools are dependent on the success of their clinics and clinic partnerships. One author cautions: "However, these creative models also may present potential political strategic risk or conflict: private practitioners may organize and protest higher than normal reimbursement schemes. Potentially, such protests could even jeopardize the very existence of such models (Dunning et al. 2009)." Notably, community health centers have historically received strong bipartisan support. For example, during the Bush administration, FQHC funding was doubled and most recently expanded through health reform legislation by the Obama administration. According to the 2017 HRSA report, more than 10,000 individual health center exists majority of which are the community health centers, that provides care to about 24.3 million people (Hasstedt 2017; Health Reform Monitoring Surveys 2014; Heisler 2017).

16.2.3 A Road to the Future

According to the Institute for Oral Health, "The group practice of the future is the dentist working with the physician" (Field and Jeffcoat 1995). The ADA reported "multidisciplinary education must become the norm and represent the meaning and purposes of primary care as it applies to dentistry. Educational sequences should include rotation strategies across discipline specialties in medicine and dentistry, clerkships and hospital rotations, and experience in faculty and residency clinics (Bailit et al. 2008; Barnett et al. 2015)." The models alluded to were school-based attempts at improving educational outcomes. Perhaps the proverbial fork in the road regarding the future of dental education leaves two paths for consideration. Is it better to travel down a road that leads a school to develop and operate a clinic? Or is the road less traveled, where a clinic becomes a school, the better of the two options? The answer, perhaps, is that a combination of both will accomplish the desired outcome. For example, didactic knowledge is measured by examination whereas competency as a practitioner is measured by clinical demonstration. At a minimum, the result must achieve learner competency, quality, and sustainability. However, the road less traveled has not been taken yet. William Gies, in his revered report written 85 years ago on the state of American dental education, wrote "Dental faculties should show the need for integrated instruction in the general principles of clinical dentistry and in its correlations with clinical medicine" (ADEAFGies Foundation 1926). Basic sciences aside, could a clinical-based educational training center have an advantage over a school-based clinical center? Soon-to-be-implemented new Commission on Dental Accreditation (CODA) standards will require schools to demonstrate competency in patient-centered care (Valachovic 2009). Might an enterprise proficient at running a successful clinical business model have an advantage running a professional, patient-centered clinical training program as compared to a pedagogical business model attempting to run a clinical training model? These questions should challenge us to reexamine why our thinking about educational models should be limited to schools being the starting point for the development of a profession that demands clinical competency, patient-centeredness, and integration as outcomes. The clinic based model may serve as an equivalent starting point and, have some distinct advantages for achieving responsiveness to recommendations and directions cited in this section.

16.2.4 A FQHC Model

Beginning in November 2002 through August 2010, the Family Health Center (FHC) of Marshfield, Inc., Marshfield, Wisconsin, launched a broad network of developing dental clinics, targeting dental professional shortage areas with the provision of dental services to the underserved communities whose dental needs were not being adequately met by the existing infrastructure.

FHC-Marshfield is a Federally Qualified Health Center (FQHC). As an FQHC, FHC receives cost-based reimbursement for its dental services to Medicaid populations. Along with the cost-based reimbursement, FQHCs are obligated to provide care to anyone regardless of their ability to pay. Presently, FHC is the nation's largest federally qualified dental health center. To date, this network of dental clinics has served over 154,153 unique patients. Notably, service was provided to a significant number of cognitively and developmentally disabled patients in special stations developed for serving patients with special needs. These patients frequently travel the furthest to get to our dental centers for care. Beginning in 2008, FHC stepped up the pace of dental clinic expansion, constructing ten dental centers until 2018. Each site has proactively included dedicated clinical and classroom training space for dental residents or students, thus laying the framework for clinic-based training of new dental professionals. In addition to the capacity for training residents and students, a dental post-baccalaureate program is being considered in partnership with regional 4 year under graduate campuses. The post-baccalaureate program is aimed at preparing students from rural and underserved areas who desire to practice in rural and underserved areas for acceptance and success in dental schools. A 1 year's dental residency program was offered in year 2015 and two dental residents completed their one year AEGD program. Moreover, this program also integrated research in their 1 year of dental residency to ensure application of evidence based practices at point-of-care (Emrick and Gullard 2013). The incorporation of research also led to publications in peer-reviewed journals (Shimpi et al. 2018, 2016a, b). Presently, FHC has partnered with Marshfield Clinic to serve as one of training clinics for A.T. Dental School to have dental students rotate through to better prepare pre-doctoral students to be successful in being responsive to rural environments which have been classically underserved. Marshfield Clinic has a long-standing history in medical student education and multiple medical residency programs.

Creating access for the underserved population was the major motivational force driving the establishment of the dental clinic network back in 2002. The findings of the IOM, Macy, and RWJF reports became the foundational framework for developing the vision of a dental education model that would realize the major recommendations found in the reports. By establishing clinical campuses in regional underserved dental health professional shortage areas, access to care where care is needed most was provided. Sustainment of a work force for provision of care across the dental clinic network is accomplished by schools contracting with FQHC's for service learning, thus circumventing challenges associated with releasing dental students at traditional dental schools to distant extramural training sites as discussed previously. This model is however not without its own set of challenges including calibration of faculty, supervision and evaluation of students in training, and achieving accreditation acceptance. However, through video connectivity and iEHR technology curriculum, learning plans, competency assessment, progression, performance, faculty development, and learner evaluations can be centrally calibrated. Additionally, this dental service-learning model based in a community health center setting offers students unique state-of-the-art exposures to alternative access models, cutting-edge informatics (including access to a combined dental-medical record) and a quality-based outcomes-driven practice.

Given the novelty of such an extended extramural dental clinical training model, there is limited data on the success of rural placement leading to retention to practice in a rural setting. The Pipeline study piloted a model for getting students into under-served communities (Andersen et al. 2005). However, that experiment was limited to 60-day rotations. Outcome driven programs may provide a predictive surrogate for purposes of comparative analysis. For example, the Rural Medical Education "RMED" program of the University of Illinois medical school at Rockford, has sustained a longstanding program in Illinois (RMED 2018). Rabinowitz et al. further reinforced that medical school rural programs have been highly successful in increasing the supply of rural physicians, with an average of 53–64% of graduates choosing to practice in rural areas. They also noted rural retention rates of 79–87% among the programs (Rabinowitz et al. 2008).

The University of Wisconsin School of Medicine and Public Health (UWSMPH) launched the Wisconsin Academy for Rural Medicine (WARM 2018). The WARM program places medical students in rural academic medical centers during their third and fourth years in medical school. Marshfield Clinic hosted the first WARM program as one of the sites. WARM students affiliating with Marshfield Clinic's system shares learning experiences with dental students, clinical rotations, team-based rounding, lectures, and exposure to a combined medical-dental patient record. In an analogous manner, the Center for Oral and Systemic Health along with Division of Education at Marshfield Clinic developed integrated computer based training materials for medical and dental providers surrounding oral and systemic health emphasizing the bi-directional association between diabetes and periodontal disease. Moreover, Smiles for Life curriculum was also implemented for training the medical providers for integrating oral health into primary practice (Douglass et al. 2007).

A secondary but not insignificant outcome of placing residents and students in clinical campuses focused on developing competency and providing care where needs are often greatest is the cost savings to taxpayers associated with the public care of patients. These savings are accomplished through the "service-learning" of the student. For example, in the model described where clinical training is embedded within the FHC clinics, the stipend resident or unpaid student learner provides the patient care as part of their service learning training while requiring oversight from one paid faculty per 4–6 learners. As a result, an academic-based clinical partnership creates a model that reduces the cost for care provided to underserved patients. An additional benefit to the community-based clinic might be realized through tuition assistance by the academic program to help support patient procedures that develop learner competencies. In educational quality and influence, dental schools should equal medical schools, for their responsibilities are similar and their tasks analogous (ADEAFGies Foundation 1926).

The Commission on Dental Accreditation (CODA) notes that one of the learning objectives of an Advanced Education General Dentistry (AEGD) Residency is to have the graduate function as a "primary care provider". To function competently in this role, the graduate needs to have a strong academic linkage to primary care medicine. At a 2010 dental deans forum, 84 years after the Gies report, Dr. Polverini made the statement "Dentistry has never been linked to the medical network but unless dentistry becomes part of the solution to the challenge of providing comprehensive patient care, it will be looked on as part of the problem, and ultimately, all dental schools will be called into question (Polverini 2012)". The use of dental informatics and an integrated record are elements essential to this competency. On 1 April 2010, FHC and Marshfield Clinic successfully transitioned all of their dental centers to a new practice management and electronic health record system that fully integrates medical and dental; one of the first such systems in the nation. CHC placement also exposes students to an integrated medical-dental care setting where learners can develop skills in system-based practice to include the interdependence of health professionals, systems, and the coordination of care. On the administrative side, dental and medical appointments can be coordinated to enhance convenience for patients and improve compliance with preventive dental visits. In 2009, Marshfield Clinic's Research Institute hired their first Dental Informatician, Dr. Amit Acharya, B.D.S., M.S., Ph.D. Dr. Acharya has been instrumental in founding the Center for Oral and Systemic Health within the Marshfield Clinic Research Institute. Along with cutting edge research, some of the key achievements towards integration of medical and dental arenas include conducting oral and systemic health conferences in the State of Wisconsin as well as attracting national and international experts to speak about medical-dental best practices to the regional medical and dental providers. With dedicated informatics and research resource centers, Marshfield Clinic has laid the groundwork for true medical/dental integration with appropriate electronic health record decision support and is positioned to develop a dental education curriculum capable of implementing the IOM recommendations. Downstream benefits of using such a curriculum are the ability of future practitioners to use informatics to improve quality of care and reduce the burden of disease.

According to an Institute of Oral Health Report (2000) it is widely accepted across the dental profession that oral health has a direct impact on systemic health, and increasingly, medical and dental care providers are building to bridge relationships to create treatment solutions. As early as 1926, William Gies recognized that "the frequency of periodic examination gives dentists exceptional opportunity to note early signs of many types of illnesses outside the domain of dentistry" (ADEAFGies Foundation 1926). The following examples show how integration of dental and medical care can impact patient outcomes, underlining the importance of this concept in dental curriculum design.

A 2017 randomized controlled trial showed that non-surgical periodontal treatment significantly improved the glycemic status of type 2 diabetic patients thus demonstrating the importance of oral health to their overall health (Mauri-Obradors et al. 2018). Another example is found in the context of preterm delivery and role of maternal periodontitis. Based on the research review conducted by Ren and Du four possible models of periodontitis in preterm birth were described and they concluded that oral health maintenance during pregnancy needs to be an integral part of the preventive care (Ren and Du 2017).

Equally important is the opportunity to develop and implement the team-based curriculum that trains future dentists and physicians in the management of chronic disease as an Accountable Care Organization (ACO) in a patient-centered environment. As an example, a study, reported that medical costs for diabetics who accessed dental care for prevention and periodontal services were significantly lower than those who didn't get dental care (Nasseh et al. 2014).

These data suggest that team based case management of prevalent chronic health conditions have considerable cost savings opportunities for government payers, third party payers, employers, and employees (Errante 2010). These economic benefits to integration as it relates to the iEHR are discussed elsewhere in this book, but begin with the ability of providers to function in a team-based environment and as such, underscore the importance of training in such an environment.

Dentists trained in a FQHC iEHR integrated educational model will be well positioned to function successfully within an ACO model. An ACO is a system where providers are accountable for the outcomes and expenditures of the insured population of patients they serve. The providers within the system are charged with collectively improving care around cost and quality targets set by the payor. Within this system, care must be delivered in a patient-centered environment. The patient-centered environment according to the National Committee for Quality Assurance (NCQA), is a health care setting that cultivates partnerships between individual patients and their personal physicians and, when appropriate, the patient's family. The ontological model developed by Sen and Sinha describes the key processes and activities using maturity concepts (Sen and Sinha 2016).

Exchange, and other means to assure that patients receive defined, timely and appropriate care while remaining cognizant of cultural, linguistic, and literacy needs of the patient being served. The model includes the opportunity to deliver patient care that is patient-centric, incorporates the patient in the care planning, considers the patient's beliefs and views, and incorporates the patient's families as needed. The model allows providers to deliver care that is inclusive of needs, attentive, and accessible. The model equips payers to purchase high quality and coordinated care among teams of providers across healthcare settings. While this describes the medical home, most dental practices also follow this process. Many dental practices function in this regard with insured populations and reflect elements of the model that medicine is creating. William Gies would be proud. Training in the delivery of accountable and patient-centered medical-dental care must be done purposefully. Commenting on the inadequate training relative to the integration of medical and dental education, Baum stated that "we need to design new curricula with meaningful core competencies for the next generation of dentists rather than apply patches to our existing ones (Baum and Scully 2015)." While this statement was made in reference to the basic sciences, the same holds true for patient-centered system-based practice competencies.

Utilizing state-of-the-art electronic medical records as a tool and the FHC infrastructure as the service venue, meaningful patient-centered system-based practice core competencies achievement becomes possible in a manner highly responsive to societal needs. By definition, FQHCs must provide primary medical care, dental care, and behavioral health. FQHC have also historically been utilized as healthcare workforce training centers and the Affordable Care Act of 2010 reinforced their role as healthcare training centers.

Specifically, this legislation serves to promote FQHCs as the entity through which the primary care workforce (including dental) will be developed and expanded. In combination, FQHCs and primary care centers are positioned to be the front runners in a medical-dental home training model which will be essential to preparing future practitioners for practice in an ACO. Critical to this success is the ability to train these practitioners on an integrated medical-dental record and informatics platform.

Use of this platform imprints most strongly during the learner's formative years of training; instructing and guiding disease management, decision making, patient care coordination, prevention, and both outcome-based and comprehensive care.

Training in this hybrid academically orientated clinically integrated setting moves dental education off its crossroads and creates the highway to its future.

16.3 Concerns

Concerns with the new models extend to their ability to integrate medical and dental disciplines at the clinical and informatics level. While the 1995 IOM report identified the need to integrate medical and dental curricula, success at the curricular and technological levels within schools, has been limited. Three major factors have contributed to the limited progress:

- **Access priorities**: Creating access to care has outranked the need to integrate care. In part, this reflects the societal need for care and public demand to reduce the burden of the "silent epidemic." Schools play an important role as a safety net to care for the uninsured and underinsured through intramural clinical service learning. Even though "dental colleges seem to be willing to bearing a large and disproportionate share of the burden in terms of access to care (Dunning et al. 2009)", schools were challenged as part of IOM, Surgeon General, and Macy reports, to expand that role. While these reports have prompted creative educational solutions to increase access, the reports understate the tremendous opportunity, quality, and cost benefits that could result from an integration of medicine and dentistry.
- **Culture of Educational Model**: It is difficult to change the culture and structure of existing schools. This is not unique to dentistry. However, the 1995 IOM report specifically recommended that schools "eliminate marginally useful and redundant courses and design an integrated basic and clinical science curriculum" The challenges with this are many. Examples include:
  - Some schools may not have other disciplines to draw from to create an integrated curriculum.
  - A number of schools use a faculty senate to determine curriculum. This can result in curriculum that preserves the current faculty structure.
  - Changing curriculum is associated with expense and can be financially prohibitive to some schools.
  - Physical changes may be needed and represent an expense and/or may, in some instances, may not be practicable based on the structure of existing facilities.
  - Public school programs may direct the final curriculum, as boards or regents one or two steps removed from the curriculum often have final authority. Conversely, private schools may specify business or mission objectives that determine final design.
  - Perhaps most germane to this text is the lack of a common technology platform between disciplines in a learning environment.

An integrated curriculum requires an integrated platform to accomplish delivery and evaluation. This is particularly essential to clinical management of the patient by professionals in training as part of a healthcare delivery team. Some progress in establishing shared basic sciences curricula has been documented in the literature. To date, no single integrated electronic health (medical-dental) record has been meaningfully adapted for educational purposes, including incorporation of assessment of the learner relative to integrated competencies, integrated case-based and problem-based curriculum, and integrated evaluation and assessment.

Another concern with new educational programs emerging in response to these reports and relative to creating a transformational integrated curriculum is that some of the programs are focusing primarily on creating clinicians with no value or emphasis on integrating training with research and/or scholarly activity. Integrated training models counter such concerns. Research will be fundamental to measuring the relative benefits and outcomes associated with treatment of patients in a shared curriculum setting and will be the catalyst for the development of integrated medical-dental informatics incorporating educational capabilities. Additionally, accreditation will also need to evaluate its response to such models.

Presently it is unclear how accrediting bodies will view an integrated cross-disciplinary curriculum. Further, due to its integrated nature, such a curriculum would lie outside of the expertise of a single traditional accrediting body focused on one particular discipline. It has yet to be determined how accrediting bodies will review and appraise such cross-disciplinary competencies.

Lastly, it is important to recognize that a successful education model with innovative informatics is only successful if its focus is patient care. Graduating learners with competency only in the use of informatics will be limited unless adapted to training and delivery programs that result in patient-centric care.

16.4 Conclusions

Research and reports over the past two decades support the need to reform dental education. First steps have been taken and lead the way for continued innovation around clinic-based education and integrated curriculum. The models identified point to a strong partnership and interrelationship with CHCs for creative, cost saving, effective, and sustainable delivery methods. Moreover, CHC's must be more involved in a training curriculum integrated with informatics. CHCs, in turn, benefit from residents and students through service-learning to help meet a societal and workforce need, while the learners benefit from increased competency. In order to train an evidence-based, patient-centered, medical-dental workforce, it is imperative that medical and dental data and record accessibility be incorporated into these training and care delivery initiatives. In order to keep moving away from the crossroads, such integration must become the pathway on which curriculum is developed and implemented.

References

AAMC. MedEdPORTAL: the journal of teaching and learning resources. 2017. https://www.mededportal.org/. Accessed 15 Jun 2018.

ADEAFGies Foundation. William J. Gies and the Gies report. 1926. http://www.adea.org/ADEAGiesFoundation/William-J-Gies-and-Gies-Report.aspx. Accessed 16 Jun 2018.

Andersen RM, Davidson PL, Atchison KA, Crall JJ, Friedman J-A, Hewlett ER, Thind A. Summary and implications of the dental pipeline program evaluation. J Dent Educ. 2009;73(2 Suppl). http://www.jdentaled.org/content/73/2_suppl/S319

Andersen RM, Davidson PL, Atchison KA, Hewlett E, Freed JR, Friedman J-A, et al. Pipeline, profession, and practice program: evaluating change in dental education. J Dent Educ. 2005;69(2):239–48.

Association of American Medical Colleges. Contemporary issues in medicine: oral health education for medical and dental S. 2008. https://aamc-meded.global.ssl.fastly.net/production/media/filer_public/14/8a/148a8d2f-6239-4876-8203-1704321f311b/oral_health_msop.pdf

Bailit HL. Organization and management of community-based dental education programs: an overview from the dental pipeline program. J Dent Educ. 2010;74(10 Suppl). http://www.jdentaled.org/content/74/10_suppl/S9

Bailit HL, Beazoglou TJ, Formicola AJ, Tedesco LA, Brown LJ, Weaver RG. U.S. state-supported dental schools: financial projections and implications. J Dent Educ. 2008;72(2 Suppl):98–109. http://www.ncbi.nlm.nih.gov/pubmed/18250386

Barnett T, Hoang H, Stuart J, Crocombe L. Non-dental primary care providers' views on challenges in providing oral health services and strategies to improve oral health in Australian rural and remote communities: a qualitative study. BMJ Open. 2015;5(10):e009341. https://doi.org/10.1136/bmjopen-2015-009341.

Baum BJ, Scully C. Training specialists in oral medicine. Oral Dis. 2015;21(6):681–4. https://doi.org/10.1111/odi.12351.

Campus News Columbia University. Macy foundation grant to explore new models for dental education—Columbia University Medical Center. 2004. http://newsroom.cumc.columbia.edu/blog/2004/07/26/macy-foundation-grant-to-explore-new-models-for-dental-education-3/. Accessed 15 Jun 2018.

Douglass AB, Gonsalves W, Maier R, Silk H, Stevens N, Tysinger J, Wrightson AS. Smiles for life: a national oral health curriculum for family medicine. A model for curriculum development by STFM groups. Fam Med. 2007;39(2):88–90. http://www.ncbi.nlm.nih.gov/pubmed/17273948

Dunning DG, Durham TM, Lange BM, Aksu MN. Strategic management and organizational behavior in dental education: reflections on key issues in an environment of change. J Dent Educ. 2009;73(6):689–95. http://www.ncbi.nlm.nih.gov/pubmed/19491346

Emrick JJ, Gullard A. Integrating research into dental student training: a global necessity. J Dent Res. 2013;92(12):1053–5. https://doi.org/10.1177/0022034513508557.

Errante. Institute for oral health – DentistryIQ. 2010. https://www.dentistryiq.com/articles/2010/07/institute-for-oral.html. Accessed 16 Jun 2018.

Field MJ, Jeffcoat MK. Dental education at the crossroads: a report by the Institute of Medicine. J Am Dent Assoc (1939). 1995;126(2):191–5. http://www.ncbi.nlm.nih.gov/pubmed/7860887

Formicola AJ, Bailit H, Beazoglou T, Tedesco LA. The Macy study: a framework for consensus. J Dent Educ. 2005;69(11):1183–5. http://www.ncbi.nlm.nih.gov/pubmed/16275682

Formicola AJ, Bailit HL, Beazoglou TJ, Tedesco LA. The Macy study: a framework for consensus. J Dent Educ. 2008;72(2 suppl):95–7. http://www.jdentaled.org/content/72/2_suppl/95

Freeman CR, Abdullah N, Ford PJ, Taing M-W. A national survey exploring oral healthcare service provision across Australian community pharmacies. BMJ Open. 2017;7(9):e017940. https://doi.org/10.1136/bmjopen-2017-017940.

Gorman C, Park A, Dell K. Health: the fires within – TIME. 2004. http://content.time.com/time/magazine/article/0,9171,993419,00.html. Accessed 15 Jun 2018.

Hasstedt K. Federally qualified health centers: vital sources of care, no substitute for the family planning safety net | Guttmacher Institute. 2017. https://www.guttmacher.org/gpr/2017/05/federally-qualified-health-centers-vital-sources-care-no-substitute-family-planning. Accessed 16 Jun 2018.
Health Reform Monitoring Surveys. Federally qualified health centers? Importance in the safety net continues for many as affordable care act implementation moves ahead. 2014. http://hrms.urban.org/briefs/federally-qualified-health-centers-importance-aca.html. Accessed 16 Jun 2018.
Hein C. Will evidence of oral-systemic interrelationships be integrated into the clinical practice of physicians and other non-dental health care providers? In: Rennie J, editors. Oral-systemic interrelationships. Sci Am. 2006. https://www.caseyhein.com/wp-content/uploads/2012/09/Oral-Systemic_Interrelationships_Will_Evidence_of_Oral-Systemic_Interrelationships_be.pdf
Hein C, Schönwetter DJ, Iacopino AM. Inclusion of oral-systemic health in predoctoral/undergraduate curricula of pharmacy, nursing, and medical schools around the world: a preliminary study. J Dent Educ. 2011;75(9):1187–99.
Heisler E. Federal health centers: an overview. 2017. https://fas.org/sgp/crs/misc/R43937.pdf
Help Wanted | The Pew Charitable Trusts. 2009. http://www.pewtrusts.org/en/research-and-analysis/reports/2009/05/28/help-wanted-a-policy-makers-guide-to-new-dental-providers. Accessed 15 Jun 2018.
ICOSH. University of Manitoba – International Centre for Oral-Systemic Health. 2007. http://www.umanitoba.ca/icosh/oshcurriculum.html. Accessed 15 Jun 2018.
Kiefer, D. Disease prevention begins in the mouth – page 1 | Life extension. 2008. http://www.life-extension.com/magazine/2008/9/Disease-Prevention-Begins-in-the-Mouth/Page-01. Accessed 15 Jun 2018.
Mauri-Obradors E, Merlos A, Estrugo-Devesa A, Jané-Salas E, López-López J, Viñas M. Benefits of non-surgical periodontal treatment in patients with type 2 diabetes mellitus and chronic periodontitis: a randomized controlled trial. J Clin Periodontol. 2018;45(3):345–53. https://doi.org/10.1111/jcpe.12858.
MdBriefCase. mdBriefCase. 2009. https://www.mdbriefcase.com/About-Us.aspx. Accessed 15 Jun 2018.
Nasseh K, Greenberg B, Vujicic M, Glick M. The effect of chairside chronic disease screenings by oral health professionals on health care costs. Am J Public Health. 2014;104(4):744–50. https://doi.org/10.2105/AJPH.2013.301644.
Oz M, Levine J. Interview: Dr. Jonathan Levine | The Dr. Oz Show. 2013. https://www.doctoroz.com/audio/interview-dr-jonathan-levine-0. Accessed 15 Jun 2018.
Piskorowski WA, Stenafac SJ, Fitzgerald M, Green TG, Krell RE. Influence of community-based dental education on dental students' preparation and intent to treat underserved populations. J Dent Educ. 2012;76(5):534–9. http://www.ncbi.nlm.nih.gov/pubmed/22550098
Polverini PJ. A curriculum for the new dental practitioner: preparing dentists for a prospective oral health care environment. Am J Public Health. 2012;102(2):e1–3. https://doi.org/10.2105/AJPH.2011.300505.
Psychology Today. When coming to a fork in the road – take it (Yogi Berra) | Psychology Today. 2011. https://www.psychologytoday.com/us/blog/look-around-and-look-within/201012/when-coming-fork-in-the-road-take-it-yogi-berra. Accessed 15 Jun 2018.
Pyle MA. New models of dental education and curricular change: their potential impact on dental education. J Dent Educ. 2012;76(1):89–97. http://www.ncbi.nlm.nih.gov/pubmed/22262553
Pyle MA, Stoller EP. Oral health disparities among the elderly: interdisciplinary challenges for the future. J Dent Educ. 2003;67(12):1327–36. http://www.ncbi.nlm.nih.gov/pubmed/14733265
Quijano A, Shah AJ, Schwarcz AI, Lalla E, Ostfeld RJ. Knowledge and orientations of internal medicine trainees toward periodontal disease. J Periodontol. 2010;81(3):359–63. https://doi.org/10.1902/jop.2009.090475.

Rabinowitz HK, Diamond JJ, Markham FW, Wortman JR. Medical school programs to increase the rural physician supply: a systematic review and projected impact of widespread replication. Acad Med. 2008;83(3):235–43. https://doi.org/10.1097/ACM.0b013e318163789b.

Ren H, Du M. Role of maternal periodontitis in preterm birth. Front Immunol. 2017;8:139. https://doi.org/10.3389/fimmu.2017.00139.

RMED. National Center for Rural Health Professions – University of Illinois College of Medicine. 2018. http://www.ncrhp.uic.edu/index.cfm?id=1053&page=Rural+Medical+Education+Program+(RMED)&b=1001. Accessed 16 Jun 2018.

Sen A, Sinha AP. An ontological model of the practice transformation process. J Biomed Inform. 2016;61:298–318. https://doi.org/10.1016/J.JBI.2016.05.001.

Shimpi N, Bharatkumar A, Jethwani M, Chyou P-H, Glurich I, Blamer J, Acharya A. Knowledgeability, attitude and behavior of primary care providers towards oral cancer: a pilot study. J Cancer Educ. 2016a;33(2):359–64. https://doi.org/10.1007/s13187-016-1084-4.

Shimpi N, Jethwani M, Bharatkumar A, Chyou P-H, Glurich I, Acharya A. Patient awareness/knowledge towards oral cancer: a cross-sectional survey. BMC Oral Health. 2018;18(1) https://doi.org/10.1186/s12903-018-0539-x.

Shimpi N, Schroeder D, Kilsdonk J, Chyou P-H, Glurich I, Penniman E, Acharya A. Medical providers' oral health knowledgeability, attitudes, and practice behaviors: an opportunity for interprofessional collaboration. J Evid Based Dent Pract. 2016b;16(1):19–29. https://doi.org/10.1016/j.jebdp.2016.01.002.

Touger-Decker R, Mobley C, Academy of Nutrition and Dietetics. Position of the Academy of Nutrition and Dietetics: oral health and nutrition. J Acad Nutr Diet. 2013;113(5):693–701. https://doi.org/10.1016/j.jand.2013.03.001.

Touger-Decker R, Mobley C, Academy of Nutrition and Dietetics. Position of the American Dietetic Association: oral health and nutrition. J Am Diet Assoc. 2003;103(5):615–25. https://doi.org/10.1053/jada.2003.50130.

U.S. Department of Health and Human Services. Oral health in America: a report of the Surgeon general. Rockville, MD: U.S. Department of Health and Human Services, National Institute of Dental and Craniofacial Research, National Institute of Health; 2000.

USDHHS. U.S. Department of Health and Human Services. The health consequences of smoking—50 years of progress: a report of the surgeon general: U.S. Department of Health and Human Services, Centers for Disease Control and Prevention, National Center. 2014.

USMLE. United States Medical Licensing Examination | Step 2 CK (Clinical Knowledge). 2018a. http://www.usmle.org/step-2-ck/. Accessed 15 Jun 2018.

USMLE. United States Medical Licensing Examination | Step 3. 2018b. http://www.usmle.org/step-3/. Accessed 15 Jun 2018.

Valachovic. Charting progress. 2009. http://www.adea.org/about_adea/Pages/ChartingProgress.aspx. Accessed 15 Jun 2018.

WARM. Wisconsin Academy for Rural Medicine (WARM). 2018. https://www.med.wisc.edu/education/md-program/warm/. Accessed 16 Jun 2018.

Chapter 17
Integrated Care Case Study: Marshfield Clinic Health System

Neel Shimpi, Ingrid Glurich, and Amit Acharya

17.1 History of the Organization

Founded in 1916 by a group of six physicians, Marshfield Clinic has expanded to become one of the largest private multispecialty group practices in the United States (MCHS 2018). This integrated and comprehensive care system serves a largely rural-dwelling population with a median low to mid-level income range in a service area that encompasses Central, Western, and Northern Wisconsin. The current infrastructure represents century-long cumulative efforts whose stated mission from inception of Marshfield Clinic was stated as: serving patients through accessible, high quality healthcare, research and education. In 2014, Marshfield Clinic and its affiliated entities prospectively underwent a corporate reorganization to become collectively incorporated as the Marshfield Clinic Health System. Presently, MCHS includes a network of 42 medical clinics, ten dental clinics served by more than 760 providers and 7600 engaged in integrated patient care delivery, research, and medical education across 57 locations throughout its service area. In addition, MCHS provides service to more than 1200 hospitals, clinics, and sites through its outreach service program. MCHS's mission remains ingrained into the organizational culture.

MCHS is comprised of Marshfield Clinic (MC), Marshfield Clinic Hospital, Marshfield Clinic Research Institute (MCRI), Marshfield Clinic Education Foundation, Security Health Plan (SHP), its health maintenance organization (HMO) and Family Health Center of Marshfield (FHC), its partnering federally qualified health center which established and oversees operational management of MCHS's dental clinic infrastructure and other community outreach initiatives to

N. Shimpi · I. Glurich · A. Acharya (✉)
Center for Oral and Systemic Health, Marshfield Clinic Research Institute,
Marshfield, WI, USA
e-mail: shimpi.neel@marshfieldresearch.org; glurich.ingrid@marshfieldresearch.org;
acharya.amit@marshfieldresearch.org

A. Acharya et al. (eds.), *Integration of Medical and Dental Care and Patient Data*,
Health Informatics, https://doi.org/10.1007/978-3-319-98298-4_17

support delivery of dental and healthcare to Medicaid and underinsured disparity populations with limited access to healthcare (Acharya 2016). The creation of a collaborative environment among MCHS entities contributes towards the common goal of providing state-of-the-art high quality, holistic healthcare access to all segments of the population within its service area and beyond. As an established accountable care organization, MCHS has also embraced evidence-based medical team and medical home models to promote availability of quality health information to patients and providers and achievement of managed care.

An overview of milestones achieved during the last 100 years towards integrated care model (Mazza 2013) at MCHS is shown below:

December 1916	Incorporation of Marshfield Clinic
1918	School of Nursing established
1922	Medical Internship program started
1943	First health insurance agreement
1944	Effort to change corporate structure to partnership
1948	Cancer screening for women instituted with pelvic, breast and papanicolau exam
1959	Marshfield Medical Foundation established
1960	First research grant for NIH-study of Farmer's lung
1970	Family practice department was established
1971	Marshfield Community Plan established computerized EKG program
1974	Family Health Center established medical residency program
1980	National Farm Medicine Center established
1987	Security Health Plan was created
1990	Merging of Marshfield Clinic Research Foundation and Marshfield Clinic
1994	Established one of the first electronic medical records in the country. Marshfield Clinic becomes recognized as a leader in medical informatics
1999	Clinic departments were organized into divisions
2000	Personalized Medicine project begins
2001	Clinic hires its first system engineer and developed department of Systems and Processes
2003	Ambulatory Surgery Center was opened Ladysmith Dental Clinic became Marshfield Clinic's first dental operation MC adopted 5-year strategic plan Clinic joined several other multispecialty clinics, hospitals, and employers as founding members of WI's first public reporting entity known as the Wisconsin Collaborative for Healthcare Quality
2004	The Center for Human Genetics was established
2005	Biomedical Informatics department was created
2014	Center for Oral and Systemic Health was established

In 1949, the MC unique patient census was 26,701 (Mazza 2013). Presently, there are more than 1.5 million unique patients seen annually including over one million patients who seek medical care and a subset exceeding 150,000 unique patients treated for dental care.

17.2 Model of Integrated Care

MCHS has been active in crafting effectiveness in integrating medical and dental domains utilizing the extensive network of healthcare providers, researchers, and a wealth of clinical expertise within MCHS. In addition, numerous efforts have been made by MCHS to eliminate health disparities among the population; and *Health Professions Education: A Bridge to Quality*, which focused on integrated, interprofessional care delivery as a potential solution established through integration of core competencies into the educational curriculum of health professionals (Medicine 2003).

MCHS was among the 106 new ACOs selected for adoption of the fee-for-service payment model for the Medicare population. MCHS has participated in the Shared Savings Program for more than a decade. Notably, MC ranked as the highest achieving organization, outperforming the ten other participating organizations of the CMS Physician Group Practice Demonstration project (Iglehart 2011). Because of the capability of its sophisticated home-grown EHR, MC demonstrated that quality improvement tracking could leverage substantial cost reduction when applied to patient care. Figure 17.1 shows the various entities affiliated with MCHS and key areas they support in facilitating integrated care delivery.

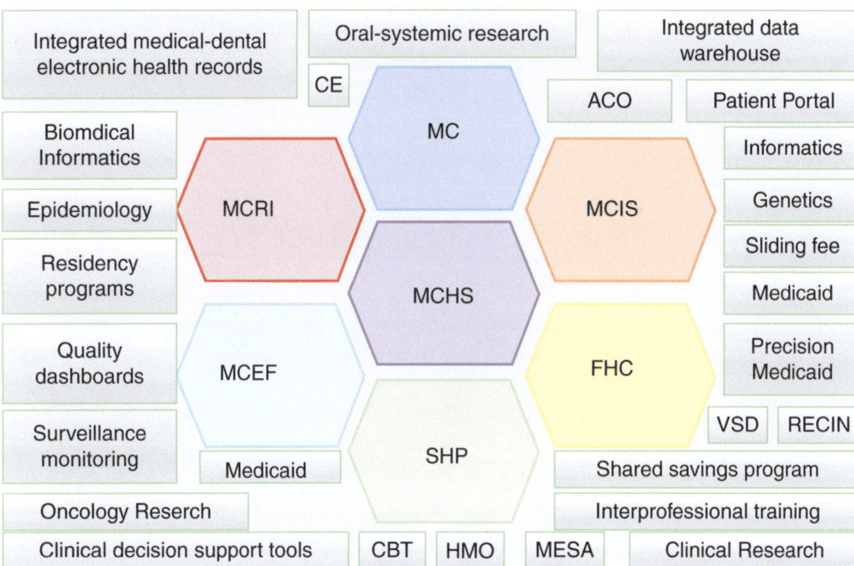

Fig. 17.1 MCHS organizational infrastructure and stakeholder roles in achieving integrated care delivery. *MCHS* Marshfield Clinic Health System, *MC* Marshfield Clinic, *MCIS* Marshfield Clinic Information System, *FHC* Family Health Center of Marshfield, Inc., *SHP* Security Health Plan, *MCEF* Marshfield Clinic Education Foundation, *MCRI* Marshfield Clinic Research Institute, *ACO* Accountable Care Organization, *HMO* Health Maintenance Organization, *CBT* Computer Based Training, *MESA* Marshfield Clinic Epidemiology Area, *VSD* Vaccine Safety Datalink, *RECIN* Registry for Effectively Communicating Immunization Needs, *CE* Continuing Education

Family Health Center of Marshfield, Inc. is a federally funded community health center that provides health care to low income, Medicaid, and uninsured populations. Family Health Center has 19 medical and ten Federally Qualified Health Center dental clinics which it operates within MCHS, an in-house pharmacy, and extensive contracts with area hospitals and other providers. To promote integrated care delivery across the dental and medical domains, MCHS features an integrated electronic health record accessible across its entire environment (Amit Acharya et al. 2012).

Figure 17.2 illustrates the unique patients treated at FHC Dental Centers across Wisconsin counties from November of 2002 to end of September, 2017.

Marshfield Clinic Information System (MCIS) is an IT company that supports the development of emerging technology and has played a key role in development of the integrated medical and dental electronic health records. MCIS is the product of Marshfield Clinic's 50-year commitment to the use of information technology to benefit patients and physicians in achieving quality health care delivery. MCIS and Marshfield Clinic jointly identified best practices for effectively assessing disease status and identifying areas in need of improvement through implementation of evidence-based guidelines (Horowitz et al. 2014; Shimpi et al. 2018). Some examples include development of patient population algorithms to allow correct identifi-

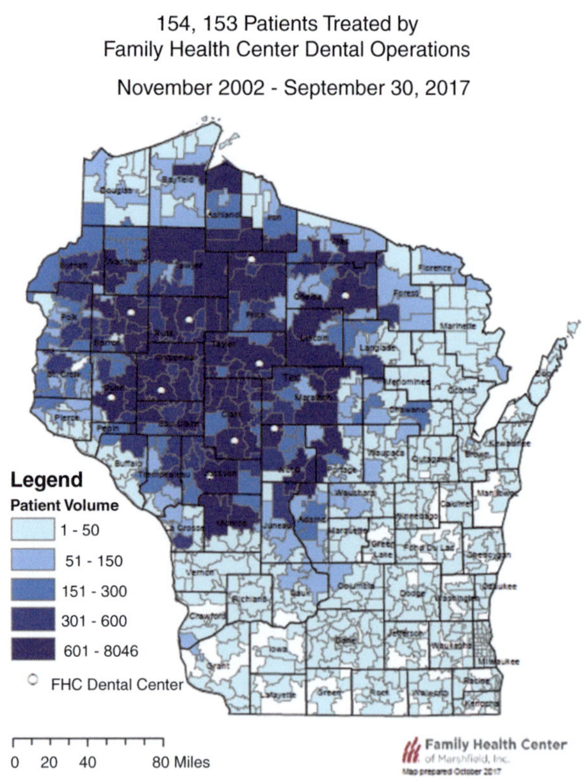

Fig. 17.2 Unique patients treated at FHC Dental Centers across Wisconsin counties

cation of patients of a given provider. Similarly patient-centric interventions were used to create standing orders that supported better care delivery.

Marshfield Clinic Research Institute (MCRI), the research arm of MCRI, consists of six research centers: Center for Clinical Epidemiology and Population Health, Center for Precision Medicine Research, Clinical Research Center, Cancer Care and Research Center, Center for Oral and Systemic Health, and National Farm Medicine Center.

Healthcare providers from Marshfield Clinic conducting clinician led research working collaboratively with scientists from MCRI have always brought a unique perspective to patient care delivery by playing a central role in advancing and translating research into clinical practice. Moreover, the Marshfield Epidemiologic Study Area (MESA) is a regional population-based health research resource that tracks all individuals (and their associated family members) who receive medical care from MCHS and reside in one of the ZIP codes that surround primary service areas in central and northern Wisconsin. This unique population health resource has helped assessing key regional oral health epidemiological questions like the prevalent periodontitis in rural parts of the country (Acharya et al. 2013). MESA has about 65,000 adult residents who receive over 90% of their inpatient and outpatient medical care from MCHS and provide a 'denominator' that permits population tracking to estimate incidence and prevalence. Over time, such collaborations have resulted in the establishment of informatics supported initiatives such as the award-winning creation of the Registry for Effectively Communicating Immunization Needs (RECIN) which allows providers to track immunization histories of their pediatric patients, featuring alerts in the EHR to trigger timely reminders that support compliance with immunization schedules that offer protection from serious childhood illnesses (McCarthy et al. 2009).

Subsequently, the Vaccine Safety Datalink (VSD) Investigational Group also created a surveillance monitoring system that could track and report any adverse events associated with vaccination (Centers for Disease Control and Prevention 2017).

In the dental arena, dental informatics researchers within the Centers for Oral Health (COSH) who also instituted the various dental component of the integrated electronic medical-dental health record, are assisting providers delivering care across the FHC of Marshfield's Dental Clinic infrastructure within MCHS through a creation of an oral health quality dashboard that tracks provider performance and dental disease outcomes and medical disease status of conditions that impact on oral health (e.g. type II diabetes mellitus) and risk assessment tools at point-of-care (Acharya et al. 2018; Acharya 2016; Hegde et al. 2017, 2018a).

Presently, more than 450 research projects are active in fields of agriculture-related safety and health, veterinary research, oncology, infectious diseases, dental and craniofacial conditions, oral-systemic conditions and health, biomedical and oral health informatics, vaccine safety, genetic bases for disease and drug interactions, treatment-based outcomes studies, development of models for the study of disease processes, pediatric health and safety, and health services research that engages healthcare providers and researchers.

17.3 Innovative Practices/Pathways

MCHS considers innovative practices an important cornerstone of patient-centered care. Several ongoing initiatives, described below, at MCHS have been accelerating and advancing improvement across medical and dental domains.

A significant barrier to accessing preventive dental care is access to dental insurance. More than half of the dental specialists in the United States refuse to treat patients enrolled in Medicaid due to insufficient reimbursement rates (U.S. Government Accountability 2010). For example, dental specialists in Wisconsin providing pediatric dental services to patients who are Medicaid enrollees are reimbursed at a rate 68.5% lower compared to the reimbursement rate received for commercially insured patients (Nasseh et al. 2014). In 2014, for the country as a whole, Medicaid only reimbursed dentists 54.07% of what commercial dental insurance agencies paid (Nasseh and Vujicic 2016). Another subpopulation of individuals experiencing access barriers are those representing the lowest middle-income population. Characteristically, this sub population earns modest wages that renders them ineligible for Medicaid, are not offered dental insurance as a component of their employee benefit package, and cannot afford out of pocket cost associated with routine annual preventive care (AHRQ 2011). This problem has been coined the challenge of the working poor; individuals receive no funding from public insurance, despite their inability to afford private insurance rates.

To improve access to dental healthcare, FHC service area has targeted care specifically to the underserved by adopting the sliding fee scale program. More importantly, the established dental clinics also represent, at point-of-care, a referral option for primary care physicians whose patients would benefit from dental care. Additional innovative practices include assessing knowledge gaps, awareness of current practices of medical and dental providers, and having cross-disciplinary training administered to the medical and dental providers through computer based trainings with respect to oral and systemic connections (Glurich et al. 2017; Shimpi et al. 2016a, b). For example the bidirectional association between diabetes and periodontal disease demonstrates the benefits of cross-disciplinary trainings.

An additional example is provided by the integrated dental-medical record (iEHR) an important resource available to medical and dental providers at MCHS that further supports the advancement of integrated care delivery. The iEHR allows the medical provider to view a patient's dental history and summary of care plans and similarly, the dental provider can track a patient's chronic health conditions and relevant care plans placed in the iEHR by their respective medical providers. Because a growing body of evidence increasingly supports bidirectional interrelations between chronic oral and systemic disease (Casanova et al. 2014; Eke et al. 2015), primary care providers (PCPs) are being considered pivotal to the establishment of integrated care models. A recent initiative piloted training of medical primary care providers in the conduct of the oral health screening examination at two of MCHS's medical clinics. In addition, initiatives to develop and offer oral health training modules for Medical providers as a continuing education initiative have been undertaken to promote holistic health care delivery.

Collectively, the northern counties of Wisconsin were experiencing a substantial shortage of mental/behavioral health professionals among a high needs population. In collaboration with MC's regional internal medicine practice and a trained mental health coordinator, a mental health surveillance screening system was developed. Screening surveys for depression were administered to patients seen in internal medicine, and a behavioral specialist works with at-risk patients and triages them for a mental health consult. The focus of this effort was to reduce incidence, severity, and duration of serious depression while concomitantly reducing related healthcare costs through prevention and early intervention.

Patients with chronic medical conditions, who are high healthcare utilizers, often seek care from multiple providers. Such patients would benefit from being assigned to internal medicine practitioners for comprehensive care management. Under the medical home model, internal medicine physicians and allied providers treat patients for their ongoing healthcare needs, provide assignments to care coordinators, and appropriately arrange care with other specialists and services such as home health agencies and nursing homes. PCMH is intended to prevent fragmented care, improve care quality, and prevent avoidable acute care visits by providing better access to health care. This has the benefit of reducing the high healthcare costs associated with fragmented care delivery and increased utilization of urgent/emergency care access among this subset of patients. FHC has been working with its healthcare partners to establish PCMH care management systems, especially for patients living in rural regions remote from specialty care access.

Moreover, the advanced access initiative at MCHS is intended to also make access to primary care providers more accessible for patients experiencing acute conditions rather than having them seen by on-call or urgent care physicians at higher cost. In this model, patients can call in and are scheduled (if possible) with their primary care physician for a same-day appointment. The basis of this approach lies in the premise that continuity of health care is important and should be available to patients and physicians. This initiative supports proactive assessment, intervention and triage, and reduces acute emergency room or urgent care visits and/or hospitalization.

17.4 Health Information Technology

MCHS has been committed to internally supporting and expanding the capabilities of its clinical information systems over the past 40 years. Home grown and a collaborative effort of physicians and biomedical and health informaticians, the iEHR represents one of the few robust integrated medical and dental electronic health records that is amenable to expansion. The medical component known as 'CattailsMD', is used by over 13,000+ users, making it one of the largest integrated, healthcare information systems in the country. Developed centrally, the iEHR supports all components of the MCHS enterprise including the clinical and hospital environments, MCRI, MCED, SHP, and Marshfield Laboratories. Marshfield Clinic informatics has been on the leading edge of health information management and information technology for decades and has been a chartless EHR environment for over 30 years (Acharya 2016). Physicians and staff anywhere within MCHS may access clinical data via laptops, tablets, and PDA's and data are backed up nightly in real time to the enterprise data warehouse. Figure 17.3 illustrates the dental dashboard component of MCHS's iEHR.

The dental component of the iEHR known as 'CattailsDental' supports the documentation and care processes in the dental domain. CattailsDental includes a dental dashboard; workflow management tools including tooth charting, periodontal charting and treatment planning; access to centralized medications, allergies, special conditions, problems list, demographics and HIPAA forms; access to medical appointments to support better coordination of care; and highly secure remote access supporting devices such as laptops and computer tablets . Both diagnoses and procedures are documented to further support integrity of the data. This capability was instituted by a redesign of CattailsDental, in 2010 supporting capture of diagnosis selection by dental providers that corresponds to the procedure (Shimpi et al. 2018).

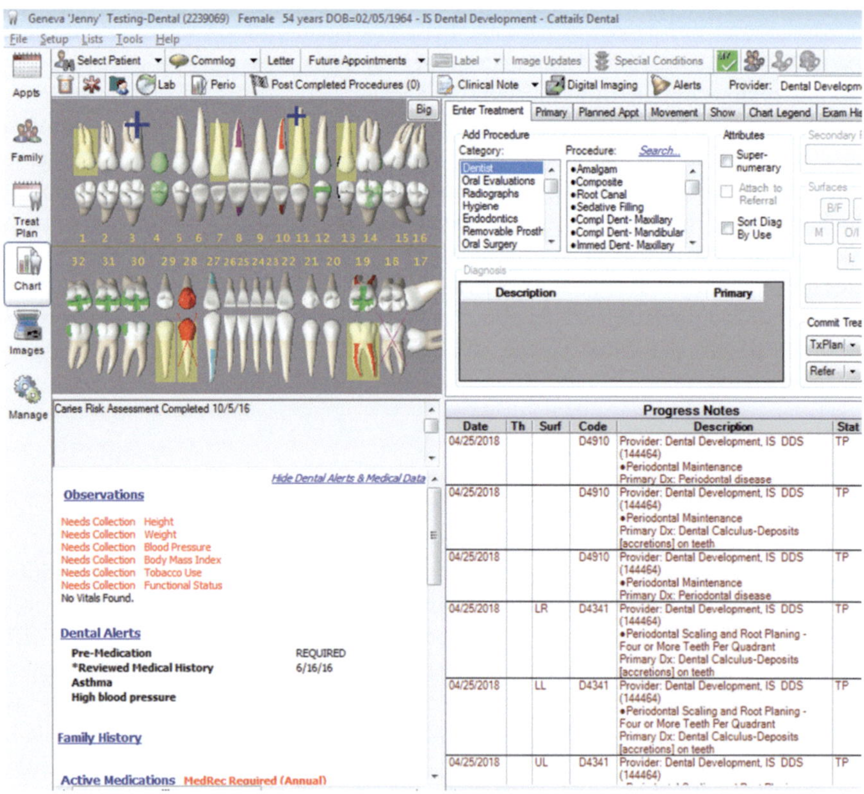

Fig. 17.3 Dental Dashboard component of MCHS's iEHR

17.4.1 Electronic Health Record and Data Warehouse Environment

The MC internally-developed iEHR is one of the oldest and most comprehensive in the country, containing coded diagnoses data back to 1960, with other coded data and digital documents back to the mid-1980s. Through its Windows©-based EMR viewer, the iEHR supports the viewing of all documents including but not limited to transcribed documents, laboratory results, vitals, and other observations. The iEHR system contains roughly 70 million text documents. MCHS informaticians have been working on acquiring actionable data points derived from clinical notes by using natural language processing (Hegde et al. 2018b).

Medication Manager supports the tracking of point-of-care integrated electronic prescribing and medication inventory system currently available for access by any MCHS provider. Any changes in the medication history is available to physicians and dentists in real-time irrespective of who made the change.

The EHR including patients' medical and dental information is supported by a high quality data repository, integrated Enterprise Data Warehouse (iEDW), which has been in existence for more than 15 years and stores diagnostic data that dates back to the early 1960s in addition to other clinical data captured at point of care. Moreover, clinical documents, narratives, and electronic transcribed documents and images from 1961 onwards are archived and available for review.

The iEDW supports over 2 TB of clinical data collected on approximately 2.6 million patients and health plan members. All data within the iEDW is highly integrated between MCHS regional clinics, SHP, and Marshfield Laboratories and individual patient records are linked by use of a unique medical record number (Patient ID), and/or hospital encounter number. The unique patient identifier supports capture of longitudinal history within the individual patient's health records. Another component of the iEDW is the research data warehouse (RDW), which contains more than 9 million patient-years of clinical data and supports research activities within MCHS.

17.5 Interprofessional Education and Practice

MCHS provides an exceptional learning environment to cultivate the necessary skills to achieve proficiency in clinical medicine, public health, education, and/or systems quality research. The residency program at MCHS offers further opportunities for outreach and advocacy for this large rural minority population. In addition, because health care is often not accessed by high-needs individuals, residents in training are exposed to a broad spectrum of diseases, often severely advanced, and encounter a rich learning environment.

The MCED also offers continuing education (CE) credits for trainings that involve interprofessional education. For example Implementation of *Smiles for Life*

Module 1 was made mandatory for the primary care physicians to provide post graduate training on oral health which is generally not offered during their professional medical training (Douglass et al. 2007). Other activities that are currently ongoing for MCHS providers include Grand Rounds, Lunch and Learn sessions, and journal clubs, among others.

MCRI strives for continuous improvement through research, conducting oral-systemic conferences, presenting at the national and international conferences, etc. Residents have a requirement to participate in research or other intellectual activity to expand their educational experience, and receive mentoring from MCED physician mentors. They present their findings by preparing posters which they present at institutional and national conferences and/or publish manuscripts on their research findings. MCRI scientists support their research through grant funded initiatives, are extensively published, and regularly attend national conferences to present their work and network with other scientists to stay in touch with cutting edge developments in their domain.

17.6 Integration Development Team Members

Team members important to integration include medical and dental providers, researchers, health educators, team leaders, administrators, policy makers, physician champions, residents, and support staff of MCHS entities as shown in Fig. 17.1.

17.7 Challenges and Next Steps

For holistic care delivery, current emphasis at MCHS is focused around:

- Achievement of the Triple Aim (improve patient care experience; improve health of people and population; and improve societal costs of disease management);
- Implementation of value-based care;
- Increase awareness of oral-systemic health associations;
- Increase acceptance and adoption of preventive services, for example HPV vaccines;
- Standardizing diagnostic codes and terminologies for dentistry (Acharya et al. 2012);
- Implementing population-based disease surveillance programs;
- Reduce costs through disease prevention programs and increase patient activation;
- Advance technological support of patient care delivery and implementation of web-based tools at point-of-care settings;
- Integration of mobile devices into clinical practices;
- Improve patient access to care.

References

Acharya A. Marshfield Clinic Health System: integrated care case study. J Calif Dent Assoc. 2016;44(3):177–81. http://www.ncbi.nlm.nih.gov/pubmed/27044239.

Acharya A, Cheng B, Koralkar R, Olson B, Lamster I, Kunzel C, Lalla E. Screening for diabetes risk using integrated dental and medical electronic health record data. JDR Clin Transl Res. 2018;3(2):188–94. https://doi.org/10.1177/2380084418759496.

Acharya A, VanWormer J, Waring S, Miller A, Fuehrer J, Nycz G. Regional epidemiologic assessment of prevalent periodontitis using an electronic health record system. Am J Epidemiol. 2013;177(7):700–7. https://doi.org/10.1093/aje/kws293.

Acharya A, Yoder N, Nycz G. An integrated medical-dental electronic health record environment: a Marshfield experience (pp. 331–351). .2012. https://doi.org/10.1007/978-1-4471-2185-5_6.

AHRQ. Access to health care. AHRQ archive. 2011. https://archive.ahrq.gov/research/findings/nhqrdr/nhqr11/chap9.html. Accessed 12 Jun 2018.

Casanova L, Hughes F, Preshaw P. Diabetes and periodontal disease: a two-way relationship. BDJ. 2014;217(8):433–7. https://doi.org/10.1038/sj.bdj.2014.907.

Centers for Disease Control and Prevention. Vaccine safety datalink (VSD). 2017. https://www.cdc.gov/vaccinesafety/ensuringsafety/monitoring/vsd/index.html. Accessed 13 Jun 2018.

Douglass A, Gonsalves W, Maier R, Silk H, Stevens N, Tysinger J, Wrightson AS. Smiles for life: a national oral health curriculum for family medicine. A model for curriculum development by STFM groups. Fam Med. 2007;39(2):88–90. http://www.ncbi.nlm.nih.gov/pubmed/17273948

Eke P, Dye B, Wei L, Slade G, Thornton-Evans G, Borgnakke W. Update on prevalence of periodontitis in adults in the United States: NHANES 2009 to 2012. J Periodontol. 2015;86(5):611–22. https://doi.org/10.1902/jop.2015.140520.

Glurich I, Schwei K, Lindeberg S, Shimpi N, Acharya A. Interdisciplinary diabetes management: qualitative assessment of medical/dental practitioners' perspectives. San Francisco, NC: International Association for Dental Research; 2017.

Hegde H, Koralkar R, Shimpi N, Glurich I, Panny A, Acharya A. Diabetes mellitus prediction using machine learning in a dental setting. AADR/CADR annual meeting. Fort Lauderdale. 2018a. https://doi.org/10.3233/THC-171127.

Hegde H, Shimpi N, Glurich I, Acharya A. Tobacco use status from clinical notes using Natural Language Processing and rule based algorithm. Technol Health Care. 2018b;26:445–56. https://doi.org/10.3233/THC-171127.

Hegde H, Steinmetz A, Theisen J, Koralkar R, Finnamore J, Halstead S. Dental quality analytics: dental measures and provider performance dashboard, vol. 96. San Francisco, CA: American Academy of Dental Research; 2017. p. 566.

Horowitz A, Robinson L, Acharya A. After visit summaries: a tool whose time has come for use in dentistry. Washington, DC: NAM; 2014. https://nam.edu/wp-content/uploads/2015/06/aftervisitsummaries.pdf

Iglehart J. Assessing an ACO prototype—Medicare's Physician Group Practice demonstration. N Engl J Med. 2011;364(3):198–200. https://doi.org/10.1056/NEJMp1013896.

Mazza J. A fifty year history of Marshfield Clinic Research Foundation: Joseph J. Mazza M.D.: 9780981570716: Amazon.com: Books. Marshfield: Marshfield Clinic Research Foundation. 2013. https://www.amazon.com/History-Marshfield-Clinic-Research-Foundation/dp/0981570712

McCarthy D, Mueller K, Klein S. Marshfield Clinic: health information technology paves the way for population health management. New York, NY: Commonwealth Fund; 2009. pub.1293. https://pdfs.semanticscholar.org/3bbc/e41b99cc33e296ec1c01d04ad7f82e46820a.pdf

MCHS. Marshfield Clinic Health System, Inc. Fact sheet. Marshfield, WI: MCHS; 2018. https://www.marshfieldclinic.org/mCorporate/Documents/MCHSFactSheet-MCHS.pdf. Accessed 12 Jun 2018.

Medicine I. Health professions education. Washington, DC: National Academies Press; 2003. https://doi.org/10.17226/10681.

Nasseh K, Vujicic M. Dental benefits coverage increased for working-age adults in 2014. Health Policy Institute Research Brief. 2016. http://www.ada.org/~/media/ADA/Scienceand Research/HPI/Files/HPIBrief_1016_2.pdf

Nasseh K, Vujicic M, Yarbrough C. A ten-year, state-by-state, analysis of medicaid fee-for-service reimbursement rates for dental care services. Health Policy Institute Research Brief. 2014.

Shimpi N, Schroeder D, Kilsdonk J, Chyou P, Glurich I, Acharya A. Assessment of dental providers' knowledge, behavior and attitude towards incorporating chairside screening for medical conditions: a pilot study. J Dent Oral Care Med. 2016a;*2*(1):1–7. https://doi.org/10.15744/2454-3276.2.102.

Shimpi N, Schroeder D, Kilsdonk J, Chyou P, Glurich I, Penniman E, Acharya A. Medical providers' oral health knowledgeability, attitudes, and practice behaviors: an opportunity for interprofessional collaboration. J Evid Based Dent Pract. 2016b;16(1) https://doi.org/10.1016/j.jebdp.2016.01.002.

Shimpi N, Ye Z, Koralkar R, Glurich I, Acharya A. Need for diagnostic-centric care in dentistry. J Am Dent Assoc. 2018;*149*(2):122–31. https://doi.org/10.1016/j.adaj.2017.09.030.

U.S. Government Accountability. Oral health: efforts under way to improve children's access to dental services, but sustained attention needed to address ongoing concerns. 2010. https://www.gao.gov/products/GAO-11-96

Chapter 18
Conclusion

Miguel H. Torres-Urquidy, Amit Acharya, Robert H. Posteraro, Valerie Powell, and Thankam Paul Thyvalikakath

18.1 Parting Words

At the beginning of the book we presented the rationale of the divide in health care where proto-barbers provided a subset of treatments that differed from those of early physicians which in turn led to dentists and physicians taking separate professional paths. As a result of those divergent paths, not only the professions but also the supporting "infrastructures" would evolve differently, having separate practices, alternative insurance offerings, and distinct regulatory frameworks that make such

M. H. Torres-Urquidy (✉)
Centers for Disease Control and Prevention, Atlanta, GA, USA
e-mail: miguel@forwardthinkingconcepts.org

A. Acharya
Center for Oral and Systemic Health, Marshfield Clinic Research Institute, Marshfield, WI, USA
e-mail: acharya.amit@marshfieldresearch.org

R. H. Posteraro
Department of Healthcare Management and Leadership, Texas Tech University Health Sciences Center School of Health Professions, Lubbock, TX, USA
e-mail: robert.posteraro@ttuhsc.edu

V. Powell
Robert Morris University, Moon Township, PA, USA
e-mail: powell@rmu.edu

T. P. Thyvalikakath
Department of Cariology, Operative Dentistry & Dental Public Health, Indiana University School of Dentistry, IUPUI, Indianapolis, IN, USA

School of Informatics and Computing, IUPUI, Indianapolis, IN, USA

Centre for Biomedical Informatics, Regenstrief Institute, Indianapolis, IN, USA
e-mail: tpt@iu.edu

A. Acharya et al. (eds.), *Integration of Medical and Dental Care and Patient Data*, Health Informatics, https://doi.org/10.1007/978-3-319-98298-4_18

separation more divergent. Because of this history, we deemed it necessary to reiterate throughout this book, the many instances where integration would be pertinent.

As described, integration of dental and medical care presents a large number of opportunities for improving our ability to deliver care, save costs, and obtain better outcomes suggesting progress towards integration in the system at large.

Harnagea et al. (2018) based on work from Valentijn et al. (2013) introduced three levels of integration between the oral and medical care systems. The first level of integration being "Macro," calls for systemic integration that includes "public oral health programs, adaptive professional regulations, public oral health insurance plans, and national oral health policies." The "Meso" level of integration calls for organizational integration including "co-location, supportive environments, and interdisciplinary networks." It also establishes professional integration by means of "interprofessional education and training and interprofessional collaboration." Finally, the "Micro" level calls for clinical integration by establishing "oral health champions, patient navigators, and interprofessional practice." With this model in mind, we can list actual examples that fit such a model:

In terms of governmental interventions several government agencies have taken notice and have established active support, through grant funding, to make integration happen (Macro level). The US federal agencies CDC (2017, 2018), CMS (2018), and HRSA (2018) all have now provided grants to establish programs that support dental and medical integration. This support comes in addition to the more traditional earlier NIH grant opportunities linking oral and systemic health (NIH 2018).

The health insurance industry is also addressing dental-medical integration (Aetna Inc. 2018; Cigna 2018; Northeast Delta Dental 2017) and it is now possible to identify efforts to achieve integration driven by financial incentives (also Macro level).

Academically, we can now find examples of formal training efforts to focus on developing awareness and expertise in the multiple aspects required for integration (Meso level). The Harvard School of Dental Medicine offers graduate programs such as a doctor of medical sciences or a master of medical sciences degree focused on integration (HSDM 2018). In addition, professional societies are also aware and calling for fostering integration as well (Rudman et al. 2010).

Throughout the book we cited examples of integration at the Micro level supported by technological innovation tied to clinical contact points.

Although these are progressive initiatives, questions still remain about the direct quantifiable impact of integration. Research by Chen et al. (2018) has found that, with the advent of Health Information Exchanges (HIEs) the number of readmissions for acute myocardial infarction (AMI) has decreased leading directly to not only improved health outcomes but also direct cost savings (about three million US dollars during the period under study in the US state of Florida and for just one clinical condition). In the case of dental and medical integration, Elani and colleagues (2018) reviewed available literature on the subject and found that further research is needed. In particular they found that of three viable reports that studied in detail the benefits of dental and medical integration, two found benefits (economically speaking) while one did not. As they state in their report, technical factors are some of the reasons that prevent a better measurement of the impact of dental-medical integration.

Further research also needs to continue on how to better and more rapidly transfer methods and findings between the dental and medical research fields. For instance, Falcettoni (2018) found that in the case of rural vs. urban medical practices, it is the rural general practitioners that see increase in income due to the surge in performing specialized procedures. The rationale for this difference is because in urban settings you are more likely to find specialists that can perform, and subsequently bill, for such procedures. However, when asked whether such findings could also be replicated among general dentists in urban areas, the response was “the problem is the data” which may not necessarily support a similar study (MHTU, personal communication). In the not so distant future, it may be possible, with a certain level of integration, to replicate studies that can shed light on the realities of clinical care that remain unexplored.

Furthermore, there are other aspects that we consider will rapidly impact healthcare and, in consequence, will likely play a role in dental and medical integration. From the technology perspective, it is difficult to predict within a short time frame what the innovations will be. On the other hand, introducing longer-term perspectives, we believe, will help the reader keep an eye on short term technological developments that are likely to influence the speed with which integration occurs.

The ongoing miniaturization of technology will likely impact the way health care is delivered where the patient’s relationship between dentists and physicians will be more symbiotic. Instead of waiting, smart devices will inform care providers of the health status of the patient, hopefully enabling more of a preventive culture and/or intercepting at a much earlier stage otherwise catastrophic conditions. Naturally, we anticipate this has the potential to address costs, which need to be addressed, hopefully also with the help of technology.

While writing this edition, we are also experiencing significant changes in aspects related to privacy and the use of data in order to obtain electronic services. Although regulations stipulate significant constraints in the case of medical information, other forms of data, which are usually not bound by the same protections, may be relevant in the context of improving our ability to reach better diagnoses and/or establish more appropriate integrated treatment plans. Knowing the eating history (type, frequency, cost) may allow for better care recommendations when a patient may want or need to lose weight as well as decrease the risk of caries. On the other hand, gaining access to such intake history may require specialized tools, falling within a different regulatory framework or even may come at a cost for either the patient or the practitioner (whether a dentist or a physician).

Further looking, we see the automation of procedures and the use of robotic technologies. Although none of these are actually new to dentistry and medicine, we anticipate that, in combination with AI, certain procedures are deemed more likely to be left for automation at the point of care. What is important to make clear here is that we do not anticipate the replacement of dentists or physicians but actually enhancing their ability to do more (faster) care or be more precise in their work when rendering treatments (Cooper et al. 2011). These tools will necessarily need to operate using integrated data.

We also anticipate an exponential growth in the ability to use genomic and proteomic based technologies to actually deliver care. As of this writing, genomic therapy has become a reality and it will be imperative to have treatments that account for both oral and systemic effects. Careful observation and surveillance will be required given the rapid evolution of such therapies and only with integrated tools will we be more likely to observe the full picture. Just to add, this will be more important if we mix other technologies such as 3D printing and new biomaterials.

New technologies are making inroads into clinical practice and will likely reshape many of our current healthcare processes (whether in the real world or in the electronic world). The introduction of Blockchain technologies allow for establishing trust in processes where trust is elusive. It also provides a mechanism to maintain a longitudinal record, which subsequently is very hard (if not impossible) to modify. These are elements that are highly applicable to the recording and managing of health data. As the biomedical community embraces Blockchain, new processes will be adapted or developed to take advantage of this new ability to keep billing, clinical, and/or research data. In the case of the goal of dental-medical integration, Blockchain may present an opportunity to amalgamate dental and medical information. Ledgers may exist where you have blocks referring to dental and medical data. Obviously, many aspects of Blockchain and healthcare still need to be worked out (privacy being a crucial element), and as Blockchain is incorporated those interested in fostering integration need to understand how this technology can expedite it.

Artificial Intelligence and expert systems more and more will play a role in healthcare. Although this is a common prediction to be found in the medical informatics literature, at the time of this writing it has seen the flourishing and socialization of tools and services that will significantly reduce the threshold to embrace such technologies. This, in turn, with the now more predominant accessibility to big datasets, will allow for easier integration, and/or discovery of new relationships between oral and systemic health.

There are further (and more speculative) advances that are on the horizon. Clinical trials using AI and synthetic data have the potential to change (and advance) the way we investigate new clinical developments (Bookbinder 2018). It is plausible, then, to envision data driven clinical trials that are highly *inclusive* measuring and advancing both dental and medical care without explicitly stating it at the beginning of a clinical trial.

The above example reminds us that there is a need to have a renewed research agenda where we identify challenges and solutions to integration. Ideally, identifying recommendations in the areas of accreditation, education, quality of care, and standards of care should lead to improved clinical, financial, socio-technical, and/or regulatory practices. Then it will be up to academic, clinical, governmental, and industrial entities to adopt these findings and start reaping such benefits.

In closing, significant inroads have been made on integration and these technologies hold great promise to achieve such a goal. Thus, we anticipate that in the next few years, with the advent of these and new unforeseen practices and tools, as well as with a better understanding of the benefits for patients and society at large, we will be able to establish and experience the full integration of dental and medical care.

Disclaimer The views presented in this chapter are solely of the author and do not necessarily represent the views of the US Government, Department of Health and Human Services and/or the Centers for Disease Control and Prevention.

References

Aetna Inc. Dental medical integration program – producers. Aetna. 2018. https://www.aetna.com/insurance-producer/dental-plans-programs/dental-medical-integration-program.html. Accessed 10 Jun 2018.

Bookbinder M. The intelligent trial: AI comes to clinical trials. Clinical Informatics News. 2018. http://www.clinicalinformaticsnews.com/2017/09/29/the-intelligent-trial-ai-comes-to-clinical-trials.aspx. Accessed 10 Jun 2018.

Centers for Disease Control and Prevention (CDC), U.S. Department of Health and Human Services. CDC-funded states, cooperative agreements, state based oral health programs, Division of Oral Health, CDC. 2017. https://www.cdc.gov/oralhealth/state_programs/cooperative_agreements/index.htm. Accessed 10 Jun 2018.

Centers for Disease Control and Prevention (CDC), U.S. Department of Health and Human Services. State actions to improve oral health outcomes (CDC-RFA-DP18–1810), Division of Oral Health, CDC. 2018. https://www.cdc.gov/oralhealth/state_programs/nofo/nofo1810states.htm. Accessed 10 Jun 2018.

Center for Medicare & Medicaid Innovation, Centers for Medicare & Medicaid Services (CMS), U.S. Department of Health and Human Services. Healthcare innovation awards round two, center for medicare & medicaid innovation. 2018. https://innovation.cms.gov/initiatives/Health-Care-Innovation-Awards/Round-2.html. Accessed 10 Jun 2018.

Chen M, Guo S, Tan X. Does health information exchange improve patient outcomes? A longitudinal study. 7th conference of the American Society of Health Economists. Atlanta, GA. 2018. https://ashecon.confex.com/ashecon/2018/webprogram/Paper5569.html. Accessed 13 Jun 2018.

Cigna. Oral Health Integration Program. Cigna. 2018. https://www.cigna.com/individuals-families/member-resources/oral-health-integration-program Accessed 10 Jun 2018.

Cooper JG, West RM, Clamp SE, et al. Does computer-aided clinical decision support improve the management of acute abdominal pain? A systematic review. Emerg Med J. 2011;28(7):553–7.

Elani HW, Simon L, Ticku S, et al. Does providing dental services reduce overall health care costs? A systematic review of the literature. J Am Dent Assoc. 2018;pii:S0002-8177(18)30203-4.

Falcettoni E. Primary care is the new specialist. Physicians' response to financial incentives. 7th conference of the American Society of Health Economists. Atlanta, GA. 2018. https://ashecon.confex.com/ashecon/2018/webprogram/Paper6187.html. Accessed 13 Jun 2018.

Harnagea H, Lamothe L, Couturier Y, et al. From theoretical concepts to policies and applied programmes: the landscape of integration of oral health in primary care. BMC Oral Health. 2018;18(1):23.

Harvard School of Medicine (HSDM). Harvard School of Dental Medicine Initiative to Integrate Oral Health and Medicine. 2018. https://hsdm.harvard.edu/integrating-oral-health-and-primary-care. Accessed 10 Jun 2018.

National Institutes of Health (NIH), U.S. Department of Health and Human Services. PAR-16-154: tailoring dental treatment for individuals with systemic diseases that compromise oral health (R01). 2018. https://grants.nih.gov/grants/guide/pa-files/PAR-16-154.html. Accessed 10 Jun 2018.

Health Resources and Services Administration (HRSA), U.S. Department of Health and Human Services. Oral health, official website of the U.S. Health Resources and Services Administration. 2018. https://www.hrsa.gov/oral-health/index.html. Accessed 10 Jun 2018.

Northeast Delta Dental. Health through oral wellness. Northeast Delta Dental – health through oral wellness – home. 2017. http://healththroughoralwellness.com/Home. Accessed 10 Jun 2018.

Rudman WJ, Hart-Hester S, Jones WA, et al. Integrating medical and dental records: a new frontier in health information management. J AHIMA. 2010;81(10):36–9.

Valentijn PP, Schepman SM, Opheij W, et al. Understanding integrated care: a comprehensive conceptual framework based on the integrative functions of primary care. Int J Integr Care. 2013;13:e010.

Appendix A

University of Detroit Mercy
School of Dentistry
8200 W. Outer Drive
Detroit, MI 48219-0900
(313) 494-6700

University of Detroit Mercy
Dental Service DRH/UHC
4201 St. Antoine
Detroit, MI 48201

Medical Consultation

Consultant: ______________________________

Address: ______________________________

______________________________ Date: ______________

Patient: ______________________________ UDM Chart Number: __________

Clinic requesting medical consultation:
Emergency/Screening 313-494-6718
Surgical Services 313-494-6739

REASON FOR CONSULTATION:

Dear Dr. ______________________________

Our patient as identified above presented to the University of Detroit Mercy School of Dentistry on ___/___/___. During the medical history review, the patient stated that he/she has Type ____ diabetes mellitus. Please provide the following information requested below so that his/her dental treatment can be initiated.

Your assistance is appreciated. Thank you.

Faculty Signature: ______________________________

RELEASE
I hereby consent to the release of my medical records to the University of Detroit Mercy School of Dentistry including any information regarding HIV status and infectious disease. I understand that this information will remain confidential.

Patient Signature: ______________________________

PHYSICIAN'S RESPONSE

1. The current HbA1c is ________% as measured on the date of ____________.
2. The glycemic control goal for this patient is HbA1c __________%

Physician Signature: ______________________________
Date: ________________

Disposition

Faculty Signature______________________________
Date______________________________

A. Acharya et al. (eds.), *Integration of Medical and Dental Care and Patient Data*, Health Informatics, https://doi.org/10.1007/978-3-319-98298-4

University of Detroit Mercy
School of Dentistry
8200 W. Outer Drive
Detroit, MI 48219-0900

University of Detroit Mercy
Dental Service DRH/UHC
4201 St. Antoine
Detroit, MI 48201

(313) 494-6700

Medical Consultation

Consultant: ______________________________

Address: ______________________________

______________________________ Date: ______________

Patient: ______________________________ UDM Chart Number: __________

Clinic requesting medical consultation:
Emergency/Screening 313-494-6718
Surgical Services 313-494-6739

REASON FOR CONSULTATION:

Dear Dr. ______________________________

Faculty Signature: ______________________________

RELEASE
I hereby consent to the release of my medical records to the University of Detroit Mercy School of Dentistry including any information regarding HIV status and infectious disease. I understand that this information will remain confidential.

Patient Signature: ______________________________

PHYSICIAN'S RESPONSE

Physician Signature: ______________________________
Date: ______________

Disposition

Faculty Signature______________________________
Date______________________________

University of Detroit Mercy
School of Dentistry
8200 W. Outer Drive
Detroit, MI 48219-0900

University of Detroit Mercy
Dental Service DRH/UHC
4201 St. Antoine
Detroit, MI 48201

(313) 494-6700

Medical Consultation

Consultant: ______________________________

Address: ______________________________

______________________________ Date: ______________

Patient: ______________________________ UDM Chart Number: __________

Clinic requesting medical consultation:
Emergency/Screening 313-494-6718
Surgical Services 313-494-6739

REASON FOR CONSULTATION:

Dear Dr. ______________________________

In compliance with the American Heart Association 2007 guidelines for infective endocarditis (IE) prevention, and to help us determine the need for antibiotic prophylaxis, please indicate which of the following condition(s) apply to this patient:

Faculty Signature: ______________________________

RELEASE

I hereby consent to the release of my medical records to the University of Detroit Mercy School of Dentistry including any information regarding HIV status and infectious disease. I understand that this information will remain confidential

Patient Signature: ______________________________

PHYSICIAN'S RESPONSE

_____ Prosthetic cardiac valve or prosthetic material used for heart valve repair
_____ Previous infective endocarditis (IE)
_____ Congenital heart disease (CHD) with findings as below
    _____Unrepaired cyanotic CHD, including palliative shunts and conduits
    _____Completely repaired CHD defect with prosthetic material or device <u>for the first 6 months after procedure</u>
    _____ Repaired CHD with residual defects at the site or adjacent to site of prosthetic patch/device which inhibit endothelialization
_____Cardiac transplantation recipients who develop cardiac valvulopathy

Physician Signature: ______________________________
Date: ______________

Disposition

Faculty Signature

UNIVERSITY OF DETROIT MERCY

University of Detroit Mercy
School of Dentistry
2700 Martin Luther King Jr Blvs
Detroit, MI 48208

University of Detroit Mercy
Dental Service DRH/UHC
4201 St. Antoine
Detroit, MI 48201

(313) 494-6700

Medical Consultation

Consultant: ______________________
Address: ______________________
______________________ Date: ______________

Patient: ______________________ UDM Chart Number: __________

Clinic requesting medical consultation:
Emergency/Screening 313-494-6718
Surgical Services 313-494-6739

REASON FOR CONSULTATION:
Dear Dr. ______________________

Ms./Mrs./Mr.________________ needs dental treatment in our dental clinic. She/He informed us that a total prosthetic joint was implanted ________years ago.
We are aware that dental procedures cause transient bacteremia that might be a risk factor for the prosthetic joint infection. We are also aware of AAOS's recommendation of antibiotic prophylaxis (AP) for dental procedures. However, we do not have complete information about her/him to assess the risk and benefit ratio for AP. Please evaluate her/him accordingly.
If you believe the benefit of AP would outweigh the risk, please provide her/him with prescriptions for antibiotics of your choice and the regimen.

Thank you for your assistance in optimizing hers/his oral health.

Faculty Signature: ______________________

RELEASE
I hereby consent to the release of my medical records to the University of Detroit Mercy School of Dentistry including any information regarding HIV status and infectious disease. I understand that this information will remain confidential.

Patient Signature: ______________________

PHYSICIAN'S RESPONSE
Please check one box below

☐ Ms./Mrs./Mr.__________'s benefit of AP outweighs the risk and I will provide the prescription.

☐ Ms./Mrs./Mr._______will not benefit from taking AP for dental procedure.

Physician Signature: ______________________
Date: ______________

Disposition

Faculty Signature______________________
Date______________________

Appendix B

Wisconsin Diabetes Mellitus Essential Care Guidelines

These guidelines furnish a model for interdisciplinary care and communication in any care environment, whether served by a paper-based patient record system or by an electronic health record (EHR) system.

- B-1 Medical-Dental: Team Referral Form (professional version): a model for communication among medical and dental providers collaborating as a team in diabetes care
- B-2 Diabetes Screening Tool for Inspection of Teeth and Gums (professional version): a tool to support medical provider oral screening examination (Oral Check)
- B-3 Oral Health (professional version): This includes sections on:
  - Visual Oral Inspection and Dental Health Education
  - Dental Exam
  - A Team Approach: Medical-Dental Collaboration
  - Identifying Undiagnosed Diabetes in the Dental Care Setting
  - Identifying Undiagnosed Periodontal Disease in the Primary Care Setting
  - Additional Resources

  Thus either the medical team or the dental team can take the initiative in referral.
- B-4 Patient Version:
  - *Recommended Care* integrates dental exam/oral check into diabetes care and states intervals
  - *Personal Diabetes Care Record* includes dental exam and oral check
- B-1. Wisconsin Diabetes Mellitus Essential Care Guidelines, http://www.dhs.wisconsin.gov/health/diabetes/PDFs/T-MedDentalTeam.pdf

- Medical-Dental: Team Referral Form (professional version)
- B-2. Wisconsin Diabetes Mellitus Essential Care Guidelines, http://www.dhs.wisconsin.gov/health/diabetes/PDFs/T-ScreenGumsTeeth.pdf
- Diabetes Screening Tool for Inspection of Teeth and Gums (professional version)
- B-3. Wisconsin Diabetes Mellitus Essential Care (professional version) Guidelines, http://www.dhs.wisconsin.gov/health/diabetes/PDFs/GL09.pdf
- Oral Health (professional version)
- B-4. Wisconsin Diabetes Mellitus Essential Care Guidelines, http://www.dhs.wisconsin.gov/publications/P4/P43081.pdf pp. 6–9 (half pages) (patient version)

Index

A. Acharya et al. (eds.), *Integration of Medical and Dental Care and Patient Data*, Health Informatics, https://doi.org/10.1007/978-3-319-98298-4

I

MIX
Papier aus verantwortungsvollen Quellen
Paper from responsible sources
FSC® C105338

If you have any concerns about our products,
you can contact us on
ProductSafety@springernature.com

In case Publisher is established outside the EU,
the EU authorized representative is:
Springer Nature Customer Service Center GmbH
Europaplatz 3, 69115 Heidelberg, Germany

Printed by Libri Plureos GmbH
in Hamburg, Germany